Update on Medical Disorders in Pregnancy

Guest Editor

JUDITH U. HIBBARD, MD

OBSTETRICS AND GYNECOLOGY CLINICS OF NORTH AMERICA

www.obgyn.theclinics.com

Consulting Editor
WILLIAM F. RAYBURN, MD, MBA

June 2010 • Volume 37 • Number 2

SAUNDERS an imprint of ELSEVIER, Inc.

W.B. SAUNDERS COMPANY

A Division of Elsevier Inc.

Elsevier, Inc. • 1600 John F. Kennedy Blvd. • Suite 1800 • Philadelphia, PA 19103-2899

http://www.theclinics.com

OBSTETRICS AND GYNECOLOGY CLINICS OF NORTH AMERICA Volume 37, Number 2
June 2010 ISSN 0889-8545, ISBN-13: 978-1-4377-1844-7

Editor: Carla Holloway

Obstetrics and Gynecology Clinics (ISSN 0889-8545) is published quarterly by Elsevier Inc., 360 Park Avenue South, New York, NY 10010-1710. Months of issue are March, June, September, and December. Periodicals postage paid at New York, NY, and additional mailing offices. Subscription price per year is $257.00 (US individuals), $431.00 (US institutions), $130.00 (US students), $309.00 (Canadian individuals), $544.00 (Canadian institutions), $191.00 (Canadian students), $376.00 (foreign individuals), $544.00 (foreign institutions), and $191.00 (foreign students). To receive student/resident rate, orders must be accompanied by name of affiliated institution, date of term, and the signature of program/residency coordinator on institution letterhead. Orders will be billed at individual rate until proof of status is received. Foreign air speed delivery is included in all *Clinics* subscription prices. All prices are subject to change without notice. POSTMASTER: Send address changes to *Obstetrics and Gynecology Clinics*, Elsevier Health Sciences Division, Subscription Customer Service, 3251 Riverport Lane, Maryland Heights, MO 63043. **Customer Service: Telephone: 1-800-654-2452 (U.S. and Canada); 314-447-8871 (outside U.S. and Canada). Fax: 314-447-8029. E-mail: journalscustomerservice-usa@elsevier.com (for print support); journalsonlinesupport-usa@elsevier.com (for online support).**

Reprints. For copies of 100 or more of articles in this publication, please contact the Commercial Reprints Department, Elsevier Inc., 360 Park Avenue South, New York, New York 10010-1710. Tel.: 212-633-3818; Fax: 212-462-1935; E-mail: reprints@elsevier.com.

Obstetrics and Gynecology Clinics of North America is also published in Spanish by McGraw-Hill Interamericana Editores S.A., P.O. Box 5-237, 06500, Mexico; in Portuguese by Reichmann and Affonso Editores, Rio de Janeiro, Brazil; and in Greek by Paschalidis Medical Publications, Athens, Greece.

Obstetrics and Gynecology Clinics of North America is covered in MEDLINE/PubMed (Index Medicus), Excerpta Medica, Current Concepts/Clinical Medicine, Science Citation Index, BIOSIS, CINAHL, and ISI/BIOMED.

Printed and bound by CPI Group (UK) Ltd, Croydon, CR0 4YY

Transferred to Digital Print 2011

GOAL STATEMENT

The goal of *Obstetrics and Gynecology Clinics of North America* is to keep practicing physicians up to date with current clinical practice in OB/GYN by providing timely articles reviewing the state of the art in patient care.

ACCREDITATION

The *Obstetrics and Gynecology Clinics of North America* is planned and implemented in accordance with the Essential Areas and Policies of the Accreditation Council for Continuing Medical Education (ACCME) through the joint sponsorship of the University of Virginia School of Medicine and Elsevier. The University of Virginia School of Medicine is accredited by the ACCME to provide continuing medical education for physicians.

The University of Virginia School of Medicine designates this educational activity for a maximum of 15 *AMA PRA Category 1 Credits*™ for each issue, 60 credits per year. Physicians should only claim credit commensurate with the extent of their participation in the activity.

The American Medical Association has determined that physicians not licensed in the US who participate in this CME activity are eligible for a maximum of 15 *AMA PRA Category 1 Credits*™ for each issue, 60 credits per year.

Category 1 credit can be earned by reading the text material, taking the CME examination online at http://www.theclinics.com/home/cme, and completing the evaluation. After taking the test, you will be required to review any and all incorrect answers. Following completion of the test and evaluation, your credit will be awarded and you may print your certificate.

FACULTY DISCLOSURE/CONFLICT OF INTEREST

The University of Virginia School of Medicine, as an ACCME accredited provider, endorses and strives to comply with the Accreditation Council for Continuing Medical Education (ACCME) Standards of Commercial Support, Commonwealth of Virginia statutes, University of Virginia policies and procedures, and associated federal and private regulations and guidelines on the need for disclosure and monitoring of proprietary and financial interests that may affect the scientific integrity and balance of content delivered in continuing medical education activities under our auspices.

The University of Virginia School of Medicine requires that all CME activities accredited through this institution be developed independently and be scientifically rigorous, balanced and objective in the presentation/discussion of its content, theories and practices.

All authors/editors participating in an accredited CME activity are expected to disclose to the readers relevant financial relationships with commercial entities occurring within the past 12 months (such as grants or research support, employee, consultant, stock holder, member of speakers bureau, etc.). The University of Virginia School of Medicine will employ appropriate mechanisms to resolve potential conflicts of interest to maintain the standards of fair and balanced education to the reader. Questions about specific strategies can be directed to the Office of Continuing Medical Education, University of Virginia School of Medicine, Charlottesville, Virginia.

The faculty and staff of the University of Virginia Office of Continuing Medical Education have no financial affiliations to disclose.

The authors/editors listed below have identified no professional or financial affiliations for themselves or their spouse/partner:

Ayub Akbari, MD; Phyllis August, MD, MPH; Emily R. Baker, MD; Tara D. Benjamin, MD; D. Ware Branch, MD; Joan Briller, MD; Bruce Cohen, MD; Meredith O. Cruz, MD, MPH, MBA; Sarah M. Davis, MD; Laura M. DiGiovanni, MD; Diana L. Fitzpatrick, MD; Abbey J. Hardy-Fairbanks, MD; Judith U. Hibbard, MD (Guest Editor); Carla Holloway (Acquisitions Editor); William Irvin, MD (Test Author); Michelle A. Kominiarek, MD; Richard H. Lee, MD; Robert Molokie, MD; Alexander Panda, MD, MPH; Britta Panda, MD; Bhuvan Pathak, MD; Tiina Podymow, MD; Sarosh Rana, MD; Laura E. Riley, MD; Dennie T. Rogers, MD; Michelle A. Russell, MD, MPH; Lili Sheibani, MD; and Michelle Silasi, MD.

The authors/editors listed below identified the following professional or financial affiliations for themselves or their spouse/partner:

Michelle A. Josephson, MD is an industry funded research/investigator and consultant for Wyeth, and is a consultant for Digitas and Bristol Myers Squibb.
S. Ananth Karumanchi, MD is a consultant for Abbott Diagnostics, Beckman Coulter, Roche Diagnostics, and Johnson & Johnson; and is employed by Beth Israel Deaconess Medical Center.
Dianne B. McKay, MD is a stockholder in Home Dialysis Therapies of San Diego.
Gabriella Pridjian, MD is on the Advisory Committee/Board for Biomarin.
William F. Rayburn, MD, MBA (Consulting Editor) is an industry funded research/investigator and a consultant for Cytokine PharmaSciences.

Disclosure of Discussion of non-FDA approved uses for pharmaceutical products and/or medical devices:

The University of Virginia School of Medicine, as an ACCME provider, requires that all faculty presenters identify and disclose any off-label uses for pharmaceutical and medical device products. The University of Virginia School of Medicine recommends that each physician fully review all the available data on new products or procedures prior to clinical use.

TO ENROLL

To enroll in the Obstetrics and Gynecology Clinics of North America Continuing Medical Education program, call customer service at 1-800-654-2452 or visit us online at *www.theclinics.com/home/cme*. The CME program is available to subscribers for an additional fee of $180.00

Contributors

CONSULTING EDITOR

WILLIAM F. RAYBURN, MD, MBA
Randolph Seligman Professor and Chair, Department of Obstetrics and Gynecology, Chief of Staff, University Hospital, University of New Mexico Health Science Center, Albuquerque, New Mexico

GUEST EDITOR

JUDITH U. HIBBARD, MD
Professor of Obstetrics and Gynecology, Division of Maternal Fetal Medicine, Department of Obstetrics and Gynecology, University of Illinois at Chicago, Chicago, Illinois

AUTHORS

AYUB AKBARI, MD
Associate Professor, Division of Nephrology, University of Ottawa, Kidney Research Center, Ottawa, Ontario, Canada

PHYLLIS AUGUST, MD, MPH
Ralph A Baer MD Professor of Research in Medicine, Professor of Obstetrics and Gynecology in Medicine, Professor of Public Health, Weill Cornell Medical College of Cornell University, New York, New York

EMILY R. BAKER, MD
Professor, Vice Chair of the Department of Obstetrics and Gynecology, Division Director of Division of Maternal and Fetal Medicine, Dartmouth-Hitchcock Medical Center, Lebanon, New Hampshire

TARA D. BENJAMIN, MD
Department of Obstetrics and Gynecology, Tulane University Medical School, New Orleans, Louisiana

D. WARE BRANCH, MD
Professor, Department of Obstetrics and Gynecology, University of Utah Health Sciences Center, Salt Lake City, Utah

JOAN BRILLER, MD
Associate Professor of Medicine, Director of the Heart Disease in Women Program, Department of Cardiology; Clinical Associate Professor, Department of Obstetrics and Gynecology, University of Illinois at Chicago, Chicago, Illinois

BRUCE COHEN, MD
Division of Maternal Fetal Medicine, Department of Obstetrics and Gynecology, Beth Israel Deaconess Medical Center, Harvard Medical School, Boston, Massachusetts

MEREDITH O. CRUZ, MD, MPH, MBA
Instructor and Fellow, Division of Maternal Fetal Medicine, Department of Obstetrics and Gynecology, University of Illinois at Chicago, Chicago, Illinois

SARAH M. DAVIS, MD
Senior Resident, Department of Obstetrics and Gynecology, University of Utah Health Sciences Center, Salt Lake City, Utah

LAURA M. DIGIOVANNI, MD
Director, The Fetal Center; Assistant Professor of Obstetrics and Gynecology and The MacLean Center of Clinical Medical Ethics; Director, Ultrasound Division; Division of Maternal-Fetal Medicine, Department of Obstetrics and Gynecology, University of Chicago, Chicago, Illinois

DIANA L. FITZPATRICK, MD
Resident, Combined Obstetrics and Gynecology and Leadership Preventive Medicine, Department of Obstetrics and Gynecology, Dartmouth-Hitchock Medical Center, Lebanon, New Hampshire

ABBEY J. HARDY-FAIRBANKS, MD
Chief Resident, Department of Obstetrics and Gynecology, Dartmouth-Hitchcock Medical Center, Lebanon, New Hampshire

JUDITH U. HIBBARD, MD
Professor of Obstetrics and Gynecology, Division of Maternal Fetal Medicine, Department of Obstetrics and Gynecology, University of Illinois at Chicago, Chicago, Illinois

MICHELLE A. JOSEPHSON, MD
Professor, Department of Medicine, Section of Nephrology, University of Chicago, Chicago, Illinois

S. ANANTH KARUMANCHI, MD
Division of Maternal Fetal Medicine, Department of Obstetrics and Gynecology; Division of Nephrology, Department of Medicine, Beth Israel Deaconess Medical Center, Harvard Medical School; Howard Hughes Medical Institute, Boston, Massachusetts

MICHELLE A. KOMINIAREK, MD
Assistant Professor, Department of Obstetrics and Gynecology, University of Illinois at Chicago, Chicago, Illinois

RICHARD H. LEE, MD
Assistant Professor of Clinical Obstetrics and Gynecology, Division of Maternal Fetal Medicine, Department of Obstetrics and Gynecology, University of Southern California, Los Angeles, California

DIANNE B. MCKAY, MD
Associate Professor, Department of Immunology and Microbial Science, The Scripps Research Institute, La Jolla; Balboa Institute of Transplantation, Sharp Memorial Hospital, San Diego, California

ROBERT MOLOKIE, MD
Associate Professor, Department of Hematology/Medical Oncology, College of Medicine; Department of Biopharmaceutical Sciences, College of Pharmacy, University of Illinois at Chicago; Department of Internal Medicine, Jesse Brown Veterans Affairs Medical Center, Chicago, Illinois

ALEXANDER PANDA, MD, MPH
Attending in Infectious Diseases, Senior Fellow in Pulmonary and Critical Care Medicine, Divisions of Pulmonary and Critical Care Medicine, and Infectious Diseases, Yale University, New Haven, Connecticut

BRITTA PANDA, MD
Fellow in Maternal Fetal Medicine, Division of Maternal Fetal Medicine, Massachusetts General Hospital, Boston, Massachusetts

BHUVAN PATHAK, MD
Fellow, Division of Maternal Fetal Medicine, Department of Obstetrics and Gynecology, University of Southern California, Los Angeles, California

TIINA PODYMOW, MD
Assistant Professor, Division of Nephrology, McGill University, Montreal, Quebec, Canada

GABRIELLA PRIDJIAN, MD
Professor and Chairman, The Ernest and Elizabeth Miller-Robin Chair, Obstetrics and Gynecology; Adjunct Professor of Pediatrics, Division of Maternal-Fetal Medicine, Department of Obstetrics and Gynecology, Tulane University Medical School, New Orleans, Louisiana

SAROSH RANA, MD
Division of Maternal Fetal Medicine, Department of Obstetrics and Gynecology, Beth Israel Deaconess Medical Center, Harvard Medical School, Boston, Massachusetts

LAURA E. RILEY, MD
Assistant Professor, Medical Director of Labor and Delivery, Division of Maternal Fetal Medicine, Massachusetts General Hospital, Boston, Massachusetts

DENNIE T. ROGERS, MD
Clinical Instructor, Department of Obstetrics and Gynecology, University of Illinois at Chicago, Chicago, Illinois

MICHELLE A. RUSSELL, MD, MPH
Assistant Professor, Department of Obstetrics and Gynecology, Dartmouth-Hitchock Medical Center, Lebanon, New Hampshire

MICHELLE SILASI, MD
Division of Maternal Fetal Medicine, Department of Obstetrics and Gynecology, Beth Israel Deaconess Medical Center, Harvard Medical School, Boston, Massachusetts

LILI SHEIBANI, MD
Resident, Division of Maternal Fetal Medicine, Department of Obstetrics and Gynecology, University of Southern California, Los Angeles, California

Contents

Although renal disease in pregnancy is uncommon, it poses considerable risk to maternal and fetal health. This article discusses renal physiology and assessment of renal function in pregnancy and the effect of pregnancy on renal disease in patients with diabetes, lupus, chronic glomerulonephritis, polycystic kidney disease, and chronic pyelonephritis. Renal diseases occasionally present for the first time in pregnancy, and diagnoses of glomerulonephritis, acute tubular necrosis, hemolytic uremic syndrome, and acute fatty liver of pregnancy are described. Finally, therapy of end-stage renal disease in pregnancy, dialysis, and renal transplantation are reviewed.

March 10th, 1958, is the birthday of the first baby born to a kidney transplant recipient. The pregnancy went to term and the baby was delivered by cesarean section for fear that a vaginal birth could adversely affect the allograft kidney sitting in the iliac fossa. Undoubtedly, this pregnancy more than 50 years ago was considered high risk because of its pioneering nature. However, given that the transplant recipient had received her kidney from her identical twin sister approximately 2 years before and was not taking any immunosuppressive medications, the pregnancy was associated with far fewer risks than most pregnancies in transplant recipients of today. Not only are immunosuppressants now available that have potential adverse affects on the developing fetus but also many kidney transplant recipients have kidney function that is suboptimal. Although thousands of women with kidney transplants have successfully delivered healthy babies, many new issues must be considered during a transplant recipient's pregnancy compared with 50 years ago. These issues are discussed in this article.

The term sickle cell disease (SSD) encompasses several different sickle hemoglobinopathies. The ability to predict the clinical course of SSD during pregnancy is difficult. This article examines pregnancy-associated complications in SSD and the management of sickle cell disorders in pregnant women. Outcomes have improved for pregnant women with SSD and nowadays the majority can achieve a successful live birth. However, pregnancy is still associated with an increased incidence of morbidity and mortality. Optimal management during pregnancy should be directed at preventing pain crises, chronic organ damage, optimization of fetal health and minimizing early maternal mortality using a multidisciplinary team approach and prompt, effective and safe relief of acute pain episodes.

Preeclampsia is a common complication of pregnancy with potentially devastating consequences to both the mother and the baby. It is the leading cause of maternal deaths in developing countries. In developed countries it is the major cause of iatrogenic premature delivery and contributes significantly to increasing health care cost associated with prematurity. There is currently no known treatment for preeclampsia; ultimate treatment involves delivery of the placenta. Although there are several risk factors (such as multiple gestation or chronic hypertension), most patients present with no obvious risk factors. The molecular pathogenesis of preeclampsia is just now being elucidated. It has been proposed that abnormal placentation and an imbalance in angiogenic factors lead to the clinical findings and complications seen in preeclampsia. Preeclampsia is characterized by high levels of circulating antiangiogenic factors such as soluble fms-like tyrosine kinase-1 and soluble endoglin, which induce maternal endothelial dysfunction. These soluble factors are altered not only at the time of clinical disease but also several weeks before the onset of clinical signs and symptoms. Many methods of prediction and surveillance have been proposed to identify women who will develop preeclampsia, but studies have been inconclusive. With the recent discovery of the role of angiogenic factors in preeclampsia, novel methods of prediction and diagnosis are being developed to aid obstetricians and midwives in clinical practice. This article discusses the role of angiogenic factors in the pathogenesis, prediction, diagnosis, and possible treatment of preeclampsia.

Update on Gestational Diabetes

Gabriella Pridjian and Tara D. Benjamin

As the rate of obesity increases in adolescent and adult women in the United States, practitioners of obstetrics see higher rates of gestational diabetes. Recent clinical studies suggest that women with gestational diabetes have impaired pancreatic beta-cell function and reduced beta-cell adaptation resulting in insufficient insulin secretion to maintain normal glycemia. Despite recent evidence that even mild hyperglycemia is associated with adverse pregnancy outcomes, controversies still exist in screening, management, and treatment of gestational diabetes. Initial studies regarding glyburide for treatment of gestational diabetes are promising. Overall, only about half of the women with gestational diabetes are screened in the postpartum period, an ideal time for education and intervention, to decrease incidence of glucose intolerance and progression to type 2 diabetes.

Cholestasis of Pregnancy

Bhuvan Pathak, Lili Sheibani, and Richard H. Lee

Intrahepatic cholestasis (ICP) of pregnancy is a disease that is likely multifactorial in etiology and has a prevalence that varies by geography and ethnicity. The diagnosis is made when patients have a combination of pruritus and abnormal liver-function tests. It is associated with a high risk for adverse perinatal outcome, including preterm birth, meconium passage, and fetal death. As of yet, the cause for fetal death is unknown. Because fetal deaths caused by ICP appear to occur predominantly after 37 weeks, it is suggested to offer delivery at approximately 37 weeks.

Ursodeoxycholic acid appears to be the most effective medication to improve maternal pruritus and liver-function tests; however, there is no medication to date that has been shown to reduce the risk for fetal death.

Although multiple mechanisms have been postulated, peripartum cardiomyopathy (PPCM) continues to be a cardiomyopathy of unknown cause. Multiple risk factors exist and the clinical presentation does not allow differentiation among potential causes. Although specific diagnostic criteria exist, PPCM remains a diagnosis of exclusion. Treatment modalities are dictated by the clinical state of the patient, and prognosis is dependent on recovery of function. Randomized controlled trials of novel therapies, such as bromocriptine, are needed to establish better treatment regimens to decrease morbidity and mortality. The creation of an international registry will be an important step to better define and treat PPCM. This article discusses the pathogenesis, risk factors, diagnosis, management, and prognosis of this condition.

The incidence of obesity is increasing rapidly, and it affects a greater proportion of women than men. Unfortunately, obesity has a negative impact on women's reproductive health, including increased adverse perinatal outcomes. Weight loss surgery, also known as bariatric surgery, is performed in many hospitals, and can allow for significant weight loss and improvement in medical comorbidities such as diabetes and hypertension. A woman who becomes pregnant after bariatric surgery usually has an uncomplicated pregnancy but requires special attention to some complications that can occur after these procedures. This article reviews the perinatal outcomes and provides recommendations for care regarding the unique issues that arise during a pregnancy after bariatric surgery.

This article reviews the impact of seasonal influenza on pregnancy with particular emphasis on the 2009 novel H1N1 pandemic. Antiviral therapy for influenza, as well as recommendations and safety data on vaccination are discussed. In addition, the impact of hepatitis A, B, and C in pregnancy is addressed with a focus on prevention and treatment strategies for hepatitis B and C.

Venous thrombosis and embolism (VTE) is one of the most common, serious complications associated with pregnancy, and now ranks as a leading cause of maternal morbidity and mortality in developed countries. Information regarding the association of VTE with acquired and heritable thrombophilias has greatly expanded in the last 20 years, adding a new layer of complexity to decisions about thromboprophylaxis. The objective of this review is to detail which patients are at clinically important increased risk for VTE, are candidates for thrombophilia screening, and warrant thromboprophylaxis. Recommended management regimens for use in specific patient subgroups are also provided.

Obstetricians must become comfortable addressing the ethical issues involved in clinical obstetrics and therefore must have an understanding of the key elements of clinical medical ethics. Balancing the principles of medical ethics can guide clinicians toward solutions to ethical dilemmas encountered in the care of pregnant women. The purpose of this article is to review the ethical foundations of clinical practice, recognize the ethical issues obstetricians face every day in caring for patients, and facilitate decision making. This article discusses the relevant ethical principles, identifies unique features of obstetrical ethics, examines ethical principles as they apply to pregnant patient and her fetus, and thereby, provides a conceptual framework for considering ethical issues and facilitating decision making in clinical obstetrics.

THE CLINICS ARE NOW AVAILABLE ONLINE!

Access your subscription at:
www.theclinics.com

Foreword

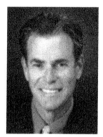

William F. Rayburn, MD, MBA
Consulting Editor

This issue of *Obstetrics and Gynecology Clinics of North America*, with Dr Judith Hibbard as Guest Editor, provides a timely update on topics pertaining to medical disorders in pregnancy. It is important that obstetricians have working knowledge of medical diseases common to women of childbearing age. It is difficult, however, to quantify accurately the broad range of medical illnesses that complicate pregnancy. Estimates have been derived from conditions warranting hospitalization. One study reported an overall antenatal hospitalization rate of 10 per 100 deliveries in their managed-care population of more than 46,000 pregnant women. About one third of those admissions were for nonobstetric conditions, such as renal, gastrointestinal, pulmonary, and infectious diseases. The care for some of these women warrants a team effort between obstetricians and specialists in either maternal-fetal medicine or internal medicine.

It is essential to be familiar with pregnancy-induced physiologic changes. Even during normal pregnancy, virtually every organ system undergoes anatomic and functional changes that can alter criteria for diagnosis and treatment of medical complications. Without such knowledge, it is nearly impossible to understand how a disease process can threaten a woman and her fetus.

On review of these articles, several fundamental principles apply to the rational approach for managing and prescribing drugs during pregnancy. (1) A woman should not be penalized for being pregnant. (2) What management plan would be recommended if she were nonpregnant? (3) What justifications are there to change such therapy because of pregnancy? (4) Individualization of care is especially important during pregnancy. (5) The healthiest mother is likely to deliver the healthiest fetus.

Practice guidelines offered here result from a formal synthesis of evidence, developed according to a rigorous research and review process. The authors' contributions offer a better understanding of evidence-based medicine, particularly as they relate to the development of guidelines. As evidence-based medicine continues to be integrated into clinical practice, an understanding of its basic elements is critical in translating the peer-reviewed literature into appropriate management of these medical

Obstet Gynecol Clin N Am 37 (2010) xv–xvi
doi:10.1016/j.ogc.2010.03.002
0889-8545/10/$ – see front matter © 2010 Elsevier Inc. All rights reserved.

obgyn.theclinics.com

conditions. The emphasis on evidence-based medicine has taken on even more importance with the accessibility of information being easier for both obstetricians and their patients.

This issue provides a fresh perspective to the treatment of commonly seen, chronic medical illnesses during pregnancy. It is our desire that this timely review activates attention to issues about such conditions in pregnancy. It is hoped that the practical information provided herein by this distinguished group of clinicians aids in the evaluation and treatment of medical complications to optimize favorable outcomes for both mother and fetus.

William F. Rayburn, MD, MBA
Department of Obstetrics and Gynecology
University of New Mexico School of Medicine
MSC 10 5580, 1 University of New Mexico
Albuquerque, NM 871310001, USA

E-mail address:
wrayburn@salud.unm.edu

Preface

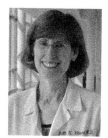

Judith U. Hibbard, MD
Guest Editor

I am delighted to have the opportunity to edit this important issue of *Obstetrics and Gynecology Clinics of North America* on the topic of Medical Complications in Pregnancy. The broad field of medicine changes rapidly, with constantly occurring new breakthroughs, approaches, and recommendations. The area of medical disorders in pregnancy encompasses a broad range of diseases; a woman may have a long-term chronic disorder that can have major implications for undertaking a pregnancy. Yet, other medical conditions are unique to pregnancy but also influence gestational outcomes. Although the obstetrician has to be knowledgeable in regard to the normal physiologic changes occurring with gestation, understanding the interplay of medical conditions with these changes on not only 1 but 2 patients, mother and fetus, can be a daunting task.

I have invited a group of outstanding physicians to author articles that are timely and clinically useful to the practicing obstetrician. Several manuscripts in this issue focus on commonly occurring illnesses but bring fresh perspective to our understanding of these disease causes, management schemes, and newer medical therapies. Other complications included are much less frequently addressed in a clear, concise article in which the obstetrician can find dependable advice for clinically managing patients. Frequently the obstetrician must make difficult management decisions that involve their 2 patients, which may lead to conflicting strategies.

The issue begins with articles on several chronic illnesses that many obstetricians encounter on a daily basis. A timely review of pregestational diabetes in pregnancy and a clinical approach to asthma in gestation begin the series. Thyroid disease in pregnancy is revisited, providing insight into issues of screening. A clinical framework for understanding renal disease in pregnancy is presented, whereas an approach to pregnant women with renal transplant, becoming more common, is provided. Sickle disease in pregnancy, seen frequently in urban centers across the country, is examined and clinical guidance offered. Several diseases unique to pregnancy present challenges for the obstetrician. A timely update on preeclampsia, clarifying the role that angiogenic factors play in the genesis and prediction of this

Obstet Gynecol Clin N Am 37 (2010) xvii–xviii
doi:10.1016/j.ogc.2010.02.016
0889-8545/10/$ – see front matter © 2010 Elsevier Inc. All rights reserved.

disease, is included. Insight is provided into newer treatment modalities in gestational diabetes, particularly oral hypoglycemic agents. Cholestasis in pregnancy is reviewed, and its medical impact as well as a management scheme is described. Newer therapies and clinical trials are described in the article on peripartum cardiomyopathy. As the incidence of obesity continues to increase, so does the number of pregnant women who have undergone previous bypass surgery; a practical approach to these gravidas is suggested. An update on the unique impact of H1N1 virus on pregnancy is reviewed. A clear, logical framework for thrombophilia screening and thromboprophylaxis in pregnancy is included. In the final article, there is an exploration of some of the ethical issues that affect mother and fetus maligned by medical diseases during gestation.

The opportunity to edit this issue of *Obstetrics and Gynecology Clinics of North America* has not only been a challenge but also an enjoyable learning experience for me. I hope you will find these articles to be as enlightening as I have found them.

Judith U. Hibbard, MD
Division of Maternal Fetal Medicine
Department of Obstetrics and Gynecology
University of Illinois at Chicago
840 South Wood Street, M/C 808
Chicago, IL 60612, USA

E-mail address:
jhibbar@uic.edu

Pregestational Diabetes

Gabriella Pridjian, MD

KEYWORDS

• Diabetes type 1 • Diabetes type 2 • Pregnancy

The number of pregnant women with preexisting diabetes is increasing, mainly from an increase in type 2[1,2] but also an increase in type 1 diabetes.[3,4] Therefore, the knowledge and management of this medical condition in pregnancy has become even more important. The epidemics of obesity and the low level of physical activity, and possibly the exposure to diabetes in utero,[5,6] are major contributors to the increase in type 2 diabetes in adults and in childhood and adolescence. Reasons for the increase in type 1 diabetes are somewhat unclear but may be related to harmful environmental conditions.

CLASSIFICATION

Diabetes in pregnancy has been traditionally grouped according to the pioneering work of Priscilla White,[7] who classified diabetes according to onset, duration, and complications to predict perinatal outcome (**Table 1**). An important distinction in classification is the existence of micro or macrovascular complications of diabetes. If no vascular complications exist, then placental growth and development are most often not impeded and the risk for intrauterine growth restriction (IUGR) is smaller. However, with vascular complications such as those noted in the lower half of **Table 1**, the risk for IUGR increases with increasing severity.[8]

Although the White's classification is still valuable, the more recent diabetes classification from the Expert Committee on the Diagnosis and Classification of Diabetes,[9] summarized in **Table 2**, may be more useful in patient management because it alerts clinicians to the type of diabetes, which may have somewhat different treatment strategies. Overall, type 1 diabetes accounts for approximately 5% to 10% of all diabetes outside of pregnancy, and type 2 diabetes for 90% to 95%.

METABOLISM IN PREGNANCY

Pregnancy itself is a diabetogenic state that exacerbates preexisting diabetes. Metabolism changes dramatically during pregnancy. Both basal and postprandial glucose

Division of Maternal-Fetal Medicine, Department of Obstetrics & Gynecology, SL11, Tulane University Medical School, 1430 Tulane Avenue, New Orleans, LA 70112, USA
E-mail address: Pridjian@Tulane.edu

Obstet Gynecol Clin N Am 37 (2010) 143–158
doi:10.1016/j.ogc.2010.02.014
0889-8545/10/$ – see front matter © 2010 Elsevier Inc. All rights reserved.

obgyn.theclinics.com

Table 1
Description of diabetes and pregnancy

Description	Class	Fetal Growth
Gestational diabetes, insulin not required	A1	No vascular disease
Gestational diabetes, insulin required	A2	Risk for macrosomia
Age of onset, ≥20 y (maturity onset diabetes)	B1	
Duration, <10 y, no vascular lesions	B2	
Age of onset, 10–19 y	C1	
Duration, 10–19 y, no vascular lesions	C2	
Age of onset, <10 y	D1	
Duration, ≥20 y	D2	
Benign retinopathy	D3	Vascular disease
Calcified arteries of legs	D4	Risk for intrauterine
Calcified arteries of pelvis	E	growth restriction
Nephropathy	F	
Many failures	G	
Cardiopathy	H	
Proliferating retinopathy	R	
Renal transplant	T	

Data from White P. Classification of obstetric diabetes. Am J Obstet Gynecol 1978;130:228–30.

metabolism gradually change over the course of pregnancy to meet the nutritional demands of the mother and fetus. As pregnancy progresses, fasting glucose decreases[10] and fasting insulin increases. Despite a decrease in fasting glucose in pregnancy, basal hepatic glucose production increases and hepatic insulin sensitivity decreases. The first and second phases of insulin secretion increase, and insulin sensitivity decreases. In women who are pregnant and obese, hepatic insulin sensitivity further decreases[11] and approaches the degree observed in type 2 diabetes.

Insulin resistance in pregnancy is likely caused by the combined metabolic effects of hormones in the maternal circulation, specifically human placental lactogen, progesterone, prolactin, and cortisol and various cytokines. The increase in insulin resistance generally parallels placental mass and the increase in placental hormones.

Table 2
Diabetes classification

	Findings	Phenotype
Type 1	Immune-mediated, genetic predisposition Insulinopenic Ketoacidosis	Begins in childhood or adolescence Thin
Type 2	Decreased insulin sensitivity Decreased insulin production Hyperosmolar coma	Often overweight Metabolic syndrome
Other specific types	Pancreatic damage: cystic fibrosis, alcoholism, mutations, etc	Various
Gestational	Diabetes first diagnosed in pregnancy (may be any of above first presenting or also diagnosed in pregnancy)	Various, usually overweight

Data from American Diabetes Association. Diagnosis and classification of diabetes mellitus. Diabetes Care 2010;33(Suppl 1):S62–9.

TREATMENT

The mainstay of treatment of preexisting diabetes in pregnancy is focused on diet, exercise, and insulin to maintain blood sugars in the physiologic range, which may vary depending on carbohydrate types (**Fig. 1**). Maternal glucose freely crosses the placenta through facilitated diffusion. Maternal hyperglycemia results in fetal hyperglycemia and hyperinsulinemia. Maternal insulin does not cross the placenta except for the small fraction bound to IgG antibody.

DIET

Medical nutrition therapy in women with diabetes should be directed by a dietician familiar with diabetes.[12] Most women with diabetes who become pregnant will likely be on nutrition therapy at the onset of pregnancy. Daily caloric requirements in pregnancy can be calculated from prepregnancy weight and are estimated to be 30 kcal/kg per day for women of normal body mass index, up to 40 kcal/kg per day for women who are underweight, 24 kcal/kg per day for overweight women, and approximately 15 kcal/kg per day for obese women. The recommended distribution of calories is 40% to 50% carbohydrate, 20% protein, and 30% to 40% fat.[13]

Monitoring carbohydrate intake is the key to achieving good glycemic control, which can be obtained through counting carbohydrates and adjusting the insulin dose required, or through maintaining a fixed amount of carbohydrates and a fixed dose of insulin per meal. Carbohydrates of low glycemic index lead to a blunted postprandial glucose level and improve ease of glycemic control (see **Fig. 1**). The U.S. Food and Drug Administration (FDA) has approved five nonnutritive sweeteners (acesulfame, aspartame, neotame, saccharin, and sucralose) and several reduced-calorie sweeteners (eg, erythritol, mannitol, sorbitol) for use in the United States, including during pregnancy. Certain women with hyperlipidemia or renal disease may require more targeted medical nutrition therapy. Diet for women with type 2 diabetes often includes a program to lose or maintain weight. However, in pregnancy, weight loss should not be a goal and following the general guidelines for weight gain in pregnancy is recommended.[14]

Women are encouraged to consume vegetables and fruits, choose whole grain foods over processed grain products, include fish approximately once a week, choose lean meats and nonfat dairy products, and drink water and calorie-free drinks (in moderation) instead of regular sugar-sweetened drinks. Women are recommended to use liquid oils for cooking instead of solid fats and cut back on high-calorie foods such as potato chips, cookies, cakes, and full-fat ice cream.

INSULIN

Several recent advances in insulin therapy have improved the management of diabetes overall and in pregnancy. In pregnancy, the goal is normal plasma glucose throughout the day with no hypoglycemia (**Table 3**). Women with preexisting diabetes in pregnancy are required to perform capillary blood glucose evaluation approximately 6 to 8 times a day, including fasting, preprandial, 1 or 2 hours postprandial, and occasionally at 2 AM.

The most efficient method to achieve optimal glycemic control is to mimic physiologic insulin levels (**Fig. 2**) through frequent administration. This entails intensive insulin treatment with delivery of basal, background insulin, and bolus insulin doses with each meal or large snack. Basal insulin is approximately 50% to 60% of the total daily insulin requirement; the remaining insulin would then be divided into injections of short-acting

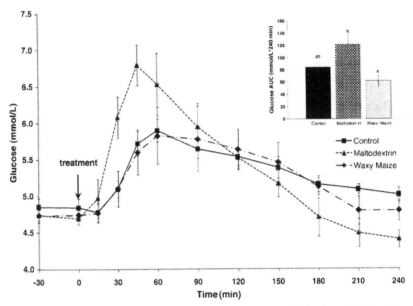

Fig. 1. Physiologic plasma glucose response depending on carbohydrate intake of various glycemic indices. The control food is white bread. (*Reprinted from* Sands AL, Leidy HJ, Hamaker BR, et al. Consumption of the slow digesting waxy maize starch leads to blunted plasma glucose and insulin response but does not influence energy expenditure or appetite in humans. Nutr Res 2009;29:387; with permission.)

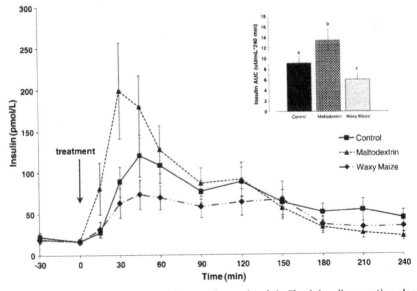

Fig. 2. Plasma insulin levels corresponding to glucose levels in **Fig. 1.** Insulin secretion closely mimics glucose levels; foods with low glycemic index will result in a more blunted insulin response. The control food is white bread. (*Reprinted from* Sands AL, Leidy HJ, Hamaker BR, et al. Consumption of the slow digesting waxy maize starch leads to blunted plasma glucose and insulin response but does not influence energy expenditure or appetite in humans. Nutr Res 2009;29:388; with permission.)

Table 3
Target plasma glucose levels

Fasting	60–95 mg/dL
Premeal	60–100 mg/dL
1 hour postprandial	<140 mg/dL
2 hours postprandial	<120 mg/dL
2–6 AM	>60 mg/dL

insulin. At minimum, women with prepregnancy diabetes require three to four injections per day or the continuous insulin pump for optimal glucose control during pregnancy.

Traditional types of insulin used for treatment of diabetes in pregnancy have been regular human and neutral protamine Hagedorn (NPH) (**Table 4**). Although these types of insulin have been widely used, their insulin profiles do not mimic the in vivo state as well as newer insulins and insulin analogs (**Fig. 3**).

Use of the newer very–short-acting insulins, lispro and aspart, better mimic postprandial insulin secretion and thus return the glucose level to normal more quickly than the traditional short-acting regular insulin. In 1999, the first prospective study of the efficacy and safety of lispro (which has the amino acid sequence in the β-chain reversed at position B28 and B29) in pregnancy was reported.[15] Lispro was shown to normalize blood glucose levels more efficaciously than human regular insulin in women with diabetes. This insulin rapidly lowered the postprandial glucose levels, thereby decreasing the A1C levels with fewer hypoglycemic episodes and without increasing the antiinsulin antibody levels. Insulin aspart was created by recombinant DNA technology so that amino acid B28, which is normally proline, is substituted with an aspartic acid residue. As with lispro, compared with regular insulin, aspart insulin reduces both postprandial plasma glucose and episodes of hypoglycemia significantly.[16] Both lispro and aspart are safe and efficacious for premeal use by pregnant women with diabetes.[16,17]

Glargine, a long-acting insulin analog, was approved by the FDA in 2000 for use as basal insulin. Insulin glargine has a glycine substitution in the α-chain at position 21 and two arginines attached to the β-chain terminal at position 30. Glargine has been shown to provide a peakless, sustained 24-hour level of insulin with once-a-day administration at bedtime or in the morning; in certain individuals glargine administered every 12 hours improves steady-state basal levels. Glargine cannot be administered in the same syringe with other insulins. Because the more natural profile of

Table 4
Insulins commonly used in women of reproductive age

Duration of Action	Type	Derivation	Onset (h)	Peak (h)
Short acting	Regular insulin[a]	Human	0.5	2–4
	Insulin lispro	Analog	0.25	1–2
	Insulin aspart	Analog	0.25	1–2.5
Intermediate-acting	Neutral protamine Hagedorn[a]	Human	1–2	5–7
	Lente[a]	Human	1–3	4–8
Long-acting	Glargine	Analog	1.1	5 (no peak)
	Determir	Analog	1–2	5 (no peak)

[a] Different manufacturers may have a slightly different profile; consult specific manufacturer's information.

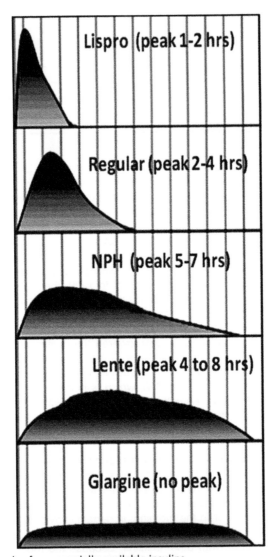

Fig. 3. Plasma levels of commercially available insulins.

glargine mimics endogenous insulin production, its use is associated with fewer nocturnal hypoglycemic episodes than NPH insulin.[18,19]

Glargine is classified as Pregnancy Category C according to the FDA. In vitro studies suggest that glargine might stimulate insulin-like growth factor 1, and use in human pregnancy has caused concern for macrosomia. However, many women treated with glargine for their basal insulin requirements have become pregnant with no adverse outcome. Several retrospective reports are now in the literature noting the safety of glargine insulin in pregnancy.

In a retrospective study, Egerman and colleagues[20] assessed outcomes in 114 pregnant patients with diabetes, of whom 65 were managed with glargine and 49 with NPH insulin as the basal insulin. Shoulder dystocia was higher in the NPH group. Gestational age at delivery, birth weight, Apgar scores, admission to the neonatal intensive care unit, respiratory distress syndrome, hypoglycemia, and congenital anomalies were similar between the groups.

In a study of glargine use as basal insulin in pregnancy in 184 gestational and 56 pre-existing women with diabetes, Henderson and colleagues[21] found that macrosomia was not increased. Fang and colleagues[22] performed a retrospective cohort study comparing 52 pregnant women treated with glargine basal insulin with 60 women treated with NPH basal insulin. Glargine was not associated with increased maternal or neonatal morbidity compared with NPH insulin, but was associated with lower rates of macrosomia, neonatal hypoglycemia, and hyperbilirubinemia.

Gallen and associates[23] reported the outcomes of 109 babies of 115 women with type 1 diabetes from United Kingdom diabetic centers who were treated with glargine in pregnancy. No unexpected adverse maternal or fetal outcome was seen.

Currently, glargine use in pregnant women with diabetes seems safe, but data are limited. Prospective, large studies confirming this finding are lacking. Glargine is easier to use than NPH and has the benefit of less hypoglycemia. Any unknown and as of yet unreported risk associated with glargine use in human pregnancy may be outweighed by its benefits. Until additional data are available, glargine could be considered in women who already use glargine with good glycemic control, have difficulty controlling their blood glucose without frequent hypoglycemia, or have difficulty incorporating the peaks of NPH into their regimen for optimal glycemic control.

DOSING REGIMENS

Dosing regimens vary according to insulins used and delivery systems. NPH and regular insulin can be dosed in three injections per day. Two thirds of the total daily dose is given in the morning in a ratio of 2:1 NPH to regular insulin. At supper, one sixth of the total daily dose is given as regular insulin and one sixth of the total daily dose is given at bedtime as NPH. The morning regular insulin is assessed using postprandial breakfast glucose level and the before-lunch glucose level. The morning NPH insulin is assessed according to the glucose result before supper; the evening regular insulin is assessed using the postprandial or bedtime levels of glucose, and the evening NPH insulin is assessed using the glucose level before breakfast the next day.

NPH and lispro or aspart can be administered in four injections per day. NPH is still dosed as 2/3 of the total daily dose. Of the 2/3 daily dose of NPH, 2/3 is given in the morning, and 1/3 at bedtime. The remaining 1/3 of the total daily dose is divided in three parts depending upon carbohydrate intake and administered 15 minutes before each meal. The dinner dose may need to be decreased to accommodate the morning NPH peak.

Glargine and aspart or lispro can be administered in four injections per day. Approximately 50% to 60% of the total daily insulin requirement is administered at bedtime as glargine, and the remaining insulin is divided into three doses with each meal. Again, the specific dose will depend on carbohydrate intake but could theoretically be divided equally for each meal.

Insulin pumps are commonly filled with lispro or aspart. Basal insulin administration is continuous through the pump and should be approximately 50% to 60% of the total daily insulin requirement; the remaining daily requirement is administered as boluses with meals and snacks. A meta-analysis of randomized controlled trials evaluating the differences between use of continuous insulin infusion versus multiple-dose insulin did not show any statistical difference in pregnancy outcome or glycemic control.[24] Other investigators found less hypoglycemic episodes with the pump.[25]

CONTINUOUS GLUCOSE MONITORING

Several companies have developed a minimally invasive technology that measures glucose continuously. Of those clinically available, one uses reverse iontophoresis, in which a low-voltage current is applied to the skin surface causing interstitial fluid (and glucose) to pass through the skin where it can be measured. The other uses a disposable subcutaneous glucose-sensing device and an electrode impregnated with glucose oxidase connected by a cable to a small monitor worn on the body. These systems measure glucose frequently, approximately every 5 minutes. Values correlate with plasma glucose laboratory values, and capillary glucose monitoring. Sensors detect trends and alarms are programmed.[26] Capillary glucose monitoring is still performed approximately 4 to 5 times a day as quality control.

Murphy and colleagues[27] analyzed the effectiveness of continuous glucose monitoring systems in 71 pregnant women with type 1 (n = 46) or type 2 (n = 25) diabetes allocated to antenatal care and continuous glucose monitoring (n = 38) or to standard antenatal care (n = 33). Women assigned to continuous glucose monitoring system devices had lower mean hemoglobin A1c (HA1c) concentrations at 32 to 36 weeks' gestation compared with women with diabetes assigned to standard antenatal care (5.8% vs 6.4%), and also had lower mean birth weight and reduced risk for macrosomia. McLachlan and colleagues[28] obtained similar findings when they analyzed the effectiveness of continuous glucose monitoring systems in 68 pregnant women with diabetes. Practically, at the current state of the art, continuous glucose monitoring systems are useful in early detection of prolonged hyperglycemia or hypoglycemia.

MATERNAL COMPLICATIONS

Medical complications of diabetes and pregnancy include those specifically related to diabetes and an increased risk for preeclampsia.

Diabetic nephropathy complicates approximately 5% of pregnancies in women with preexisting diabetes. Most affected pregnancies are in women with type 1 diabetes, but diabetic nephropathy can occur in those with type 2, and generally progresses less quickly. Disease progression is characterized by hypertension and deteriorating glomerular filtrations rate. Progression of diabetic nephropathy can be attenuated by aggressive treatment of hypertension and intensive glycemic control.[29]

Some women with diabetic nephropathy display the expected increase in glomerular filtration noted in normal pregnancy; others do not experience a significant increase. Women with overt diabetic nephropathy experience increased proteinuria in pregnancy. The greater the proteinuria at the onset of pregnancy, the greater its increase during the pregnancy. Protein excretion can double or triple in the third trimester compared with the first, and can confuse the diagnosis of preeclampsia. Overall, with close evaluation and management, pregnancy outcomes in women with diabetic nephropathy have been good, but not completely without risk.

Approximately 50% of women deliver preterm iatrogenically because of maternal or fetal indications, 15% have fetuses with intrauterine growth restriction (IUGR), and preeclampsia occurs in approximately 50%. Women with a prepregnancy creatinine of greater than 1.5 mg/dL have the highest perinatal complication rate.[30,31] Antihypertensive therapy delays progression of diabetic nephropathy. Angiotensin-converting enzyme inhibitors or angiotensin receptor blockers have clearly been shown to be superior in slowing progression of microalbuminuria in women with diabetes with and without hypertension.[32,33] Unfortunately, these medications are teratogenic throughout pregnancy and cannot be used during pregnancy.[34]

Diabetic retinopathy, still one of the leading causes of blindness and visual disability in the world, is most often associated with long-standing type 1 diabetes. Evidence shows that diabetic retinopathy advances with pregnancy,[35,36] at least for the short term. However, pregnancy does not seem to have long-term consequences on diabetic retinopathy. Controversy exists over whether the microvascular changes in the eye are from pregnancy itself or the rapid improvement of glycemic control that occurs in some women when pregnancy is discovered.[37,38]

Factors associated with progression of diabetic retinopathy in pregnancy are the duration of type 1 diabetes, presence of chronic hypertension or preeclampsia, the degree of hyperglycemia, poor glycemic control at conception, and the stage of disease at onset of pregnancy.[39] Fluid retention, vasodilation, and increased blood flow in pregnancy are believed to accelerate the loss of autoregulatory function of the retinal capillary bed.[40,41] Diabetic retinopathy can be classified as background, preproliferative, or proliferative, depending on progression. Progression from nonproliferative to proliferative retinopathy ranges from 6% to 30% depending on severity.[42] The treatment of diabetic retinopathy using laser photocoagulation is as effective in pregnancy as outside of pregnancy and should not be delayed.

Diabetic neuropathy in pregnancy has not been well studied. A short-term increase in distal symmetric polyneuropathy may occur in association with pregnancy, but at least in one study the increase appeared to be transient.[43] Women with diabetic gastroparesis may experience more protracted nausea and vomiting of pregnancy. This complication should be considered and treated.

Coronary artery disease is not commonly seen in pregnant women with diabetes. Information related to the incidence of coronary artery disease in pregnant women with diabetes is sparse and only case reports exist in the literature. Data are insufficient to extrapolate recommendations. However, women with preexisting angina or myocardial infarction should generally not be encouraged to become pregnant, particularly if they have diminished cardiac function.

Diabetic ketoacidosis (DKA) is an uncommon occurrence in treatment-compliant women with type 1 diabetes, despite the increased risk for this complication associated with the ketogenesis of normal pregnancy. However, DKA is a common complication in undiagnosed diabetes.[44] Any pregnant woman with vomiting or dehydration and blood sugars greater than 200 mg/dL should have electrolytes, plasma bicarbonate, and serum acetone levels measured to confirm DKA diagnosis. Arterial blood gasses should be obtained if the plasma bicarbonate is low and acetone is present. Several management algorithms are available.[45,46]

The precipitant of DKA is often infection, which should be diagnosed and treated promptly. Resolution of DKA can be slower in pregnancy. DKA is often associated with a nonreassuring fetal heart rate tracing, which in most cases resolves once the metabolic acidosis improves. However, despite improved management, DKA remains an important cause of fetal loss in diabetic pregnancies.[47]

FETAL COMPLICATIONS

Women with diabetes are subject to an increased risk for first trimester miscarriage, congenital malformations, IUGR, macrosomia, birth trauma, stillbirth, and iatrogenic preterm delivery. The neonate is at risk for hypoglycemia, hypocalcemia, hyperbilirubinemia, polycythemia, and morbidity and mortality from congenital malformations or severe prematurity. Children of mothers with diabetes are at risk for obesity, glucose intolerance, and cardiovascular disease later in life.

Diabetic embryopathy occurs in approximately 6% to 10% of diabetic pregnancies and is directly related to HA1c levels during organogenesis.[48,49] The risk for malformations in a fetus of a mother with a normal HA1c level is only slightly greater than that for the general population; newborns of women with a conception HA1c greater than 10% have an approximately 22% probability of having congenital malformations. Most malformations occur during embryogenesis[49] and are seen with all types of preexisting diabetes.[50] Several investigators have documented the decrease in congenital malformation risk in women who had preconception care.[51,52]

The stillbirth rate in women with diabetes has decreased recently to approximately 5.8 of every 1000 births.[53] Approximately half of these stillbirth or fetal deaths are related to hyperglycemia, and the remainder caused by infection or congenital anomalies.[54] Studies with fetal blood sampling confirm that hyperglycemia has been associated with fetal hypoxia and acidosis.[55]

Kjos and colleagues[56] described obstetric outcomes in 2134 women with all types of diabetes after participation in an antepartum fetal surveillance program of twice weekly nonstress tests (NSTs) with amniotic fluid volume determinations. They found that no stillbirth occurred within 4 days of the last antepartum testing, and that 85 women required cesarean delivery for fetal distress. Predictive factors for emergent cesarean delivery for nonreassuring fetal tracings included spontaneous decelerations, nonreactive NSTs, and both findings together. Using this testing scheme, these investigators were able to decrease the stillbirth rate to 1.4 of every 1000.

In a meta-analysis, Balsells and colleagues[57] compared type 1 and 2 diabetes and found that women with type 2 had lower HA1c at the first visit but a higher rate of perinatal mortality (odds ratio, 1.50; 95% CI, 1.15–1.96). Despite a milder glycemic disturbance, women with type 2 diabetes had no better perinatal outcomes than those with type 1.

MANAGEMENT
Preconception

In the preconception period, insulin regimens can be modified to improve glycemic control, cholesterol-lowering medications should be discontinued, and angiotensin-converting enzyme inhibitors should be discontinued or changed to a calcium channel blocker. Folic acid supplementation is instituted. Baseline renal function can be assessed to evaluate risk in a pregnancy and an ophthalmologic evaluation performed. Other health or genetic risks should also be addressed. Counseling regarding specific risks and expectations in a diabetic pregnancy should be provided.

The First Trimester

Women who present in the first trimester with poorly controlled diabetes require rapid normalization of blood sugar to try to prevent congenital malformations and hypoglycemia. Hospitalization may be required to reevaluate diet, modify insulins, and adjust blood sugars expeditiously. Education regarding the importance of dietary intake and glycemic control to the health of the fetus can be helpful to motivate women who do not have their diabetes under control.

Women with type 2 diabetes with good glycemic control may not need a further increase in insulin until the second trimester. However, on average, women with type 1 diabetes will require an additional 0.9 units of insulin per kilogram of body weight.[58] The need for increased insulin in women with type 1 diabetes in the first trimester should be individualized depending on glycemic control, food intake, and consideration of the transient drop of insulin requirement that may occur in some women the late first trimester.[59]

Anorexia, nausea, and vomiting during the first trimester can decrease oral intake and predispose to hypoglycemia. Severe hypoglycemia in pregnancy is most common in the first trimester.[60] Changes in timing or dose of insulin may be required. Glycemic disturbance is usually less severe in pregnant women with type 2 diabetes than in those with type 1. If not done in the preconception period, medications should be modified as noted earlier.

Initial evaluation of women with diabetes includes the usual prenatal laboratory studies performed for nonpregnant women. In addition, laboratory studies should be obtained to assess organ damage and determine a baseline for the risk for preeclampsia later in pregnancy. These tests include liver enzymes, renal function, HA1c, and a 24-hour urine for protein and creatinine clearance. Asymptomatic bacteriuria should also be assessed similar to other pregnant women. Clinical judgment dictates whether a chest radiograph, electrocardiogram, or maternal echocardiogram should also be obtained. Certainly further assessment of the heart is warranted in women who have hypertension, history of pulmonary edema, angina, or myocardial infarction. Ophthalmologic examination with assessment of the retina should be performed at least in each trimester. Obstetric ultrasound to document viability early in the evaluation should be obtained.

First trimester screening is particularly useful in women with preexisting diabetes. Nuchal translucency can be used for early screening for not only chromosomal abnormalities but also complex congenital heart disease.[61]

The Second Trimester

Insulin requirements increase notably in the second trimester, and frequent adjustments may be needed. Targeted ultrasound for congenital anomalies and fetal echocardiogram should be performed with subsequent ultrasound for fetal growth every 3 to 4 weeks. Maternal serum screening can be helpful in screening for open fetal defects.

The Third Trimester

Insulin requirements to maintain good glycemic control continue to increase and may reach 140% of prepregnancy doses. Hospitalization for glucose control may be required, particularly for noncompliant women at highest risk for stillborn.

Twice-weekly NST[56,62] should be initiated by 32 weeks' gestation. In women with hypertension and IUGR, testing can begin at 28 gestational weeks. The contraction stress test and biophysical profile are generally used when the NST is nonreactive. Doppler assessment of umbilical artery waveforms should be reserved for further assessment of suspected IUGR fetuses.

Women with well-controlled diabetes, normal antenatal testing, and normally grown fetuses can go into spontaneous labor, with induction reserved until approximately 40 weeks' gestation. Early delivery without maternal or fetal indication in women with diabetes is no longer the norm unless fetal lung maturity is documented. Cesarean delivery should be reserved for other obstetric indications, fetal compromise, or estimated fetal weight greater than 4000 to 4500 g.

Intrapartum

Tight glycemic control in labor helps decrease neonatal hypoglycemia in women with preexisting diabetes.[63] This degree of control is best accomplished with an intravenous insulin infusion during labor. Women should be instructed to not take their basal or long-acting insulin when in labor or the day of labor induction, and to begin an

Table 5
Intrapartum intravenous insulin infusion

Capillary Blood Glucose (mg/dL)	Insulin Infusion Rate (U/h[a])	Intravenous Fluids (125 mL/h)
<80	Off	D5 lactated ringer
81–100	0.5	D5 lactated ringer
101–140	1.0	D5 lactated ringer
141–180	1.5	Normal saline
181–220	2.0	Normal saline
>220	2.5	Normal saline

[a] Standard drip: 100 units regular insulin per 100 mL 0.9% sodium chloride (1 unit per 1 mL). Total intravenous fluid rate may need adjustment in preeclampsia or cardiac disease. Preload for neuraxial anesthesia should be performed with normal saline. Capillary glucose levels performed every hour and insulin infusion adjusted accordingly.

insulin infusion similar to that used at Tulane University (**Table 5**). The infusion parameters may need to be increased in women with insulin-resistant type 2 diabetes. After delivery, the infusion can be discontinued or, if a cesarean delivery was needed and full diet not instituted, it can be continued but insulin decreased. One postpartum algorithm decreases the infusion rate by 0.5 U/h, so that normal saline is used if the blood sugar is 81 to 100 mg/dL, 0.5 U/h if the blood sugar is 101 to 140 mg/dL, 1.0 U/h if the blood sugar is 141 to 180 mg/dL, and so forth.

Postpartum

Insulin requirements decrease quickly after delivery of the placenta. Insulin dosing can either be decreased by 40% to 50% or can be changed to prepregnancy doses. Women with diabetes who breastfeed have lower daily blood glucose levels and generally require less insulin. Breastfeeding may also have a protective effect against the development of type 1 diabetes in childhood.[64,65]

SUMMARY

Diabetes can be a challenge in pregnancy, but with education, close monitoring, and newer therapeutic modalities, these women can have healthy newborns. Close attention to diet, glycemic control, metabolic stresses, and early diagnosis and monitoring of complications can make pregnancy a successful experience for women with diabetes.

REFERENCES

1. Narayan KM, Boyle JP, Geiss LS, et al. Impact of recent increase in incidence on future diabetes burden. Diabetes Care 2006;29(9):2114–6.
2. Zimmet P, Alberti KG, Shaw J. Global and societal implications of the diabetes epidemic. Nature 2001;414:782–7.
3. The DIAMOND Project Group. Incidence and trends of childhood type 1 diabetes worldwide 1990–1999. Diabet Med 2006;23:857–66.
4. Dabelea D. The accelerating epidemic of childhood diabetes. Lancet 2009;373: 2027–33.

5. Barker DJ, Hales CN, Fall CH, et al. Type 2 (non-insulin-dependent) diabetes mellitus, hypertension and hyperlipidaemia (syndrome X): relation to reduced fetal growth. Diabetologia 1993;36(3):267–8.
6. Whincup PH, Kaye SJ, Owen CG, et al. Birth weight and risk of type 2 diabetes: a systematic review. JAMA 2009;300(24):2886–97.
7. White P. Classification of obstetric diabetes. Am J Obstet Gynecol 1978;130:228–30.
8. Haeri S, Khoury J, Kovilam O, et al. The association of intrauterine growth abnormalities in women with type 1 diabetes mellitus complicated by vasculopathy. Am J Obstet Gynecol 2008;199:278 e1–5.
9. American Diabetes Association. Diagnosis and classification of diabetes mellitus. Diabetes Care 2010;33(Suppl 1):S62–9.
10. Catalano PM, Tyzbir ED, Roman NM, et al. Longitudinal changes in insulin release and insulin resistance in nonobese pregnant women. Am J Obstet Gynecol 1991;165:1667–72.
11. Sivan E, Chen X, Homko, et al. Longitudinal study of carbohydrate metabolism in healthy obese pregnant women. Diabetes Care 1997;20:1470–5.
12. American Diabetes Association. Standards of medical care in diabetes—2008. Diabetes Care 2008;31:S12–54.
13. Jovanovic L, Peterson CM. Dietary manipulation as a primary treatment strategy for pregnancies complicated by diabetes. J Am Coll Nutr 1990;9:320–5.
14. Obesity in pregnancy, ACOG Committee Opinion No. 315. American College of Obstetricians and Gynecologists. Obstet Gynecol 2005;106:671–5.
15. Jovanovic L, Ilic S, Pettitt DJ, et al. The metabolic and immunologic effects of insulin lispro in gestational diabetes. Diabetes Care 1999;22:1422–6.
16. Home PD, Lindholm A, Hylleberg B, et al. Improved glycemic control with insulin aspart: a multi-center randomized double-blind crossover trial in type 1 diabetic patients. UK Insulin Aspart Study Group. Diabetes Care 1998;21:1904–9.
17. Singh C, Jovanovic L. Insulin analogues in the treatment of diabetes in pregnancy. Obstet Gynecol Clin North Am 2007;34:275–91.
18. Rosenstock J, Dailey G, Massi-Benedetti M, et al. Reduced hypoglycemia risk with insulin glargine: a meta-analysis comparing insulin glargine with human NPH insulin in type 2 diabetes. Diabetes Care 2005;28:950–5.
19. Horvath K, Jeitler K, Berghold A, et al. Long-acting insulin analogues versus NPH insulin (human isophane insulin) for type 2 diabetes mellitus. The Cochrane Library 2009;2:CD005613. DOI:10.1002/14651858.CD005613.pub3.
20. Egerman RS, Ramsey RD, Kao LW, et al. Perinatal outcomes in pregnancies managed with antenatal insulin glargine. Am J Perinatol 2009;26(8):591–5.
21. Henderson CE, Machipalli S, Marcano-Vasquez H, et al. A retrospective review of glargine use in pregnancy. J Reprod Med 2009;54(4):208–10.
22. Fang YM, MacKeen D, Egan JF, et al. Insulin glargine compared with neutral protamine Hagedorn insulin in the treatment of pregnant diabetics. J Matern Fetal Neonatal Med 2009;22(3):249–53.
23. Gallen IW, Jaap A, Roland, et al. Survey of glargine use in 115 pregnant women with type 1 diabetes. Diabet Med 2008;25:165–9.
24. Mukhopadhyay A, Farrell T, Fraser RB, et al. Continuous subcutaneous insulin infusion vs intensive conventional insulin therapy in pregnant diabetic women: a systematic review and metaanalysis of randomized, controlled trials. Am J Obstet Gynecol 2007;197:447–56.

25. Gabbe SG, Holing E, Temple P, et al. Benefits, risks, costs, and patient satisfaction associated with insulin pump therapy for the pregnancy complicated by type 1 diabetes mellitus. Am J Obstet Gynecol 2000;182:1283–91.
26. Yogev Y, Hod M. Use of new technologies for monitoring and treating diabetes in pregnancy. Obstet Gynecol Clin North Am 2007;34:241–53.
27. Murphy HR, Rayman G, Lewis K, et al. Effectiveness of continuous glucose monitoring in pregnant women with diabetes: randomized clinical trial. BMJ 2008;337: a1680.
28. McLachlan K, Jenkins A, O'Neal D. The role of continuous glucose monitoring in clinical decision-making in diabetes in pregnancy. Aust N Z J Obstet Gynaecol 2007;47(3):186–90.
29. Jovanovic R, Jovanovic L. Obstetric management when normoglycemia is maintained in diabetic pregnant women with vascular compromise. Am J Obstet Gynecol 1984;149:617–23.
30. Gordon M, Landon MB, Samuels P, et al. Perinatal outcome and long-term follow-up associated with modern management of diabetic nephropathy (Class F). Obstet Gynecol 1996;87:401–9.
31. Feig DS, Razzaq A, Sykora K, et al. Trends in deliveries, prenatal care, and obstetrical complications in women with pregestational diabetes: a population-based study in Ontario, Canada, 1996–2001. Diabetes Care 2006;29:232–5.
32. Ravid M, Brosh D, Levi Z, et al. Use of Enalapril to attenuate decline in renal function in normotensive, normoalbuminuric patients with type 2 diabetes mellitus. Ann Intern Med 1998;128:982–8.
33. Kasiske BL, Kalil RS, Ma JZ, et al. Effect of antihypertensive therapy on the kidney in patients with diabetes: a meta-regression analysis. Ann Intern Med 1993;118: 129–38.
34. Cooper WO, Hernandez-Diaz S, Arbogast PG, et al. Major congenital malformations after first trimester exposure to ACE inhibitors. N Engl J Med 2006;354: 2443–51.
35. Rosenn B, Miodovnik M, Kranias G, et al. Progression of diabetic retinopathy in pregnancy. Am J Obstet Gynecol 1992;166:1214–8.
36. Laatikainen L, Larinkari J, Teramo K, et al. Occurrence and prognostic significance of retinopathy in diabetic pregnancy. Metab Pediatr Ophthalmol 1980;4:191–5.
37. Rosenn BM, Miodovnk J. Medical complications of diabetes mellitus in pregnancy. Clin Obstet Gynecol 2000;43:17–31.
38. Chew EY, Mills JL, Metzger BE, et al. for the National Institute of Child Health and Human Development—diabetes in early pregnancy study. Metabolic control and progression of retinopathy: the diabetes in early pregnancy study. Diabetes Care 1995;18:631–7.
39. Lovestam-Adrian M, Agardh CD, Aberg A, et al. Pre-eclampsia is a potent risk factor for deterioration of retinopathy during pregnancy in type I diabetic patients. Diabet Med 1997;14:1059–65.
40. Kaaja R, Loukovaara S. Progression of retinopathy in type 1 diabetic women during pregnancy. Curr Diabetes Rev 2007;3:85–93.
41. Grunwald JE, DuPont J, Riva CE. Retinal haemodynamics in patients with early diabetes mellitus. Br J Ophthalmol 1996;80:327–31.
42. Chang S, Fuhrmann M, Jovanovich L. The diabetes in early pregnancy study group (DIEP): pregnancy, retinopathy normoglycemia. A preliminary analysis. Diabetes 1985;35(Suppl):3A.
43. Hemachandra A, Ellis D, Lloyd CE, et al. The influence of pregnancy on IDDM complications. Diabetes Care 1995;18:950–4.

44. Montoro MN, Myers VP, Mestman JH, et al. Outcome of pregnancy in diabetic ke-
    toacidosis. Am J Perinatol 1993;10:17–20.
45. Gabbe SG, Carpenter LB, Garrison EA. New strategies for glucose control in
    patients with type 1 and type 2 diabetes mellitus in pregnancy. Clin Obstet Gyne-
    col 2007;50:1014–24.
46. Carroll MA, Yeomans ER. Diabetic ketoacidosis in pregnancy. Crit Care Med
    2005;339:S347–53.
47. Schneider MB, Umpierrez GE, Ramsey RD, et al. Pregnancy complicated by
    diabetic ketoacidosis, maternal and fetal outcomes. Diabetes Care 2003;26:
    958–9.
48. Miller E, Hare JW, Cloherty JP, et al. Elevated maternal hemoglobin A1c in early
    pregnancy and major congenital anomalies in infants of diabetic mothers. N Engl
    J Med 1981;304:1331–4.
49. Mills JL, Baker L, Goldman A. Malformations in infants of diabetic mothers occur
    before the seventh gestational week: implications for treatment. Diabetes 1979;
    23:292–3.
50. Schaefer-Graf UM, Buchanan TA, Xiang A, et al. Patterns of congenital anomalies
    and relationship to initial maternal fasting glucose levels in pregnancies compli-
    cated by type 2 and gestational diabetes. Am J Obstet Gynecol 2000;182:
    313–20.
51. Steel JM, Johnstone FD, Hepburn DA, et al. Can prepregnancy care of diabetic
    women reduce the risk of abnormal babies? BMJ 1990;301:1070–4.
52. Willhoite MB, Bennert HW, Palomaki GE, et al. The impact of preconception coun-
    seling in pregnancy outcomes. The experience of the Maine Diabetes in Preg-
    nancy Program. Diabetes Care 1993;16:450–5.
53. Mondestin MA, Ananth CV, Sumulian JC, et al. Birth weight and fetal death in the
    United States: the effect of maternal diabetes during pregnancy. Am J Obstet
    Gynecol 2002;187:922–6.
54. Dudly D. Diabetic-associated stillbirth: incidence, pathophysiology, and preven-
    tion. Obstet Gynecol Clin 2007;34:293–307.
55. Bradley RJ, Brudenell JM, Nicolaides KH. Fetal acidosis and hyperlacticaemia
    diagnosed by cordocentesis in pregnancies complicated by maternal diabetes
    mellitus. Diabet Med 1991;8:464–8.
56. Kjos SL, Leung A, Henry OA, et al. Antepartum surveillance in diabetic preg-
    nancies: predictors of fetal distress in labor. Am J Obstet Gynecol 1995;173:
    1532–9.
57. Balsells M, Garcia-Patterson A, Gich I, et al. Maternal and fetal outcome in
    women with type 2 versus type 1 diabetes mellitus: a systematic review and
    metaanalysis. J Clin Endocrinol Metab 2009;94(11):4284–91.
58. Langer O, Anyaegbunam A, Brustman L, et al. Pregestational diabetes:
    insulin requirements throughout pregnancy. Am J Obstet Gynecol 1988;159:
    616–21.
59. Jovanovic L, Mils JL, Knopp RH, et al. The National Institute of Child Health and
    Human Development—Diabetes in Early Pregnancy Study Group. Declining
    insulin requirements in the late first trimester of diabetic pregnancy. Diabetes
    Care 2001;24:1130–6.
60. Nielsen LR, Johansen M, Pedersen-Bjergaard U, et al. Predictors and role of
    metabolic control. Diabetes Care 2009;31:9–14.
61. Hyett J, Perdu M, Sharland G, et al. Using fetal nuchal translucency to screen for
    major congenital heart defects at 10-14 weeks of gestation: population based
    cohort study. BMJ 1999;318:81–5.

62. Barrett JM, Salyer SL, Boehm FH. The nonstress test: an evaluation of 1000 patients. Am J Obstet Gynecol 1981;141:153–8.
63. Curet LB, Izquierdo LA, Gilson GJ, et al. Relative effects of antepartum and intrapartum maternal blood glucose levels on incidence of neonatal hypoglycemia. J Perinatol 1997;17:113–5.
64. Sadauskaite-Kuehne V, Ludvigsson J, Padaiga Z, et al. Longer breastfeeding is an independent protective factor against development of type 1 diabetes mellitus in childhood. Diabetes Metab Res Rev 2004;20:150–7.
65. Stuebe AM, Rish-Edwards JW, Willett WC, et al. Duration of lactation and incidence of type 2 diabetes. JAMA 2005;294(20):2601–10.

Asthma in Pregnancy: Pathophysiology, Diagnosis and Management

Abbey J. Hardy-Fairbanks, MD[a],*, Emily R. Baker, MD[b]

KEYWORDS

- Peak expiratory flow rate • Bronchoconstriction
- Exacerbation • Inhaled corticosteroids

Asthma is a common, potentially serious, even life-threatening, chronic medical condition seen amongst nearly all groups of patients, regardless of ethnicity and socioeconomic circumstances. This article addresses the group of pregnant women with symptomatic asthma as well as those whose asthma is asymptomatic as a result of good control. The incidence, the pathophysiologic changes of pregnancy, and the interplay between these changes and asthma are reviewed in this article. The classification of these patients and appropriate management strategies are discussed.

Overall, the prevalence and morbidity of asthma are increasing, although mortality rates have decreased.[1] Asthma complicates 3.7% to 8.4% of all pregnancies, between 200,000 and 376,000 pregnancies annually in the United States.[2–4] Acute exacerbations that necessitate emergency care or hospitalization have been reported in 9% to 11% of pregnant women cared for by asthma specialists. Most women with asthma have an uneventful pregnancy course; however, some may experience life-threatening exacerbations requiring hospitalization, intubation, intensive care management, and, rarely, preterm delivery.[5]

Treatment varies, based on the severity classification of each individual patient's asthma and includes avoidance of triggers, medications, and close monitoring. The ultimate goal of therapy is to reduce the number of hypoxemic episodes (ie, acute exacerbations and chronic symptoms) in the mother.

[a] Department of Obstetrics and Gynecology, Dartmouth-Hitchcock Medical Center, 1 Medical Center Drive, Lebanon, NH 03756, USA
[b] Division of Maternal and Fetal Medicine, Dartmouth-Hitchcock Medical Center, 1 Medical Center Drive, Lebanon, NH 03756, USA
* Corresponding author.
E-mail address: Abbey.J.Hardy-Fairbanks@hitchcock.org

Obstet Gynecol Clin N Am 37 (2010) 159–172
doi:10.1016/j.ogc.2010.02.006
0889-8545/10/$ – see front matter © 2010 Elsevier Inc. All rights reserved.

obgyn.theclinics.com

PHYSIOLOGIC CHANGES OF RESPIRATORY FUNCTION IN PREGNANCY

Multiple changes in maternal physiology interact with the pathophysiologic activities of asthma. Increased estrogen levels increase mucosal edema and hypervascularity in upper airways.

As the uterus grows, it elevates the diaphragm approximately 4 to 5 cm, and with this comes a reduction in the functional residual capacity of about 18% (approximately1.7–1.35 L) because of a progressive decrease in expiratory reserve volume. Pregnancy also results in a 20% increase in oxygen consumption to support a 15% increase in maternal metabolic rate.[6] To compensate for the increased demands of pregnancy, minute ventilation is increased by 40% to 50%. This relative hyperventilation results not from increased respiratory rate, but from increasing tidal volume. These changes are secondary to progesterone-mediated stimulation of the respiratory center to a set point to accept a lower partial pressure of carbon dioxide (**Fig. 1, Table 1**).

This natural hyperventilation of pregnancy causes arterial blood gases (ABG) to reveal a respiratory alkalosis that is compensated for by a metabolic acidosis. Typical blood gases have a pH of 7.40 to 7.45, and a P_{CO_2} of 28 to 32 mm Hg. There is a mild increase in P_{O_2} of 106 of 110 mm Hg. Increased pH is compensated for by increased renal excretion of bicarbonate (which accounts for polyuria in early pregnancy).[5] The P_{O_2} in the umbilical veins is lower than that in the placental venous channels; thus, maternal hypoxemia will quickly result in a decreased oxygen content supplied to the fetus. Chronic hypoxemia could lead to intrauterine growth restriction and low birth weight. A low P_{CO_2} is essential to fetal acid-base balance, and increased maternal P_{CO_2} will affect the fetus' ability to excrete acid and cause fetal acidosis.[5] When interpreting the ABG of the pregnant patient, a normal-appearing P_{CO_2} actually reflects a degree of carbon dioxide retention and possible impending respiratory failure. The hypercarbic environment in maternal asthma that is poorly controlled can exist even without an acute exacerbation – as a chronic state. Hence optimal control of asthma symptoms is essential for the health of the pregnant woman and her fetus.

Pregnancy does not have an effect on the forced expiratory volume in 1 second (FEV_1) or peak expiratory flow rate (PEFR). Although these respiratory measurements are preserved in pregnancy, they are negatively affected by asthma symptoms and exacerbations, making them an ideal method of monitoring asthma severity in pregnancy. A FEV1 measurement requires spirometry equipment not usually available in the OB/GYN office. A peak flow meter (**Fig. 2**) is an easy inexpensive way to monitor patients at their prenatal visit or while they are at home. To measure peak flow, the patient should stand up straight and take as deep a breath as possible. She should

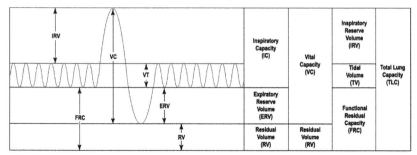

Fig. 1. Lung volumes. (*From* Lung volumes. Wikipedia: The Free Encyclopedia. Wikimedia Foundation, Inc. Available at: http://en.wikipedia.org/wiki/1/2Q17_File:LungVolume.jpg.)

Table 1
Lung volume descriptions and changes during pregnancy

Lung Capacity Measurement	Description	Physiologic Change in Pregnancy
Functional residual capacity	Volume of air left in the lungs after a tidal breath out. The amount of air that stays in the lungs during normal breathing	↓17%–20% (300–500 mL)
Respiratory rate	Number of breaths per minute	Unchanged
Residual volume	Amount of air left in the lungs after maximum exhalation	↓20%–25% (200–300 mL)
Tidal volume	Normal volume of air displaced between normal inhalation and exhalation with no extra effort	↑ 30%–50%
Expiratory reserve volume	Amount of additional air that can be pushed out after the end expiratory level of normal breathing	↓ 5%–15% (100–300 mL)
FEV_1	Volume of air exhaled during the first second of a forced expiratory maneuver	Unchanged
PEFR	Maximal flow (or speed) achieved during maximally forced expiration initiated at full inspiration; measured in L/s	Unchanged
Minute volume/ ventilation	Volume of air that can be inhaled or exhaled in 1 min	↑ 30%–50%

Abbreviations: FEV_1, forced expiratory volume in one second; PEFR, peak expiratory flow rate.

then close her lips around the mouthpiece and exhale as fast and hard as possible. She should repeat this 3 times, recording each value, the highest of which is considered the current peak flow. A baseline best value should be acquired at the first prenatal visit, or even better at a preconceptual visit. This value provides a reference for comparison to diagnose an exacerbation or need for added treatment.

PATHOPHYSIOLOGY OF ASTHMA

Asthma is characterized by paroxysmal or persistent symptoms of bronchoconstriction including breathlessness, chest tightness, cough, and sputum production. Diagnosis requires improvement in symptoms as well as objective changes in pulmonary function tests such as FEV_1 or PEFR with administration of a β agonist. Diagnosis of

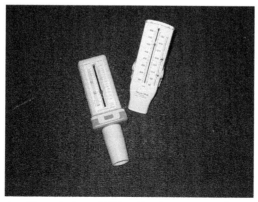

Fig. 2. Peak flow meter. (*From* Asthma. Wikipedia: The Free Encyclopedia. Wikimedia Foundation, Inc. Available at: http://en.wikipedia.org/wiki/File:Two_Peak_Flow_Meters.jpg.)

Table 2
Diagnosis of asthma

Symptoms	Wheezing, cough, shortness of breath, chest tightness
Signs	Wheezing on auscultation Absence does not exclude diagnosis
Temporal relationships	Worsening at night, fluctuating intensity
Diagnosis confirmation	Demonstration of airway obstruction that is at least partially reversible Greater than 12% increase in FEV_1 after bronchodilator administration

asthma in pregnancy is no different from that in the nonpregnant patient. Typical signs and symptoms of asthma are seen in **Table 2**. The most common cause of respiratory symptoms such as shortness of breath in pregnancy is physiologic dyspnea of pregnancy and not asthma or other pathology. However, dyspnea of pregnancy does not typically have the associated cough, tightness, or obstructive signs seen with asthma. Consideration must also be given to gastroesophageal reflux disease, pneumonia, postnasal drip caused by allergic rhinitis, or bronchitis as alternate diagnoses. If the clinical picture is consistent with asthma, but reversibility of airway obstruction cannot be demonstrated, then a trial of asthma treatment can be used for diagnosis in pregnancy.[1]

Interactions of Pregnancy and Asthma

Overall, the effect that pregnancy has on any one patient's asthma is unpredictable, and the likely intricate interaction of the immune changes of asthma on pregnancy is unclear. Possible mechanisms include maternal hormone changes and altered β-adrenergic receptor responsiveness. Even fetal sex may play a role, with some data showing increased severity of symptoms in pregnancy with a female fetus.[7,8] A large prospective study by Schatz and colleagues[9] reported that asthma symptoms improved in pregnancy in 23% and worsened in 30%. This widely held rule of thirds (one-third of patients with asthma in pregnancy improving, one-third worsening, and one-third with no change) makes asthma in pregnancy the very definition of unpredictable.

In a large prospective study, rates of asthma exacerbation and hospitalization in pregnant patients with asthma were found to be directly proportional to the degree of severity classification (**Table 3**). Patients with mild asthma were found to have an incidence of exacerbations at 12.6% with a hospitalization rate of 2.3%. Women with moderate asthma had an exacerbation rate of 25.7% and hospitalization rate of 6.8%. Women with severe asthma had an exacerbation rate of 51.9% and a hospitalization rate of 26.9%.[9] Thus, knowing the classification of a patient's asthma is important in assessing her risk of exacerbation.

Initial investigations of asthma in pregnancy via retrospective studies showed an association with many adverse outcomes of pregnancy including, but not limited to, low birth weight, preterm delivery, preeclampsia, cesarean delivery, and hyperemesis.[1,10–12] These older studies had many inadequacies in their methodology. Several large prospective studies have refuted these findings and showed that asthma was not associated with many of these outcomes.[4,13] Most recently, in large controlled studies, severe asthma was associated with gestational diabetes and delivery before 37 weeks.[13] Preterm delivery, gestational diabetes, preeclampsia, preterm labor, oligohydramnios, or low birth weight were not associated with asthma of any severity.

Table 3
Asthma severity classification system and management strategies in pregnancy

Asthma Severity	Mild Intermittent Asthma	Mild Persistent Asthma	Moderate Persistent Asthma	Severe Asthma
Overall control	Well controlled	Not well controlled	Not well controlled	Very poorly controlled
Symptoms classification	• Symptoms twice per week or less • Nocturnal symptoms twice per month or less • FEV_1 80% of predicted or more, varies less than 20%	• Symptoms more than twice per week, but not daily • Nocturnal symptoms more than twice per month • FEV_1 80% of predicted, variability of 20%–30%	• Daily symptoms • Nocturnal symptoms more than once per week • FEV_1 more than 60% to less than 50% predicted. Variability more than 30% • Regular medications necessary to control symptoms	• Continuous symptoms • Nocturnal symptoms are frequent • FEV_1 60% or less of predicted, variability greater than 30% • Regular oral corticosteroids necessary to control symptoms
Preferred management	• No daily medications, albuterol as needed	• Low-dose inhaled corticosteroid	• Low-dose inhaled corticosteroid AND salmeterol OR • Medium-dose inhaled corticosteroid and salmeterol if needed	• High-dose inhaled corticosteroid and salmeterol AND oral corticosteroid if needed
Alternative management		• Cromolyn OR • Leukotriene receptor antagonist OR • Theophylline	• Low-dose or (if needed) medium-dose inhaled corticosteroid and EITHER leukotriene receptor antagonist or theophylline	• High-dose inhaled corticosteroid AND theophylline AND if needed oral corticosteroid

For acute symptoms: Albuterol 2–6 puffs as needed for FEV_1 less than 80%, exposure to allergens or exercise should supplement all treatment plans. May repeat in 20 minutes. If no response then patient should seek medical attention.

Adapted from National Heart, Lung, and Blood Institute, National Asthma Education and Prevention Program. Expert panel report: guidelines for the diagnosis and management of asthma. NIH Publication No. 05-5236. Bethesda (MD): NHLBI. Available at: http://www.nhlbi.nih.gov/health/prof/lung/asthma/astpreg/astpreg_full.pdf.

Two studies, with a total of 2403 pregnancies, showed increased risk of pregnancy-induced hypertension, but only in those with moderate to severe daily symptoms.[4,14] The outcomes for pregnant patients with asthma requiring corticosteroid therapy were associated with decreased gestational age at delivery, preeclampsia, and small-for-gestational-age infants.[4,13] These data point toward poor perinatal outcomes being associated with poorly controlled asthma and not with treatment medications.

The mechanism of the effect of asthma on the developing fetus is poorly understood. Many studies have suggested that maternal hypoxia, inflammation, smoking, and altered placental function may contribute to poor outcomes in patients with asthma.[10,11] Reduced Po_2 in maternal blood is a feature of severe chronic asthma, asthma exacerbations, and status asthmaticus. Even a small decrease in maternal Po_2 can put the fetus at risk of hypoxemia; but also, increases in maternal Pco_2 affect the fetal ability to excrete acid waste, resulting promptly in fetal acidosis. These maternal blood gas aberrations can have serious effects on the fetus.[15] Despite the lack of precise knowledge of the pathophysiologic interactions of asthma with the fetus, it is clear that with worsening severity of asthma comes the risk of increasingly negative fetal and maternal outcomes.

CLASSIFICATION OF ASTHMA SEVERITY AND CONTROL

Classification of a patient's asthma severity is important to help predict the possible risk of severe exacerbation and the need for maintenance therapy. Patients with mild asthma, who require regular medications, have the same number and severity of exacerbations as those with moderate asthma.[9] Thus, the generalist obstetrician should be familiar with the classification, evaluation, and management of asthma in pregnancy.

Patients should be assessed at the first prenatal visit for history of exacerbations, hospitalizations, the use of oral steroids in the past, and the need for mechanical ventilation. For multiparous women, their asthma history in previous pregnancies should be reviewed. Schatz and colleagues[16] noted that when subjects were assessed in successive pregnancies, 60% of them followed the same course with their asthma symptoms. Instruction in the use of a peak flow meter and recording of a baseline value should also be done at this early stage in pregnancy. If the patient is already aware of her personal best value, it should be recorded.

Table 3 presents the National Institutes of Health classification system for asthma severity.[17] The preferred and alternative management strategies for each class of asthma in pregnancy are also included in this table. These classifications should be seen as a dynamic system in which, during a pregnancy, a patient may change classes and treatments several times. Knowing and applying the classification system is essential to selecting appropriate management as well as anticipating complications during pregnancy. Patients with mild intermittent asthma, patients with mild persistent asthma, and selected patients with moderate persistent asthma can be treated adequately by the generalist obstetrician. Patients with severe asthma and those with moderate asthma that is increasingly complex require referral to a pulmonologist and a maternal-fetal medicine specialist for shared management of pregnancy and asthma.

Importance of Adequate Asthma Treatment

Studies to investigate pregnancy outcomes in patients with asthma have had inconsistent results. Many of these studies lack power, had small sample sizes, and were lacking controls. Two recent, large, multicenter, prospective cohort studies evaluated the effects of asthma on perinatal outcomes. First, Bracken and colleagues[4] prospectively followed 2205 pregnancies and showed that preterm delivery was not associated with asthma; however, requirement of theophylline or oral corticosteroids was associated with a statistically significant reduction in gestational age at delivery. Small-for-gestational-age infants and preeclampsia were associated with moderate asthma or those with daily symptoms. These data suggest that poor control of maternal asthma negatively affects perinatal outcome.

In the second study, Dombrowski and colleagues,[13] as part of a large multicenter, prospective, observational cohort study, showed that there was no association between asthma and delivery before 32 weeks' gestation. Of all the other outcomes investigated, only cesarean delivery was associated with moderate to severe asthma. Patients with asthma requiring oral corticosteroid therapy were associated with delivering before 37 weeks and having infants weighing less than 2500 g.

Data from the latter study did demonstrate a relationship between a lower FEV_1 at prenatal visits and increased risk of prematurity and low birth weight infants; however, this was not statistically significant.[18] Both studies were consistent with suboptimal control of asthma being associated with increased risk of adverse pregnancy outcome.[4,13]

Multiple other smaller prospective studies consistently demonstrate that maternal and neonatal outcomes in women with mild or moderate asthma are excellent. In 1993, the National Asthma Education and Prevention Program (NAEPP) of the National Institutes of Health, Heart, Lung and Blood Institute recommended antiinflammatory treatment for all pregnant women with moderate or severe asthma. Since that recommendation was published, studies have demonstrated fewer adverse effects on fetal outcome in women with asthma,[19] further supporting the important concept that optimal and aggressive control of asthma of all severity can ameliorate the possible adverse outcomes. It is essential that providers pay close attention to the severity classification of a patient's asthma and treat accordingly. It would be a mistake, with potentially severe consequences, to decrease or discontinue any asthma medications because of a newly diagnosed pregnancy.

ASTHMA MANAGEMENT

The ultimate goal of asthma therapy is to prevent hypoxic episodes to preserve continuous fetal oxygenation; improved maternal and perinatal outcomes are achieved with optimal control of asthma. One-third of women with asthma develop worsening of control during pregnancy, therefore close monitoring and reevaluation are essential. There are 4 important aspects of asthma treatment to ensure optimal control: close monitoring, education of patients, avoidance of asthma triggers, and pharmacologic therapy. Patients who are not responding adequately to treatment should have their level of treatment accelerated.

Monitoring Asthma in Pregnancy

The reliability of subjective measures by patient or physician for asthma severity has not proven dependable. FEV_1 has been shown to be a reliable objective measure of airway obstruction and correlates with pregnancy outcome.[18] FEV_1 measurement requires a spirometer, which is not available in most physicians' offices. The measurement of PEFR can easily be performed in the office at a prenatal visit using a peak flow meter. PEFR should be performed with the patient standing and taking a maximum inspiration. The best value of 3 attempts is used for comparison with previous numbers.

Typical PEFR in pregnancy should be 380 to 550 L/min. Each individual patient should establish her personal best and that number should be recorded in the prenatal chart at the earliest prenatal visit. The caregiver can then provide the patient with a peak flow meter marked with 80%, 50% to 80%, and less than 50% of the patient's personal best.[1] Patients should be advised that 80% or more of PEFR is considered good control; however, optimal control in pregnancy is 90% to 100% of personal best. The pregnant woman should be advised that if PEFR is within the 50% to 80% range she should arrange an appointment to see her physician or obtain advice regarding changes in medication. At less than 50%, she should be seen immediately in the emergency department if necessary.

Patient Education

Patient education should begin at the first prenatal visit. Explanation of the importance of optimal asthma control and the risks of poor control for the patient and the fetus should be discussed early in pregnancy. Patients should be taught how to do peak flow measurements, how to record the results, and what values should be of concern, as well as who to contact in emergent situations. Patients should be observed using their inhalers and peak flow meters and correct use reinforced. Frank discussion about the importance of continuing asthma medications and the possible severe consequences for the patient and her fetus with discontinuation is vital.

Avoidance of Triggers

Up to 80% of patients with asthma have positive skin tests to allergens, the most common being animal dander, dust mites, cockroach antigens, pollens, and molds. There are nonimmune triggers as well, including strong odors, tobacco smoke, air pollutants, and drugs such as aspirin and β-blockers. For exercise-triggered asthma, the use of a bronchodilator 5 to 60 minutes before exercise may reduce symptoms. Avoidance of these allergens and triggers can significantly reduce the need for medication and the occurrence of exacerbations during and after pregnancy. All patients should be strongly encouraged to stop smoking, but especially those with asthma because they are at increased risk for worsening chronic and acute asthma sequelae.

Pharmacotherapy

Medical therapy includes a stepwise approach in an attempt to use the least amount of medication necessary to control a patient's asthma and keep her severity in the mild range. Goals of therapy include having normal or near-normal pulmonary function and minimal or no chronic symptoms, exacerbations, or limitations on activities. The final goal is to minimize the adverse effects of treatment.

It is safer for pregnant women with asthma to be treated with asthma medications than to have exacerbations or asthma symptoms.[17] It is assumed that asthma medications are as effective in the pregnant patient as in the nonpregnant woman; however, there may be physiologic changes in pregnancy that affect many aspects of the pharmacokinetics of these medications.

The mainstay of therapy is to treat airway inflammation to reduce hyperresponsiveness and prevent symptoms. Secondary therapy is aimed at treatment of exacerbations with bronchodilator therapy. At least twice during pregnancy, treatment should be reviewed and stepped up if symptoms are persistent; or, if symptoms are well controlled, therapy can be maintained or even decreased.[17]

Inhaled Corticosteroids

Inhaled corticosteroids (ICS) are preferred for the management of all levels of persistent asthma in pregnancy.[17] Corticosteroids are the most effective treatment for the airway inflammation of asthma and reduce the hyperresponsiveness of airways to allergens and triggers. These medications have also been shown to decrease the incidence of exacerbations by more than threefold compared with those who do not use ICS.[1] Concern for risk of congenital malformations with ICS exposure in the first trimester has proved unfounded; multiple studies have confirmed their safety regardless of dose.[20] **Table 4** reviews the most commonly used available inhaled and oral corticosteroids for asthma treatment.

A meta-analysis by Murphy and colleagues[12] investigated the association between asthma in pregnancy and low birth weight, defined as less than 2500 g, and grouped patients by inhaled corticosteroid use. In 4 studies in which these medications were not used, their risk of low birth weight was significantly increased (risk ratio [RR] 1.55).

In a review of more than 6000 pregnant women who used ICS there was no association with congenital malformations or adverse perinatal outcomes.[17] A Swedish Birth

Table 4
Doses for corticosteroids in the management of asthma

Corticosteroid	Amount Per Dose	Low Dose	Medium Dose	High Dose
Inhaled Corticosteroids[a]				
Beclomethasone CFC	42 or 84 μg/puff	168–504 μg	504–840 μg	>840 μg
Beclomethasone HFA	40 or 80 μg/puff	80–240 μg	240–480 μg	>480 μg
Budesonide[b]	200μg/INH	200–600 μg	600–1200 μg	>1200 μg
Flunisolide	250 μg/puff	500–1,000 μg	1,000–2,000 μg	>2,000 μg
Fluticasone HFA	44 μg/puff 110 μg/puff 220 μg/puff	88–264 μg	264–660 μg	>660 μg
Fluticasone DPI	50 μg/INH 100 μg/INH 250 μg/INH	100–300 μg	300–750 μg	>750 μg
Oral Corticosteroids				
Methylprednisolone	2, 4, 8, 16, 32 mg tablets	• 7.5–60 mg daily in a single dose in a.m. or every other day as needed for control		
Prednisone	5 mg tablets	• Short-course burst to achieve control: 40–60 mg/d as a single dose or divided doses for 3–10 days; no taper needed		
Prednisosolone	1, 2.5, 5, 10, 20, 50 mg tablets			

Abbreviations: CFC, chlorofluorocarbon; DPI, dry powder inhaler; HFA, hydrofluoroalkane; INH, inhalation.
[a] Total daily puffs is usually divided into twice daily dosing regimen.
[b] Budesonide is the preferred ICS in pregnancy.
Data from National Heart, Lung, and Blood Institute as part of the National Institute of Health and the Department of Health and Human Services National Asthma Education and Prevention Program. Expert panel report: guidelines for the diagnosis and management of asthma. NIH Publication No. 05-5236. Bethesda (MD): NHLBI. Available at: http://www.nhlbi.nih.gov/health/prof/lung/asthma/astpreg/astpreg_full.pdf.

Registry of 2014 infants who had been exposed to budesonide in early pregnancy showed no adverse effects.[21] Because there are more data regarding this medication than other corticosteroids, budesonide is considered the preferred medication by the NAEPP and is US Food and Drug Administration (FDA) pregnancy category B. All other corticosteroids are category C. However, if a woman's asthma is well controlled on a different inhaled steroid, it is recommended that the regimen be continued.[19]

Inhaled β2 Agonists

Inhaled β2 agonists are recommended for asthma treatment for all classes of severity. Albuterol is the first-line rescue inhaler for the rapid relief of symptoms of acute bronchospasm. It should be noted that metered dose inhalers have recently been revised by manufacturers to eliminate chlorofluorocarbons, and to now use hydrofluoroalkane (HFA) as a propellant. Because of this change, many commonly used inhalers have new brand names, and generic forms may not be available (eg, Proventil to Proventil HFA, Schering-Plough Corporation).

It is important to inquire at each prenatal visit how often the patient has needed to use her β2 agonist inhaler. Based on the NAEPP review of 6 published studies that included 1599 pregnant women with asthma and a prospective study of 1828 pregnant women with asthma who used β2 agonists in pregnancy, there was no association with adverse outcome.[17,22] If a patient requires more than 2 inhalation treatments with a β agonist per week, this indicates the need for an additional antiinflammatory agent such as ICS.

Another large prospective study of 1828 women with asthma confirmed the lack of relationship between the use of inhaled β agonists and adverse maternal or fetal outcome.[22] In nonpregnant individuals, reliance on β agonists alone, when inhaled corticosteroids are indicated, has been reported to increase mortality, and cessation of corticosteroid therapy was also associated with increased mortality.[23] Although pregnant women were not studied, the findings of this later trial certainly would suggest the importance of adequate treatment of asthma by severity in pregnancy with the addition of ICS to β agonists when indicated.

Leukotriene Moderators, Cromolyn and Theophylline

Leukotrienes are arachidonic acid metabolites that have been implicated in the bronchospasm cascade of asthma exacerbations by increasing vascular permeability. Both zafirlukast and montelukast are pregnancy category B; however, there are very few data on their efficacy or safety in human pregnancy. Leukotriene antagonists are an alternative treatment for mild persistent asthma and can be used as an adjunct for moderate to severe asthma for improved control of symptoms (see **Table 2**).

Cromolyn and theophylline are alternative treatments for mild persistent asthma and adjunctive treatments for moderate and severe persistent asthma, but are not the preferred regimen. Cromolyn blocks early and late bronchospasm and response to asthma triggers.[24] It functions to relax smooth muscle and has some antiinflammatory properties. Cromolyn does appear to be safe during pregnancy[17]; however, experience with dosing by many providers may be lacking. Theophylline is useful only for chronic therapy and is not helpful in acute exacerbations. Theophylline is associated with several adverse effects such as insomnia, heartburn, palpitations, and nausea. Theophylline has many significant drug interactions because the rate of theophylline clearance is altered, resulting in increased theophylline levels and possible toxicity. Some of these medications include cimetidine, lorazepam, and erythromycin. Serum levels should be maintained between 5 and 12 μg/mL during pregnancy.

Management of an Acute Asthma Exacerbation in Pregnancy

An asthma exacerbation in a pregnant woman places mother and fetus at increased risk for a negative outcome because of the risk of severe hypoxemia during these events. The most important management of an acute exacerbation is prevention; however, Schatz and colleagues[9] noted that 52% of patients with severe asthma have an exacerbation during pregnancy, and many of these women require hospitalization.

Murphy and colleagues[25] followed 146 women with asthma prospectively throughout their pregnancies and found that 8% of women with mild asthma, 47% with moderate asthma, and 65% with severe asthma had severe exacerbations, for an overall rate of 65%. The mean gestational age at exacerbation was 25.1 weeks. Twenty-nine percent of exacerbations in this cohort were associated with noncompliance with ICS. It is of vital importance that all obstetric providers, even those caring for women with mild asthma, know the evaluation and treatment for an acute exacerbation.

Murphy and colleagues[25] also found in this study that the rate of low birth weight in male infants was significantly increased and that male infants weighted approximately 300 g less when mothers experienced at least 1 severe asthma exacerbation in pregnancy. The magnitude of this decrease in birth weight was greater than the effect of maternal smoking on birth weight, emphasizing the importance of exacerbation prevention with adequate chronic asthma treatment.

Fig. 3[17] summarizes the treatment strategies for acute exacerbations of asthma in pregnancy. Initial evaluation in the emergency department or labor and delivery should be the same as for acute asthma in the nonpregnant state: measurement of PEFR and comparison with predicted or previously recorded best. Oxygen should be given and oxygen saturation kept higher than 95%. Possible differential diagnoses of a severe exacerbation unresponsive to initial treatment should include pulmonary edema, pulmonary embolism, cardiomyopathy, and amniotic fluid embolism.

The goal of hospital management is reversal of bronchoconstriction with inhaled β2 agonists and corticosteroids, prevention and correction of hypoxemia, or reduction of hypercarbia. Intensive care unit admission or intubation is indicated in those with life-threatening asthma, in those with P_{CO_2} higher than 40 to 45 mm Hg on arterial blood gas, mental status changes, maternal exhaustion, respiratory acidosis, or fetal distress.

Initial treatment for acute asthma exacerbation	Assess Patient Response	Further evaluation and care
1) Give supplemental inhaled oxygen to keep O₂ saturation >95%. 2) Administration of inhaled albuterol via nebulizer driven by oxygen every 20 minutes, up to three doses in the first hour. 3) If no improvement (or if severe exacerbation) give IV or oral corticosteroids. 4) Continuous external fetal monitoring for those >24 weeks gestation.	**Good response:** PEFR 70% or more and sustained for 60 minutes. Normal exam, no distress, reassuring fetal status.	Discharge to home
	Incomplete response: PEFR 50-69%. Continued mild or moderate symptoms.	Continue to monitor, add iprotropium bromide. Continue oxygen and inhaled albuterol. Individualize plan for further observation or hospitalization. Consider systemic steroids.
	Poor response: PEFR less than 50%, pCO₂>40-42mmHg	Continue fetal assessment. Consult intensive care unit for admission. IV corticosteroids.

Fig. 3. Treatment for acute exacerbations of asthma in pregnancy. (*Data from* National Asthma Education and Prevention Program expert panel report. Managing asthma during pregnancy: recommendations for pharmacologic treatment-2004 update. Available at: http://www.nhlbi.nih.gov/health/prof/lung/asthma/astpreg/astpreg_full.pdf.)

Refractory status asthmaticus is defined as a severe exacerbation of asthma that is unresponsive to bronchodilators and corticosteroids and that requires intensive care unit admission and typically mechanical ventilation. In patients who require intensive care unit admission and intubation and who continue to have refractory life-threatening asthma despite aggressive treatment, delivery should be considered a therapeutic option; however, this is rarely required. A cesarean delivery is most likely necessary because of the urgency of the need for delivery. Information about the management of refractory status asthmaticus in obstetric patients is minimal and only available in the form of case series reports. Review of 3 case reports with a total of 10 cases, 2 of which were past 32 weeks, revealed 2 patients who underwent cesarean delivery and improved dramatically after the procedure.[14,26,27]

Improvement in a severe asthma exacerbation after delivery may result from several physiologic factors, including reduced pressure on the diaphragm and decreased oxygen consumption.[5] Vaginal delivery may be possible during an acute exacerbation in the setting of progressive active labor, normal maternal oxygenation, absence of hypercapnea, adequate neuraxial anesthesia, and use of operative vaginal delivery. If delivery is being considered for maternal reasons at a gestational age between 24 and 34 weeks, then betamethasone should be given before delivery for fetal lung maturity if at all possible.

Management of Asthma During Labor and Delivery

Asthma medications should not be discontinued or delayed during labor and delivery. Although asthma during labor is typically quiescent, consideration should be given to obtaining a peak flow measurement on admission and then every 12 hours or as needed to monitor for asthma exacerbation. Monitoring is likely only necessary in those women who have a history of exacerbations during pregnancy. Neuraxial anesthesia decreases oxygen requirements and minute ventilation and thus can be helpful for control of asthma symptoms during labor. If systemic (oral or intravenous) corticosteroids have been used in the previous 4 weeks for treatment, then the patient should receive stress-dose steroids to prevent an adrenal crisis. Usually, this regimen begins with hydrocortisone 100 mg every 8 hours, continued for 24 hours post partum, and then stopped. Tapering stress steroids is not necessary.

Medications typically used for tocolysis, induction of labor, and during delivery can have an influence on asthma symptoms, especially in the most severe or medication-sensitive asthmatic patients. Prostaglandins E2 or E1 can be used for cervical ripening, for post partum hemorrhage or to induce abortion without significant adverse reaction.[28] In these cases, respiratory status of the patient should be monitored in a routine fashion.[29] Carboprost (prostaglandin F2α), ergonovine, and methylergonovine can cause bronchospasm, especially in the aspirin-sensitive patient.[30] For these patients, choosing a medication such as misoprostol, which is an E1, may be more appropriate.

Magnesium sulfate is a bronchodilator, and should not have a deleterious effect on asthma, but indomethacin can induce bronchospasm in an asthmatic patient with known aspirin sensitivity. No formal studies on calcium channel blockers in the asthmatic gravid patient have been published, but bronchospasm has not been observed with the wide clinical use of these medications for tocolysis.

Breastfeeding

Asthma medications are excreted in small and varying amounts into breast milk. The NAEPP found that there was no contraindication for the use of prednisone, theophylline, cromolyn, antihistamines, ICS, or inhaled β agonist for breastfeeding.[17] Patients should be instructed, and strongly encouraged, to continue their asthma medications post partum with or without breastfeeding.

SUMMARY

Asthma is a chronic illness that complicates a significant number of pregnancies. Generalist obstetricians should be familiar with its diagnosis, classification, treatment, and possible complications in pregnancy. Providers should instruct and strongly urge patients to remain on asthma medications during pregnancy because one-third of patients have worsening of their asthma, including those women with mild asthma. There are proven negative effects from exacerbations and poor control on pregnancy outcome, whereas there are clear benefits of good control. Patient education about the importance of good asthma control is essential for improving compliance and self-monitoring.

REFERENCES

1. Dombrowski M, Schatz M. Asthma in pregnancy: ACOG practice bulletin. Obstet Gynecol 2008;111:457–64.
2. Alexander S, Dodds L, Aromson BA. Perinatal outcomes in women with asthma during pregnancy. Obstet Gynecol 1998;92:435–40.
3. Kwon HL, Belanger K, Bracken MB. Asthma prevalence among pregnant and childbearing-aged women in the United States: estimates from national health surveys. Ann Epidemiol 2003;13:317–24.
4. Bracken MD, Triche EW, Belandger K, et al. Asthma symptoms, severity, and drug therapy: a prospective study of effects on 2205 pregnancies. Obstet Gynecol 2003;102:739–52.
5. Hanania N, Belfort M. Acute asthma in pregnancy. Crit Care Med 2005;33: S319–24.
6. Nelson-Piercy C, Waldron M, Moore-Gillon J. Respiratory disease in pregnancy. Br J Hosp Med 1994;51(8):398–401.
7. Clifton V. Maternal asthma during pregnancy and fetal outcomes: potential mechanisms and possible solutions. Curr Opin Allergy Clin Immunol 2006;6:307–11.
8. Beecroft N, Cochrane GM, Milburn HJ, et al. Effect of sex of fetus on asthma during pregnancy: blind prospective trial. Br Med J 1998;317(7162):856–7.
9. Schatz M, Dombrowski MP, Wise R, et al. Asthma morbidity during pregnancy can be predicted by severity classification. J Allergy Clin Immunol 2003; 112(2):283.
10. Liu S, Wen SW, Demissie K, et al. Maternal asthma and pregnancy outcomes: a retrospective cohort study. Am J Obstet Gynecol 2001;184(2):90–6.
11. Demissie K, Breckenridge MB, Rhoads GG. Infant and maternal outcomes in the pregnancies of asthmatic women. Am J Respir Crit Care Med 1998;158(4): 1091–5.
12. Murphy VE, Gibson PG, Smith R, et al. Asthma during pregnancy: mechanisms and treatment implications. Eur Respir J 2005;25(4):731–50.
13. Dombrowski MP, Schatz M, Wise R, et al. Asthma during pregnancy. Obstet Gynecol 2004;103(1):5–12.
14. Lurie S, Mamet Y. Caesarean delivery during maternal cardiopulmonary resuscitation for status asthmaticus. Emerg Med J 2003;20(3):296–7.
15. Beck SA. Asthma in the female: hormonal effect and pregnancy. Allergy Asthma Proc 2001;22(1):1–4.

16. Schatz M, Harden K, Forsythe A, et al. The course of asthma during pregnancy, post partum, and with successive pregnancies: a prospective analysis. J Allergy Clin Immunol 1988;81(3):509–17.
17. National Asthma Education and Prevention Program expert panel report. Managing asthma during pregnancy: recommendations for pharmacologic treatment-2004 update. J Allergy Clin Immunol 2005;115(1):34–46. Available at: http://www.nhlbi.nih.gov/health/prof/lung/asthma/astpreg/astpreg_full.pdf. Accessed January 21, 2010.
18. Schatz M, Dombrowski MP, Wise R, et al. Spirometry is related to perinatal outcomes in pregnant women with asthma. Am J Obstet Gynecol 2006;194(1):120–6.
19. Dombrowski MP. Asthma and pregnancy. Obstet Gynecol 2006;108(3 Pt 1):667–81.
20. Blais L, Beauchesne MF, Rey E, et al. Use of inhaled corticosteroids during the first trimester of pregnancy and the risk of congenital malformations among women with asthma. Thorax 2007;62(4):320–8.
21. Kallen B, Rydhstroem H, Aberg A. Congenital malformations after the use of inhaled budesonide in early pregnancy. Obstet Gynecol 1999;93(3):392–5.
22. Schatz M, Dombrowski MP, Wise R, et al. The relationship of asthma medication use to perinatal outcomes. J Allergy Clin Immunol 2004;113(6):1040–5.
23. Suissa S, Ernst P, Benayoun S, et al. Low-dose inhaled corticosteroids and the prevention of death from asthma. N Engl J Med 2000;343(5):332–6.
24. Cockcroft DW, Murdock KY. Comparative effects of inhaled salbutamol, sodium cromoglycate, and beclomethasone dipropionate on allergen-induced early asthmatic responses, late asthmatic responses, and increased bronchial responsiveness to histamine. J Allergy Clin Immunol 1987;79(5):734–40.
25. Murphy VE, Gibson P, Talbot PI, et al. Severe asthma exacerbations during pregnancy. Obstet Gynecol 2005;106(5 Pt 1):1046–54.
26. Elsayegh D, Shapiro JM. Management of the obstetric patient with status asthmaticus. J Intensive Care Med 2008;23(6):396–402.
27. Gelber M, Sidi Y, Gassner S, et al. Uncontrollable life-threatening status asthmaticus—an indicator for termination of pregnancy by cesarean section. Respiration 1984;46(3):320–2.
28. Towers CV, Briggs GG, Rojas JA. The use of prostaglandin E2 in pregnant patients with asthma. Am J Obstet Gynecol 2004;190(6):1777–80 [discussion: 80].
29. Crawford JS. Bronchospasm following ergometrine. Anaesthesia 1980;35(4):397–8.
30. Stenius-Aarniala B, Piirila P, Teramo K. Asthma and pregnancy: a prospective study of 198 pregnancies. Thorax 1988;43(1):12–8.

Diagnosis and Management of Thyroid Disease in Pregnancy

Diana L. Fitzpatrick, MD[a],*, Michelle A. Russell, MD, MPH[b]

KEYWORDS

• Thyroid • Pregnancy • Management

Thyroid disease is common, affecting 1% to 2% of pregnant women. Pregnancy may modify the course of thyroid disease, and pregnancy outcomes can depend on optimal management of thyroid disorders. Consequently, obstetric providers must be familiar with thyroid physiology and management of thyroid diseases in pregnancy. Following a brief overview of physiology, this article provides an in-depth review of diagnosis and management of the spectrum of thyroid disease occurring in pregnancy. Recommendations for screening and treatment of hypo- and hyperthyroidism are summarized. Specific attention is given to the limitations of current research and the status of ongoing work.

THYROID PHYSIOLOGY IN PREGNANCY

Thyroid physiology is governed by the hypothalamic-pituitary axis. The hypothalamus continuously stimulates the pituitary via thyroid releasing hormone (TRH), the levels of which are inversely related to those of thyroid hormone. TRH modulates pituitary production of thyroid-stimulating hormone (TSH), and TSH in turn stimulates thyroid release of thyroid hormones, thyroxine (T_4) and triiodothyronine (T_3). TSH levels are controlled by TRH and negative feedback of T_3 and T_4 on the hypothalamic-pituitary axis.

Thyroid physiology is notable for 3 events during pregnancy[1]:

- Increased estrogen results in a two- to threefold increase in thyroxine-binding globulin (TBG), which lowers free thyroid hormone and stimulates the hypothalamic-pituitary-thyroid axis.

[a] Combined Obstetrics and Gynecology and Leadership Preventive Medicine, Department of Obstetrics and Gynecology, Dartmouth-Hitchock Medical Center, One Medical Center Drive, Lebanon, NH 03756, USA
[b] Department of Obstetrics and Gynecology, Dartmouth-Hitchock Medical Center, One Medical Center Drive, Lebanon, NH 03756, USA
* Corresponding author.
E-mail address: Diana.L.Fitzpatrick@Hitchcock.org

Obstet Gynecol Clin N Am 37 (2010) 173–193
doi:10.1016/j.ogc.2010.02.007
0889-8545/10/$ – see front matter © 2010 Elsevier Inc. All rights reserved.

- Human chorionic gonadotropin (hCG) and TSH have identical α subunits. Because of its similarity to TSH, hCG stimulates release of T_3 and T_4, which then act as negative pituitary feedback and cause a transient TSH decrease in weeks 8 to 14.
- Increased peripheral metabolism of thyroid hormone occurs primarily in the second and third trimester, resulting from elevation in placental type II and type III deiodinases. Type II deiodinase converts T_4 to T_3, and type III deiodinase converts T_4 to reverse triiodothyronine (rT_3), as well as converting rT_3 to 3,3'-diiodothyronine (T2). The fetus is dependent on the type II conversion of T_4 to T_3.[2]

The placenta transfers a small amount of maternal T_3 and T_4. This maternally derived thyroid hormone supports fetal development during critical organogenesis. Production of T_4 by the fetus is detectable by 14 weeks' gestational age (wga). Full fetal thyroid activity is present by midgestation and concentrations of thyroid hormone increase until term.

Thyroid Function Testing in Pregnancy

The physiologic changes in pregnancy make interpretation of laboratory tests difficult. The increase in TBG leads to increased measured levels of total T_4 (TT_4) and T_3 (TT_3), limiting their diagnostic usefulness. Free T_4 (FT_4) and free T_3 (FT_3) levels are generally believed to reflect thyroid function during pregnancy better than TT_4 or TT_3 but may also be altered by TBG.[3] FT_3 measurement is rarely necessary. Resin T_3 uptake (RT_3U) decreases in pregnancy but can be used to calculate the free T_4 index (FT_4I). The FT_4I accounts for increased TBG and is an indirect measure of FT_4 ($FT_4I = TT_4 \times RT_3U$). The reported reference values for FT_4I are 4.5 to 12.5 μg/dL.[3] TSH and FT_4 or FT_4I are used to assess and follow thyroid diseases in pregnancy.[4]

Although pregnancy-induced changes in thyroid physiology and their effects on laboratory interpretation have long been known, uncertainty remains regarding reference ranges for thyroid tests. To date, no universally accepted ranges exist. Whereas the reference range for TSH in the general population is 0.45 to 4.5 mU/L, several studies have described ranges for thyroid testing in pregnancy but have shown variation by gestational age, number of fetuses, population studied, laboratory, and testing method (**Table 1**).[5–11] Adding to the difficulty of setting reference ranges, the median TSH is lowest in the first trimester, with wider variation than in later trimesters.[12,13] Some have proposed using gestational age–specific nomograms for TSH reported as multiples of the median, similar to the reporting of analytes used in aneuploidy screening programs; however, this is not yet clinically available. A large population-based study of pregnant women defined the reference range (2.5–97.5th centile) for TSH in the first half of pregnancy as 0.08 to 2.99 mU/L.[7,14] Providers performing thyroid function testing and managing thyroid diseases during pregnancy should be aware of the areas of uncertainty.

Thyroid Screening and Pregnancy

There is controversy surrounding routine thyroid screening in pregnancy. **Table 2** contrasts the opinions of vested professional organizations regarding screening. The American College of Obstetrics and Gynecology (ACOG) does not recommend routine screening in patients without history or symptoms consistent with thyroid disease.[4] In keeping with these recommendations, a 2004 survey of 441 obstetricians indicated that 80% do not perform routine screening in pregnancy. The Endocrine Society also recommends case finding based on risk factors (**Box 1**).[15]

Table 1
Summary of studies and pregnancy-specific ranges for thyroid function tests among singleton gestations

Authors	Sample Population	Method	Test (units)	Gestational Age-Specific Ranges 2.5–97.5th Centiles			TPO + TG ab +
Bocos-Terraz, 2009[10]	n = 1198 Spain	High-performance immunoassay	TSH (mU/mL) FT4 (ng/dL) FT3 (pg/mL)	≤20 wk 0.03–2.65 0.77–1.34 2.24–4.43	>20 wk 0.12–3.56 0.17–1.17 2.25–4.18	–	14.7%
Cleary-Goldman, 2008[9]	n = 10990 United States	Chemiluminescent immunoassay	TSH (mU/L) FT4 (ng/dL)	~11–14 wk 0.036–4.28 0.72–1.46	~16–18 wk 0.213–3.93 0.72–1.32	–	15%
Casey, 2007[6]	n = 13599 Texas	Third-generation immunoassay	TSH (mU/L) FT4 (ng/dL)	<20 wk 0.08–3.0 0.85–1.9		–	Not measured
Stricker, 2007[11]	n=2272 Switzerland	High throughput immunoassay	TSH (mU/L) FT4 (ng/dL) FT3 (pg/mL) TT4 (nmol/L) TT3 (nmol/L)	<6–12 wk 0.088–2.83 0.82–1.42 2.29–4.04 72.3–171.2 1.25–2.72	12–24 wk 0.2–2.79 0.74–1.22 2.2–3.75 94.8–182.5 1.43–3.16	24–term 0.31–2.9 0.67–1.05 2.16–3.62 94.9–193.4 1.4–3.16	Excluded
Haddow, 2004[8]	n = 1005 Maine	Third-generation immunoassay	TSH (mU/L)	<14 wk nc–3.61	15–21wk nc–3.71	–	Excluded

Abbreviations: FT3, free triiodothyronine; FT4, free thyroxine; mU/L, milliunits per liter; nc, not calculated; ng/dL, nanograms per deciliter; nmol/L, nanomoles per liter; pg/mL, picograms per milliliter; TG ab+, thyroglobulin antibody positive; TPO+, thyroperoxidase antibody positive; TSH, thyroid-stimulating hormone; TT3, total triiodothyronine; TT4, total thyroxine.

Table 2
Opinions of professional organizations regarding thyroid disease screening and treatment in pregnancy

Organization	Thyroid Screening with TSH	Goal TSH During Treatment (mU/L)	Treatment of Subclinical Hypothyroidism
ACOG[4]	Case finding	Not specified	Not recommended
USPSTF[96]	Case finding	Not specified	Not specified
TES[15,a]	Case finding	2.5 in first trimester 3.0 in second, third trimesters	Recommended
AACE[97,98]	Routine	0.3–3.0	Recommended
BTA[99,b]	Case finding	0.4–2.0	Recommended

Abbreviations: AACE, American Association of Clinical Endocrinologists; ACOG, American College of Obstetricians and Gynecologists; ATA, American Thyroid Association; BTA, British Thyroid Association; mU/L, milliunits per liter; RCOG, Royal College of Obstetricians and Gynaecologists; TES, The Endocrine Society; TSH, thyroid-stimulating hormone; USPTF, United States Preventive Services Task Force.

[a] Guidelines cosponsored by AACE, Asia & Oceana Thyroid Association (AOTA), ATA, European Thyroid Association (ETA), Latin American Thyroid Association (LATA).

[b] Joint statement supporting BTA guidelines by The Royal College of Physicians, The Association for Clinical Biochemistry, The Society of Endocrinology, BTA, The British Thyroid Foundation Patient Support Group, The British Society of Pediatric Endocrinology and Diabetes and endorsed by Royal College of General Practitioners. *Data from* The Diagnosis and Management of Primary Hypothyroidism: statement on behalf of The Royal College of Physicians in particular its Patient and Carer Network and the Joint Specialty Committee for Endocrinology & Diabetes, The Association for Clinical Biochemistry, The Society for Endocrinology, The British Thyroid Association, British Thyroid Foundation Patient Support Group, The British Society of Pediatric Endocrinology and Diabetes, endorsed by The Royal College of General Practitioners. November 19, 2008. Available at: http://www.british-thyroid-association.org/news/Docs/hypothyroidism_statement.pdf. Accessed December 31, 2009.

Box 1
Increased risk for thyroid disease with greater than or equal to 1[a]

Signs or symptoms of thyroid under- or overfunction

Goiter

History of hyperthyroid disease, hypothyroid disease, postpartum thyroiditis, or thyroid surgery

Previous therapeutic head or neck irradiation

Type 1 diabetes mellitus or other autoimmune disorder

Family history of thyroid disease

Infertility

History of miscarriage or preterm delivery

Thyroid antibodies (when known)

Unexplained anemia or hyponatremia

Increased cholesterol level

[a] Pregnant patient needs evaluation with serum TSH.

It remains unclear whether routine screening can improve pregnancy outcomes compared with case finding. To begin to answer this question, a prospective observational study is underway to evaluate the effects of instituting screening for thyroid dysfunction in pregnancy. Planned data collection includes the prevalence of undiagnosed thyroid deficiency, treatment compliance, pregnancy outcomes, and postpartum course of thyroid disease (NCT00818896).

HYPOTHYROIDISM AND PREGNANCY

Hypothyroidism is an underproduction of thyroid hormones. It affects 1% to 2% of women in the United States and complicates 0.3% of pregnancies.[16] The symptoms are vague and are similar to pregnancy concerns including fatigue, constipation, cold intolerance, muscle cramps, insomnia, weight gain, carpal tunnel syndrome, hair loss, voice changes, and slowed thinking. Other findings may include dry skin, periorbital edema, and prolonged relaxation of deep tendon reflexes. Presence of thyroid enlargement is variable. Given that symptoms of hypothyroidism can be confused with those of pregnancy, there should be a low threshold for thyroid testing. Serum TSH on a third-generation assay is the initial test for hypothyroidism. Laboratory values associated with hypothyroidism include increased TSH, low FT_4 or FT_4l, and variable presence of thyroperoxidase antibodies (TPO). **Fig. 1** reviews the diagnosis and management of a pregnant patient with hypothyroidism and emphasizes confirmation of diagnosis with a second set of laboratory values.

Hypothyroidism is associated with premature birth, preeclampsia, abruption, low birth weight (LBW), postpartum hemorrhage, and impaired neuropsychological

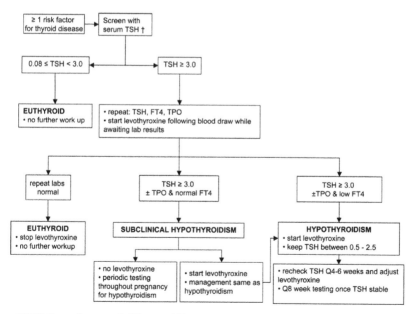

† Gestational age specific nomograms for TSH recommended for screening; however, TSH level of 3.0mU/L is sufficiently low to have high screening sensitivity. TSH Thyroid Stimulating hormone (mU/L), FT4 free thyroxine,TPO thyroperoxidase antibody

Fig. 1. Diagnosis and management algorithm for pregnant woman with greater than or equal to 1 risk factor (see **Box 1**) for thyroid disease without prior diagnosis of hypothyroidism. (See **Fig. 2** for hyperthyroidism algorithm.)

development in childhood.[17,18] Based on limited data, treatment may improve pregnancy outcomes. Hallengren and colleagues[19] found that fetal loss among hypothyroid women occurred in 29% of untreated, compared with 6% of levothyroxine-treated, patients. In another study of pregnant hypothyroid women, Haddow and colleagues[14] found that children born to untreated mothers had intelligence quotient (IQ) scores that were 7 points lower than treated peers, and 19% had IQ scores less than 85 compared with 5% of treated.

Treatment of Hypothyroidism in Pregnancy

Women with preexisting hypothyroidism should have early assessment of TSH to adjust medications. During the first trimester there is an estimated 30% to 50% increase in the levothyroxine requirement. Some suggest hypothyroid women increase their dose by 30% as soon as they are pregnant.[20] Preconception counseling is an opportunity to educate, optimize treatment, and provide an additional 25-µg prescription of levothyroxine to start with a positive pregnancy test. Women diagnosed with hypothyroidism during pregnancy should start with 1 to 2 µg/kg/d of levothyroxine. An initial dose ranges between 100 and 150 µg/d with adjustments in 25- to 50-µg increments.[16] TSH should be reassessed 4 to 6 weeks following a dose change, with a treatment goal in pregnancy between 0.5 and 2.5 mU/L.[21] Once stable, TSH can be checked every 8 weeks.

The bioavailability of levothyroxine can be affected by medications or foods. Carafate, cholestyramine, ferrous sulfate, and calcium carbonate reduce its absorption. Phenytoin and carbamazepine increase its clearance. In addition, pregnant patients should space their levothyroxine and prenatal vitamin by 2 to 3 hours.

Postpartum, most hypothyroid women can have the levothyroxine dose decreased. Those who entered pregnancy on an adequate dose can resume their prepregnancy dose. For those with a new diagnosis of hypothyroidism during pregnancy, reduction can be accomplished by decreasing their dose by ~30% (often a decrease of 25 µg). TSH should be reassessed at 6 weeks postpartum.

Causes of Hypothyroidism in Pregnancy

Primary hypothyroidism

In adult women, 95% of hypothyroidism results from primary disease of the thyroid gland, most commonly the autoimmune condition Hashimoto thyroiditis.[22] Autoimmune thyroid disease is common among women with type 1 diabetes mellitus, Sjögren syndrome, Addison disease, or pernicious anemia. Up to 25% of patients with type 1 diabetes will develop postpartum thyroid disease.[23] Other causes of primary hypothyroidism include subacute thyroiditis, endemic iodine deficiency, suppurative thyroiditis, history of thyroidectomy or radioiodine ablation, and medication exposure.

Thyroiditis

Hashimoto thyroiditis Hashimoto thyroiditis, also known as lymphadenoid thyroiditis and chronic lymphocytic thyroiditis, is the most common cause of hypothyroidism in iodine-sufficient populations. The incidence increases with age and is common in women, with a rate of 4 per 1000.[24] In Hashimoto, antithyroid-specific antibodies damage the thyroid gland.[25] TPO antibodies are present in almost all patients. The antibody-mediated injury of the thyroid gland may present initially as a transient hyperthyroidism that usually evolves insidiously into hypothyroidism. Along with thyromegaly, myxedema is one of the few clinical signs that leads a provider to suspect Hashimoto specifically.

Subacute thyroiditis There are 2 forms of subacute thyroiditis: subacute granulomatous thyroiditis and subacute lymphocytic thyroiditis. Although the causes differ, these subacute diseases have a similar course, starting with transient hyperthyroidism followed by transient hypothyroidism.[26] The disease course may last just 4 to 6 weeks or as long as 9 months. The recovery rate is more than 90%, and only 10% of patients have persistent goiter and mild hypothyroidism.[26]

Subacute granulomatous thyroiditis, also known as subacute painful thyroiditis, is believed to be caused by viral infection. The onset is sudden, with fever, myalgia, and neck pain. On physical examination, a painfully enlarged thyroid is the hallmark.

Subacute lymphocytic thyroiditis, also known as subacute painless thyroiditis, includes postpartum thyroiditis. Subacute lymphocytic thyroiditis is distinguished from subacute granulomatous thyroiditis by the presence of a painlessly enlarged thyroid gland. Suspicion of thyroiditis should be increased during puerperium because it affects approximately 5% of postpartum women. Recurrence is as high as 80% for subsequent gestations.[27] Recurrence may be even more common in women with positive TPO antibodies.

The hyperthyroid phase of thyroiditis can be differentiated from Graves disease by the lack of radioiodine uptake during a thyroid scan.[28] The management of thyroiditis hyperthyroidism is supportive, with β-adrenergic blockers for palpitations and tremors and nonsteroidal antiinflammatory agents or corticosteroids in severe cases. Antithyroid medications are generally not needed because the hyperthyroidism is transient. Women with a history of postpartum thyroiditis should be monitored annually for hypothyroidism and treated accordingly.[15,27]

Iodine deficiency

Iodine deficiency affects more than 38% of the world's population.[29] Although iodine sufficiency is improving, it remains a public health concern in 47 of 130 countries surveyed.[30,31] Southeast Asia and Europe are the most affected populations under the World Health Organization (WHO).[30] Iodine deficiency is assessed at the population level, because in individuals there is a large day-to-day variation in urinary iodine (UI) excretion, and this variation is muted with a large sample size.[32] Iodine sufficiency in a population is determined through measuring median UI excretion. In the United States there was a decrease in median UI excretion from 320 µg/L in the 1970s to a new steady state of 140s-160s, most recently 168 µg/L in 2002.[33,34] National Health and Nutrition Examination Survey (NHANES) III data show that the median UI excretion in pregnant women is 141 µg/L.[33] This raises concern that, although the general population of the United States is iodine sufficient, there are subpopulations at risk for iodine deficiency such as immigrants from endemic regions, groups with dietary restrictions, and pregnant women.[35]

Iodine deficiency in pregnancy The most devastating outcomes of iodine deficiency in pregnancy include perinatal mortality and congenital cretinism (growth failure, mental retardation, and other neuropsychological deficits).[4] Iodine deficiency remains the leading cause of preventable mental retardation worldwide.[36,37] A meta-analysis of 19 studies conducted in iodine deficient areas found that deficiency is responsible for a mean IQ loss of 13.5 points.[38] Decreases in maternal FT_4 due to mild deficiency may have adverse effects on cognitive function of offspring.[15] The median UI concentration for a population of pregnant women is considered insufficient if less than 150 µg/L and for lactating women if less than 100 µg/L. Iodine needs increase in pregnancy as a result of renal clearance as well as fetal and placental uptake. The recommended nutrient intake for iodine during pregnancy and lactation should average 250 µg/d.[39]

In most populations, iodized salt and seafood are the major sources of iodine. In the United States, table salt is iodized with potassium iodide at 100 parts per million.[40] Iodized table salt is chosen by about 50% to 60% of the Unites States population; however, approximately 70% of ingested salt comes from processed foods that are not prepared with iodized salt.[41,42] Pregnant women should be counseled that although they may be limiting their intake of fish for concerns of mercury levels, they should include other sources of iodine in their diet and make sure their prenatal vitamins are fortified with iodine. Iodine-rich foods include seaweed, seafood, potato (baked with peel), cow's milk, turkey breast (baked), navy beans, and eggs.[43]

Secondary hypothyroidism

Secondary hypothyroidism is rare. It has been described as the result of damage to the hypothalamus or pituitary from tumor, surgery, radiation, Sheehan syndrome, and lymphocytic hypophysitis.

Sheehan syndrome and lymphocytic hypophysitis are rare conditions unique to pregnancy. Sheehan syndrome is pituitary necrosis from vascular hypoperfusion. It has been reported to occur following severe pregnancy-related hemorrhage or hypotension. The presentation can vary from insidious, with failure to lactate or resume menses, to acute panhypopituitarism with high morbidity. When the diagnosis is suspected, evaluation requires stimulation testing and intracranial imaging, which often shows an empty sella turcia. Up to 90% develop secondary hypothyroidism.[44] Management consists primarily of hormone replacement.[45]

Lymphocytic hypophysitis occurs in the peripartum period. It is believed to be an autoimmune disorder leading to anterior pituitary destruction. The most common presentation involves mass effect with headache and visual field changes and endocrine dysfunction that can vary from panhypopituitarism to single-hormone deficiency.[46] Intracranial imaging typically shows an enhancing sellar turcica mass that is indistinguishable from a pituitary macroadenoma. Corticosteroids have been effective, but surgical debulking is indicated in the presence of mass effect. Management of this rare condition can be difficult when the symptoms are not severe, at which time the pros and cons of expectant management versus tissue diagnosis must be weighed.[47] Multidisciplinary management should involve neurosurgery and endocrinology.

Subclinical thyroid disorders

The diagnosis and management of subclinical thyroid disorders is controversial, and the clinical significance in pregnancy is debated.

Subclinical hypothyroidism in pregnancy Subclinical hypothyroidism is defined as increased TSH with normal concentrations of FT_4 and FT_3. The prevalence of subclinical hypothyroidism during pregnancy is estimated to be 2% to 5%.[48–50] Women with subclinical hypothyroidism are more likely than euthyroid women to have antibodies for TPO; 31% compared with 5%.[6] Half of these women progress to hypothyroidism within 8 years.[51] Subclinical hypothyroidism, like hypothyroidism, is seen more frequently in women with autoimmune diseases. The association of TPO antibodies with subclinical hypothyroidism, and the tendency of this group to progress to hypothyroidism, support the belief that it is part of a spectrum of autoimmune hypothyroid disease. In contrast, TPO antibodies are no more common in women with isolated hypothyroxinemia than in women with normal thyroid function. This finding causes some to question the significance of isolated hypothyroxinemia as a pertinent biologic entity.[6]

By definition, subclinical hypothyroidism during pregnancy is an asymptomatic condition. The diagnosis is made by laboratory testing with a TSH greater than 3.0 mU/L and normal FT_4. Concerns have been raised regarding the effect of mild maternal thyroid hormone deficiency on fetal neurodevelopment. Haddow and colleagues[14] concluded from their case-control study that decreases in childhood intellectual performance can occur even when a pregnant woman's hypothyroidism is mild and probably asymptomatic. Allan and colleagues[52] showed that pregnant women with TSH more than 10 mU/L experience significantly more stillbirths, although this study population may not reflect subclinical hypothyroidism because it did not differentiate hypothyroidism from subclinical hypothyroidism. A study by Casey and colleagues[13] found an increased risk of preterm delivery from 2.5% in euthyroid women compared with 4% in women with subclinical hypothyroidism, as well as a threefold higher risk of abruption. The incidence of gestational hypertension, preeclampsia, and stillbirth was not significantly different. Refuting these findings, a secondary analysis of First and Second Trimester Evaluation of Risk (FaSTER) Trial data did not show an association between subclinical hypothyroidism and preterm labor, abruption, or any adverse pregnancy outcome.[9] It has not yet been shown that treatment of subclinical hypothyroidism with levothyroxine can prevent or modify any of the associated outcomes. As such, routine screening and treatment of subclinical hypothyroidism in pregnancy is not universally recommended or accepted practice.

Isolated hypothyroxinemia and pregnancy

Isolated hypothyroxinemia is defined as a low FT_4 and normal TSH. Isolated hypothyroxinemia can be found in approximately 1% to 2% of pregnancies and is defined as low FT_4 with normal TSH.[6] Pop and colleagues[53,54] found that, during pregnancy, maternal FT_4 less than 10th percentile at 12 wga was associated with an increased risk of impaired psychomotor development in infants evaluated at 10 months and 2 years of age. Casey and colleagues[6] evaluated the outcomes of 17,298 pregnancies and found that isolated maternal hypothyroxinemia in the first half of pregnancy has no adverse affects on pregnancy outcome. Supporting this, adverse pregnancy outcomes were not consistently associated with first or second trimester isolated maternal hypothyroxinemia in a large cohort enrolled in the FaSTER Trial.[9] To date, there are no studies showing benefit from levothyroxine treatment of isolated hypothyroxinemia during pregnancy on pregnancy outcome or subsequent infant development.

Clinicians providing care for pregnant women are left with uncertainty regarding issues of screening for, and management of, subclinical hypothyroid disorders, although studies are underway. A prospective observational study is recruiting subjects to examine the neurodevelopmental outcome of children born to women with isolated hypothyroxinemia (NCT00147433). In addition, a large multicenter randomized double-blinded placebo controlled trial is in progress to examine the effect of levothyroxine treatment in women with subclinical hypothyroidism or hypothyroxinemia on the neurodevelopmental outcome of their children (NCT00388297).

HYPERTHYROIDISM IN PREGNANCY

Hyperthyroidism is the result of an excess of thyroid hormones that complicates less than 1% of pregnancies.[4] Recognition of hyperthyroidism during pregnancy can be elusive because signs overlap with pregnancy symptoms such as nausea and vomiting, increased appetite, heat intolerance, insomnia, changes in bowel habits, fatigue, and irritable or anxious mood. Symptoms uncommon in normal pregnancy, but found in hyperthyroidism, are weight loss or failed weight gain despite increased dietary intake, resting tachycardia, hypertension, tremor, eye stare, eyelid lag, proptosis, and thyroid enlargement or nodule.

There are few high-quality studies to guide the management of hyperthyroidism in pregnancy. As such, management of hyperthyroidism in pregnancy reflects the standard of care for the general population with a few exceptions. Treatment options in pregnancy include antithyroid medications and thyroidectomy. In all but the mildest cases of hyperthyroidism, treatment is advised because there may be an association between uncontrolled hyperthyroidism and pregnancy complications. These complications include spontaneous abortion, minor congenital anomalies, preeclampsia, preterm birth, LBW, abruption, neonatal thyroid dysfunction, and perinatal mortality.[55-57] Maternal complications of uncontrolled hyperthyroidism are primarily related to thyroid storm, including arrhythmia and congestive heart failure.[58] Subclinical hyperthyroidism, in which TSH is low but FT_4 is normal, does not affect pregnancy outcomes and treatment is unnecessary.[59] To avoid fetal exposure to the complications of hyperthyroidism and its treatment options, preconception treatment is preferred, although not always possible.

Diagnosis of suspected hyperthyroidism can be confirmed by laboratory testing showing low TSH on a third-generation assay and high FT_4 or FT_4I. FT_3 is only used to exclude rare cases of T_3 thyrotoxicosis when the serum TSH is low and FT_4 or FT_4I is normal.

Treatment of Hyperthyroidism in Pregnancy

Antithyroid medications

As described in **Fig. 2**, the first line of treatment of hyperthyroidism is antithyroid medication, of which there is 1 class, the thionamides. This class comprises 3

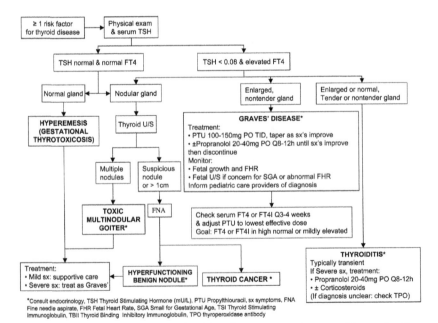

Fig. 2. Diagnosis and management algorithm for pregnant woman with greater than or equal to 1 risk factor (see **Box 1**) for thyroid disease without prior diagnosis of hyperthyroidism. (See **Fig. 1** for hypothyroidism algorithm.)

medications: propylthiouracil (PTU), methimazole, and carbimazole, which work by inhibiting the production of T_4. PTU also blocks the conversion of T_4 to T_3. Currently, PTU is used more frequently than methimazole, because methimazole may be teratogenic. There have been numerous case reports describing cutis aplasia and congenital abnormalities (choanal atresia, gastrointestinal, and facial) in pregnancies treated with methimazole.[60] Although a causal relationship between methimazole and cutis aplasia or the spectrum of birth defects is not certain, the reports have led to the avoidance of methimazole in early pregnancy.[61] Carbimazole is unavailable in the United States.

In addition to teratogenic concerns, all antithyroid medications cross the placenta and can cause iatrogenic fetal hypothyroidism. To reduce this risk, the lowest dose of antithyroid medication to achieve a maternal FT_4 or FT_4I in the upper third of the normal range or slightly more than normal should be used.[62] One approach would be to use the Casey and colleagues[6] pregnancy-specific reference range for FT_4 (0.85–1.9 ng/dL) or FT_4I (4.5–12.5 μg/dL) as goals.[3] A typical PTU dose to achieve this is 300 to 450 mg/d given in 3 oral doses of 100 to 150 mg each. Occasionally doses of 600 mg daily are necessary. β-Adrenergic blockers inhibit conversion of T_4 to T_3 and can be used as an adjunctive treatment to antithyroid medications to reduce tachycardia, palpitations, and tremors. Propranolol 20 to 40 mg orally every 8 to 12 hours may be used while awaiting response to the antithyroid medications. PTU dose adjustments are based on FT_4 or FT_4I testing performed every 3 to 4 weeks. TSH is not helpful in treatment monitoring because it remains low. Improvement in symptoms occurs after 3 to 4 weeks of treatment but a full response may take 8 weeks. Antithyroid medications can and should be tapered as pregnancy progresses, but there is controversy as to whether they should be discontinued or maintained through delivery. Block and replace therapy, combining high doses of antithyroid medication with levothyroxine, is not advised in pregnancy because the antithyroid medications readily cross the placenta but levothyroxine does not, which increases the risk of fetal hypothyroidism.[62] The fetus should be monitored for signs of hypothyroidism by clinical examination for growth and fetal heart tones for baseline bradycardia. Approximately 10% of those exposed to PTU will develop fetal or neonatal hypothyroidism.[63] Ultrasound is not routinely recommended but has been advocated by some to assess fetal biometry and for evidence of fetal goiter.[4] The normal fetal thyroid can be difficult to see on routine ultrasound examination, but a goiter is suspected if there is a symmetric paratracheal mass, neck hyperextension, and polyhydramnios. Case reports describe confirmation of suspected fetal hypothyroidism in women on antithyroid medications by percutaneous umbilical blood sampling. Treatment has consisted of decreasing the maternal antithyroid medication or weekly intra-amniotic instillation of thyroid hormone.[64] Because of the potential complications of percutaneous umbilical blood sampling and repeat amniocentesis, this management approach should not be routine.

A rare but serious side effect of the thionamides is agranulocytosis, which occurs in 0.1% of patients. Before initiating therapy, a baseline assessment of white blood cell count should be performed. Women must be instructed to call for evaluation if they experience a sore throat or febrile illness. In such an event, a complete blood count is performed immediately and, if agranulocytosis is diagnosed, all antithyroid medications are permanently discontinued. In addition, PTU and methimazole have been implicated in rare cases of fatal hepatic failure.[65,66] Antithyroid medications can be continued postpartum as there is minimal excretion into breast milk. The American Academy of Pediatrics and WHO support the compatibility of breastfeeding and all antithyroid medications.[67,68]

Surgery

Subtotal or near-total thyroidectomy is the surgical management for women with complications of severe refractory hyperthyroidism, intolerance of medications, agranulocytosis, noncompliance, or malignant thyroid cancer. Ideally, surgery is delayed until postpartum, but it can be performed in pregnancy when necessary. If surgery is required during pregnancy it is best accomplished in the second trimester to avoid possible anesthesia complications such as potential teratogenicity and preterm birth. Other concerns regarding thyroid surgery in pregnancy are airway management and recurrent laryngeal nerve injury. Surgical risks of total thyroidectomy include 2% to 4% risk of injury of the recurrent laryngeal nerve and 1% risk of hypoparathyroidism following inadvertent resection of parathyroid glands. Complications, costs, and length of stay associated with thyroid surgery may be increased in pregnancy.[69] Thyroidectomy for Graves disease with subsequent discontinuation of antithyroid medications can lead to fetal hyperthyroidism if thyroid-stimulating antibodies are present.[70]

Radioiodine ablation

Radioiodine ablation using iodine 131 (^{131}I) is contraindicated during pregnancy and lactation. All sexually active, childbearing-age women with a uterus should have a pretreatment pregnancy test to avoid inadvertent administration during gestation.[71] The ^{131}I crosses the placenta and, although early exposure may have little effect on the fetus, after 12 wga the fetal thyroid is capable of concentrating the ^{131}I and is susceptible to the ablative effects. Case series of fetal exposure to ^{131}I after 10 to 12 wga show at least a 3% rate of congenital hypothyroidism and neurologic abnormalities.[72–74] In an attempt to prevent fetal thyroid ablation by blocking ^{131}I uptake, some have prescribed PTU and potassium iodide 5 to 10 gtts orally twice daily within 7 to 10 days after inadvertant ^{131}I administration.[75] Because of the possible increased risk of adverse pregnancy outcomes after ^{131}I ablative therapy, effective contraception is recommended for at least 3 months, and some recommend postponing conception for 1 year following therapy.[76] More recently, Garsi and colleagues[77] recommended postponing conception until stable serum TSH levels are achieved on levothyroxine. There has also been concern that prior maternal gonadal exposure to ^{131}I may be associated with later adverse reproductive outcomes, but there seems to be no increase in fetal malformation, spontaneous abortion, stillbirth, or preterm birth in women who have undergone prior radioiodine ablation.[77]

Causes of Hyperthyroidism in Pregnancy

The most common cause of clinically significant hyperthyroidism in pregnancy is Graves disease, but the differential includes hyperemesis gravidarum/gestational transient thyrotoxicosis, solitary hyperfunctioning nodule, and thyroiditis. In addition, there are some other causes to consider, including toxic multinodular goiter, exogenous thyroid hormone (iatrogenic or factitious), gestational trophoblastic disease, metastatic thyroid cancer, struma ovarii, pituitary tumor, iodine induced, and medication associated.

Hyperemesis gravidarum/gestational transient thyrotoxicosis

Transient biochemical features of hyperthyroidism may be observed in 2% to 15% of women in early pregnancy.[78,79] In these cases, unlike Graves disease, there is no antecedent history or symptoms of hyperthyroidism. Women with hyperemesis gravidarum have intractable nausea and vomiting leading to dehydration, electrolyte disturbance, and weight loss. Routine assessment of thyroid function is not recommended in the evaluation of hyperemesis gravidarum unless there is suspicion of clinical hyperthyroidism.[4,80] If assessed, serum TSH is frequently low and FT_4 or FT_4I is high. The cause of the transient hyperthyroidism is believed to be a result of cross-reactivity between hCG and TSH at the thyroid receptor. Supportive therapy with anti-emetics, hydration, electrolyte replacement, and nutrition is recommended. In nearly all cases, spontaneous resolution occurs by 18 wga without treatment.[81] Antithyroid medications should be avoided unless there is persistence of hyperthyroid symptoms and thyroid function abnormalities beyond 18 to 20 wga because this may indicate Graves disease and should be treated.[27]

Graves disease

Graves disease is an autoimmune disorder occurring in 0.5% of the population. It accounts for more than 90% to 95% of hyperthyroidism associated with pregnancy. Unlike transient gestational thyrotoxicosis, the symptoms of Graves disease often antedate pregnancy. Graves disease is due to antibodies that stimulate thyroid receptors, producing thyroid hypertrophy and hyperfunction. Accordingly, the thyroid gland is enlarged on examination. In addition, abnormal eye findings of proptosis and extra-ocular muscle palsy are common. Several antibodies can be associated with Graves disease, including TPO, thryoglobulin, microsomal, and thyroid receptor antibodies (TRAbs). The activity of the TRAbs can be measured via tests for thyroid-stimulating immunoglobins (TSI) or thyrotropin-binding inhibitory immunoglobulins (TBII). TRAbs are specific to Graves disease, but measurement is not necessary to make the diagnosis.[4] The diagnosis is made by clinical examination and low serum TSH, high FT_4 or FT_4I, and, if measured, higher FT_3 compared with FT_4. Management with antithyroid medications is standard during pregnancy, reserving surgery for complicated cases. Surgery ultimately provides the most durable treatment option. Relapse rates after surgery are 5% compared with 40% after antithyroid medication, and TRAbs are more likely to decrease after surgery.[70,82] Graves disease is known to exacerbate in the first trimester and to improve in the second and third trimesters of pregnancy, allowing tapering of medications. Close monitoring in the postpartum period is important, as disease flares have been reported. Women who are weaned from antithyroid medications should have thyroid function testing at the 6-week postpartum visit. Care of women with Graves disease in pregnancy should be multidisciplinary and involve an obstetrician familiar with the management of maternal medical conditions, an endocrinologist, and often an ophthalmologist. Women with proptosis or other eye findings should be referred to an ophthalmologist for evaluation and management of ophthalmopathy, which may be present in as many as half the cases of Graves disease.

Neonatal Graves disease occurs in about 1% to 5% of babies born of women with the condition.[83] Regardless of the maternal thyroid status, TRAbs can remain after treatment by surgery or radioiodine ablation, and the fetus may be affected by their transplacental passage. Affected fetuses may exhibit in utero and neonatal hypothyroidism or hyperthyroidism. Some have recommended measurement of maternal TRAbs at 28 to 32 wga in all women with active or treated Graves disease to determine the risk of fetal and neonatal thyroid dysfunction.[15] ACOG does not recommend routine TRAb testing, because management is rarely changed by the results.[4] Fetal hypothyroidism from TBII may manifest as bradycardic baseline fetal heart rate (FHR), goiter, and intrauterine growth restriction (IUGR). Findings associated with fetal hyperthyroidism from TSI include tachycardic baseline FHR, goiter, IUGR, craniosynostosis, premature skeletal maturation, cardiac failure, and hydrops.[83,84] There are case reports describing percutaneous umbilical blood sampling to confirm the diagnosis of suspected fetal hypothyroidism or hyperthyroidism. Treatment of the hyperthyroid fetus has been reported by means of administering maternal PTU concurrently with levothyroxine. Treatment of the hypothyroid fetus by means of serial intra-amniotic instillation of levothyroxine has also been reported.[85] These approaches are isolated to case reports, and series and should not be used in routine practice; referral to a maternal fetal medicine specialist is advised. Pediatric care givers should be informed of all cases of past and present maternal Graves disease, as well as antithyroid medications and presence of maternal TRAbs.

Thyroid Nodules in Pregnancy

Thyroid nodules occur in 1% to 2% of young women. The chance of having a palpable thyroid nodule increases with age. Among reproductive-age women, most palpated nodules of the thyroid are benign. Evaluation of a thyroid nodule includes a serum TSH and an ultrasound assessment of the neck and thyroid gland. Multinodular goiter is defined as the presence of 2 or more nodules. Thyroid nodules are described as functional or nonfunctional depending on whether they produce thyroid hormone. Functional nodules are less likely to be malignant, but this is not absolute. Autoimmune thyroid diseases may increase the risk of thyroid cancer, and coexistent Graves disease or Hashimoto thyroiditis must be considered if the serum TSH is low or high, respectively. Fine-needle aspiration of thyroid nodules during pregnancy is recommended to exclude cancer if they are growing, suspicious (microcalcifications, hypoechoic, increased vascularity, infiltrative margins), or larger than 1 cm.[15,65] Management of hyperthyroidism in pregnancy resulting from a hyperfunctioning solitary nodule or multinodular goiter consists of antithyroid medications, β-adrenergic blockers, and thyroid surgery.[15]

THYROID CANCER IN PREGNANCY

Thyroid cancer is the most commonly diagnosed endocrine malignancy. The incidence of this cancer is rising, likely as a result of increased detection of early-stage cases in a reservoir of subclinical disease.[86] Among United States reproductive-age women in 2002 to 2006, the age-specific annual incidence rates of invasive thyroid cancer ranged from 7 to 23 cases in 100,000 persons (http://SEER.cancer.gov). Accordingly, it affects approximately 14 out of 100,000 pregnant women.[87] Thyroid cancer is likely to be asymptomatic and diagnosed by a palpable nodule found on prenatal examination.[88] The histologic types of thyroid cancer include differentiated (papillary and follicular), medullary, Hurthle cell, and anaplastic. Papillary thyroid cancer is the most common histologic type diagnosed during pregnancy and it has an excellent long-term prognosis. The approach to diagnosis in a pregnant woman with a palpable thyroid nodule is similar to that in the nonpregnant woman. Serum TSH and ultrasound assessment of the neck and thyroid gland with fine-needle aspiration for suspicious nodules are recommended. With concerns that pregnancy hormones may influence tumor behavior, uncertainty exists about the optimal timing of surgical treatment in those with suspicious biopsy results. Timing of treatment should be based on the tumor histology and clinical presentation. If localized, differentiated thyroid cancer is diagnosed in the second or third trimester, it may be acceptable to delay surgery until postpartum.[89] There is no apparent increase in adverse pregnancy outcomes in women diagnosed with differentiated thyroid cancer who receive subtotal or total thyroidectomy during pregnancy or postpartum compared with the baseline obstetric population. The 10-year survival rate for differentiated thyroid cancer diagnosed during pregnancy is 99% and is not different from that diagnosed in age-matched nonpregnant women.[89] Women who undergo surgical treatment during pregnancy require monitoring of thyroid function and need replacement levothyroxine. Many will require postsurgical medical management of thyroid cancer with doses of levothyroxine to achieve suppressed TSH levels.[90] Careful monitoring for clinical symptoms of hyperthyroidism due to overtreatment is important during pregnancy. The 10-year recurrence rate of thyroid cancer is ~15% to 20%, and ultrasound surveillance of the neck for local or nodal recurrence may be indicated depending on the histology and stage of disease.[91] Thyroglobulin levels are measured after completion of surgical treatment and are predictive of persistent or recurrent disease.[92] Postsurgical ^{131}I whole-body scintigraphy and radioiodine remnant ablation are contraindicated during pregnancy and lactation. Because of the increasing incidence of thyroid cancer in young adults, the excellent long-term survival in this population, and the increasingly common choice to delay childbearing, many obstetricians will provide obstetric care for women with previously treated and newly diagnosed thyroid cancer. Multidisciplinary care involving the obstetrician, endocrinologist, and medical or surgical oncologist is essential in managing women with a history of thyroid cancer or those with thyroid cancer diagnosed during pregnancy.

THYROID STORM

Thyroid storm, an acute exacerbation of hyperthyroidism, is a rare but critical medical complication. It may present as unexplained fever, tachycardia, neurologic changes, arrhythmias, and cardiac failure in the setting of poorly controlled or undiagnosed

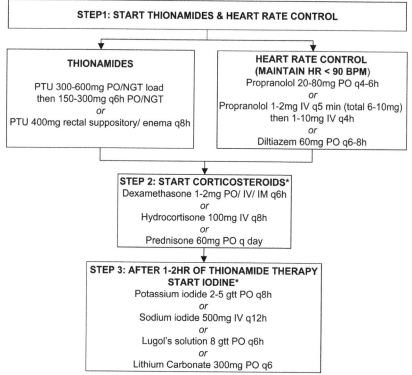

Fig. 3. Stepwise approach to medication management of thyroid storm in pregnancy.

hyperthyroidism. Characteristic laboratory values are consistent with hyperthyroidism and may also include leukocytosis, transaminitis, and hypercalcemia. Inciting factors include infection, surgery, medical complications, preeclampsia, and delivery. A high index of suspicion, low threshold for evaluation, and prompt treatment are essential to avoid adverse outcomes. Intensive monitoring may require intensive care unit admission, especially if there is evidence of cardiac decompensation. Initial stabilization requires intravenous fluid and electrolyte replacement. Once the diagnosis is established or highly likely, an antithyroid medication must be started to block further production of T_4. The maternal heart rate should be controlled. β-Adrenergic blocking agents also impede the conversion of T_4 to T_3. Iodine blocks release of T_4 and can be commenced after an initial 1 to 2 hours of stabilization with the antithyroid medication. Corticosteroids are often given to further reduce the peripheral conversion of T_4 to T_3. Specific recommendations for medications and doses vary slightly in the literature but most have thionamide, β-adrenergic blockers, corticosteroids, and iodide in common (**Fig. 3**). Supportive therapy may be needed to treat fever and hypoxia. Maternal telemetry, central monitoring, and arterial monitoring may be indicated, depending on clinical circumstances. The inciting factor should be sought and treated if possible. Consultation with an endocrinologist and an obstetrician familiar with the management of critically ill pregnant women is appropriate. If the fetus is of a viable gestational age, fetal monitoring should be considered. Intervention on behalf of the fetus should not be undertaken until the maternal condition is stabilized, because vaginal or cesarean delivery may exacerbate thyroid storm.[1,4,93–95]

SUMMARY POINTS

- Thyroid disease is common in pregnancy.
- Hypothyroidism and hyperthyroidism are associated with adverse pregnancy outcomes, and treatment may improve these outcomes.
- Untreated hypothyroidism during pregnancy may be associated with impaired intellectual development in childhood.
- It is unclear whether subclinical thyroid disorders are associated with adverse pregnancy or childhood outcomes, or whether treatment is beneficial.
- Routine screening for thyroid disease in women without risk factors is not recommended or accepted practice.
- Normal reference ranges for thyroid function tests in pregnancy are not established.

REFERENCES

1. Nader S. Maternal-fetal medicine. In: Creasy R, Resnik R, Iams J, editors. Thyroid diseases and pregnancy. 5th edition. Philadelphia (PA): W.B. Saunders; 2004.
2. Fisher DA. Hypothyroxinemia in premature infants: is thyroxine treatment necessary? Thyroid 1999;9(7):715–20.
3. Lee RH, Spencer C, Mestman JH, et al. Free T4 immunoassays are flawed during pregnancy. Am J Obstet Gynecol 2009;200(3):260, e1–6.
4. American College of Obstetricians and Gynecologists, Committee on Practice Bulletins. ACOG Practice Bulletin. Clinical management guidelines for obstetrician-gynecologists. Number 37, August 2002 (replaces practice Bulletin Number 32, November 2001). Thyroid disease in pregnancy. Obstet Gynecol 2001;98(5 Pt 1): 879–88.
5. Surks M, Ortiz E, Daniels GH, et al. Subclinical thyroid disease. JAMA 2004;291: 228–38.

6. Casey BM, Dashe JS, Spong CY, et al. Perinatal significance of isolated maternal hypothyroxinemia identified in the first half of pregnancy. Obstet Gynecol 2007; 109(5):1129–35.

7. Dashe JS, Casey BM, Wells CE, et al. Thyroid-stimulating hormone in singleton and twin pregnancy: importance of gestational age-specific reference ranges. Obstet Gynecol 2005;106(4):753–7.

8. Haddow J, Knight G, Palomak G, et al. The reference range and within-person variability of thyroid stimulating hormone during the first and second trimesters of pregnancy. J Med Screen 2004;11:170–4.

9. Cleary-Goldman J, Malone FD, Lambert-Messerlian G, et al. Maternal thyroid hypofunction and pregnancy outcome. Obstet Gynecol 2008;112(1):85–92.

10. Bocos-Terraz J, Izquierdo-Álvarez S, Bancalero-Flores J, et al. Thyroid hormones according to gestational age in pregnant Spanish women. BMC Res Notes 2009;2:237.

11. Stricker R, Echenard M, Eberhart R, et al. Evaluation of maternal thyroid function during pregnancy: the importance of using gestational age-specific reference intervals. Eur J Endocrinol 2007;157:509–14.

12. Gilbert RM, Hadlow NC, Walsh JP, et al. Assessment of thyroid function during pregnancy: first trimester (weeks 9–13) reference intervals derived from Western Australian women. Med J Aust 2008;189(5):250–3.

13. Casey BM, Dashe JS, Wells CE, et al. Subclinical hypothyroidism and pregnancy outcomes. Obstet Gynecol Feb 2005;13:105(2):239–45.

14. Haddow JE, Palomaki GE, Allan WC, et al. Maternal thyroid deficiency during pregnancy and subsequent neuropsychological development of the child. N Engl J Med 1999;341(8):549–55.

15. Abalovich M, Amino N, Barbour LA, et al. Management of thyroid dysfunction during pregnancy and postpartum: an Endocrine Society clinical practice guideline. J Clin Endocrinol Metab 2007;92(8 Suppl):S1–S47.

16. Casey BM, Leveno KJ. Thyroid disease in pregnancy. Obstet Gynecol 2006;108: 1283–92.

17. Burman KD. Controversies surrounding pregnancy, maternal thyroid status, and fetal outcome. Thyroid 2009;19(4):323–6.

18. Davis LE, Leveno KJ, Cunnigham FG. Hypothyroidism complicating pregnancy. Obstet Gynecol 1988;72:108–12.

19. Hallengren B, Lantz M, Andreasson B, et al. Pregnant women on thyroxine substitution are often dysregulated in early pregnancy. Thyroid 2009;19(4):391–4.

20. Alexander EK, Marquessee E, Lawrence J, et al. Timing and magnitude of increase in levothyroxine requirements during pregnancy in women with hypothyroidism. N Engl J Med 2004;351:241–9.

21. Dickey RA, Wartofsky L, Feld S. Optimal thyrotropin level: normal ranges and reference intervals are not equivalent. Thyroid 2005;15:1035–9.

22. Wartofsky L, Van Nostrand D, Burman KD. Overt and 'subclinical' hypothyroidism in women. Obstet Gynecol Surv 2006;61:535–42.

23. Alvarez-Marfany M, Roman SH, Drexler AJ, et al. Long-term prospective study of postpartum thyroid women with insulin dependent diabetes mellitus. J Clin Endocrinol Metab 1994;79:10–6.

24. Fauci AS, Kasper DL, Brauwald E, et al, editors. Harrison's online: featuring the complete contents of Harrison's principles of internal medicine. 17th edition. Available at: http://www.accessmedicine.com. Accessed December 30, 2009.

25. Roitt IM, Campbell PN, Doniach D. The nature of thyroid auto-antibodies present in patients with Hashimoto's thyroiditis (lymphadenoid goiter). Biochem J 1958; 69:249–56.

26. Hamburger JI. The various presentations of thyroiditis. Ann Intern Med 1986;104: 219–24.
27. Cooper DS. Hyperthyroidism. Lancet 2003;362(9382):459–68.
28. Slatosky J, Shipton B, Wahba H. Thyroiditis: differential diagnosis and management. Am Fam Physician 2000;61(4):1047–52, 1054.
29. Pearce EN. Iodine in pregnancy: is salt iodization enough? J Clin Endocrinol Metab 2008;93(7):2466–8.
30. Assessment of iodine deficiency disorders and monitoring their elimination: a guide for programme managers. 3rd edition. World Health Organization; 2007.
31. de Benoist B, Andersson M, Egli I, et al. Iodine status worldwide: WHO global database on iodine insufficiency. Geneva (Switzerland): World Health Organization; 2004.
32. Borak J. Adequacy of iodine nutrition in the United States. Conn Med 2005;69: 73–7.
33. Hollowell JG, Staehling NW, Hannon WH, et al. Iodine nutrition in the United States. Trends and public health implications: iodine excretion data from National Health and Nutrition Examination Surveys I and III (1971–1974 and 1988–1994). J Clin Endocrinol Metab 1998;83:3401–8.
34. Caldwell KL, Jones RL, Hollowell JG. Urinary iodine concentration – United States National Health and Nutrition Examination Survey (2001–2002). Thyroid 2005; 15(7):692–9.
35. Andersson M, de Benoist B, Delange F, et al. Prevention and control of iodine deficiency in pregnant and lactating women and in children less than 2 years old: conclusions and recommendations of the technical consultation. Public Health Nutr 2007;10(12A):1606–11.
36. Xue-Yi C, Xin-Min J, Zhi-Hong D, et al. Timing of vulnerability of the brain to iodine deficiency in endemic cretinism. N Engl J Med 1994;331:1739–44.
37. DeLong GR, Stanbury JB, Fierro-Benitez R. Neurological signs in congenital iodine-deficiency disorder. Dev Med Child Neurol 1985;27:317–24.
38. Bleichrodt N, Born MP. A meta-analysis of research on iodine and its relationship to cognitive development. In: Stanbury JB, editor. The damaged brain of iodine deficiency. New York: Cognizant Communication; 1994. p. 195–200.
39. WHO. Prevention and control of iodine deficiency in pregnant and lactating women and children less than two years old. Geneva (Switzerland): World Health Organization; 2007. Public Health Nutrition.
40. Centers for Disease Control and Prevention. National report on biochemical indicators of diet and nutrition in the U.S. population 1999–2002. Available at: http://www.cdc.gov/nutritionreport/part_4a.html#ref. Accessed December 22, 2009.
41. Institute of Medicine, Food and Nutrition Board. Dietary reference intakes: vitamin A, vitamin K, arsenic, boron, chromium, copper, iodine, iron, manganese, molybdenum, nickel, silicon, vanadium, and zinc. Washington, DC: National Academy Press; 2001.
42. The Public Health Committee of the American Thyroid Association. Iodine supplementation for pregnancy and lactation — United States and Canada: recommendations of the American Thyroid Association. Thyroid 2006;16:949–51.
43. Pennington JAT, Schoen SA, Salmon GD, et al. Composition of core foods of the US food supply, 1982–1991. III. Copper, manganese, selenium, and iodine. J Food Compost Anal 1995;8:171–217.
44. Dökmeta HS, Kilicli F, Korkmaz S, et al. Characteristic features of 20 patients with Sheehan's syndrome. Gynecol Endocrinol 2006;22(5):279–83.

45. Garner PR, Burrow GN. Medical complications during pregnancy. In: Burrow G, Duffy T, Copel JA, editors. Pituitary and adrenal disorders of pregnancy. 6th edition. Philadelphia (PA): WB Saunders Company; 2004. p. 163–80.
46. Molitch ME, Gillam MP. Lymphocytic hypophysitis. Horm Res 2007;68(Suppl 5): 145–50.
47. Ng WH, Gonzales M, Kay AH. Lymphocytic hypophysitis. J Clin Neurosci 2003; 10(4):409–13.
48. Klein RZ, Haddow JE, Faix JD, et al. Prevalence of thyroid deficiency in pregnant women. Clin Endocrinol (Oxf) 1991;35:41–6.
49. Woeber KA. Subclinical thyroid dysfunction. Arch Intern Med 1997;157:1065–8.
50. Canaris GH, Manowitz NR, Mayor G, et al. The Colorado thyroid disease prevalence study. Arch Intern Med 2000;160:526–34.
51. Jayme JJ, Ladenson PW. Subclinical thyroid dysfunction in elderly. Trends Endocrinol Metab 1994;5:79–86.
52. Allan WC, Haddow JE, Palomaki GE, et al. Maternal thyroid deficiency and pregnancy complications: implications for populations screening. J Med Screen 2000; 7:127–30.
53. Pop VJ, Kuijpens JL, van Baar AL, et al. Lowe maternal free thyroxine concentrations during early pregnancy are associated with impaired psychomotor development in infancy. Clin Endocrinol (Oxf) 1999;50:149–55.
54. Pop VJ, Brouwers EP, Vader HL, et al. Maternal hypothyroxinaemia during early pregnancy and subsequent child development: a 3-year follow-up study. Clin Endocrinol (Oxf) 2003;59:282–8.
55. Millar LK, Wing DA, Leung AS, et al. Low birth weight and preeclampsia in pregnancies complicated by hyperthyroidism. Obstet Gynecol 1994;84(6):946–9.
56. Momotani N, Ito K, Hamada N, et al. Maternal hyperthyroidism and congenital malformation in the offspring. Clin Endocrinol 1984;20:695–700.
57. Momotani N, Ito K. Treatment of pregnant patients with Basedow's disease. Exp Clin Endocrinol 1991;97(2–3):268–74.
58. Davis LE, Lucas MJ, Hankins GD, et al. Thyrotoxicosis complicating pregnancy. Am J Obstet Gynecol 1989;160(1):63–70.
59. Casey BM, Dashe JS, Wells CE, et al. Subclinical hyperthyroidism and pregnancy outcomes. Obstet Gynecol 2006;107(2 Pt 1):337–41.
60. Johnsson E, Larsson G, Ljunggren M. Severe malformations in infant born to hyperthyroid woman on methimazole. Lancet 1997;350(9090):1520.
61. Diav-Citrin O, Ornoy A. Teratogen update: antithyroid drugs-methimazole, carbimazole, and propylthiouracil. Teratology 2002;65(1):38–44.
62. Patil-Sisodia K, Mestman JH. Graves hyperthyroidism & pregnancy: a clinical update. Endocr Pract 2010;16(1):118–29.
63. Rosenfeld H, Ornoy A, Shechtman S, et al. Pregnancy outcome, thyroid dysfunction and fetal goitre after in utero exposure to propylthiouracil: a controlled cohort study. Br J Clin Pharmacol 2009;68(4):609–17.
64. Van Loon AJ, Derksen JT, Bos AF, et al. In utero diagnosis and treatment of fetal goitrous hypothyroidism, caused by maternal use of propylthiouracil. Prenat Diagn 1995;15(7):599–604.
65. Cooper D, Doherty G, Haugen B, et al. Revised American Thyroid Association Management Guidelines for patients with thyroid nodules and differentiated thyroid cancer. Thyroid 2009;11(19):1167–214.
66. Williams KV, Nayak S, Becker D, et al. Fifty years of experience with propylthiouracil-associated hepatotoxicity: what have we learned? J Clin Endocrinol Metab 1997;82(6):1727–33.

67. Policy Statement. Committee on Drugs. American Academy of Pediatrics: the transfer of drugs and other chemicals into breast milk. Pediatrics 2001;108:766–89.
68. The WHO Working Group, Bennet PN, editors. Drugs and human lactation. New York: Elsevier; 1988. p. 194–5.
69. Kuy S, Roman SA, Desai R, et al. Outcomes following thyroid and parathyroid surgery in pregnant women. Arch Surg 2009;144(5):399–406.
70. Laurberg P, Bournaud C, Karmisholt J, et al. Management of Graves' hyperthyroidism in pregnancy: focus on both maternal and foetal thyroid function, and caution against surgical thyroidectomy in pregnancy. Eur J Endocrinol 2009; 160(1):1–8.
71. America College of Radiology. ACR standard for the performance of therapy with unsealed radionuclide sources. In: Standards 1999–2000. Reston (VA): American College of Radiology; 1999. p. 265–70.
72. Berg GE, Nyström EH, Jacobsson L, et al. Radioiodine treatment of hyperthyroidism in a pregnant women. J Nucl Med 1998;39(2):357–61.
73. Stoffer SS, Hamburger JI. Inadvertent 131I therapy for hyperthyroidism in the first trimester of pregnancy. J Nucl Med 1976;17(02):146–9.
74. Evans PM, Webster J, Evans WD, et al. Radioiodine treatment in unsuspected pregnancy. Clin Endocrinol (Oxf) 1998;48(3):281–3.
75. Gorman CA. Radioiodine and pregnancy. Thyroid 1999;9(7):721–6.
76. Schlumberger M, De Vathaire F, Ceccarelli C, et al. Exposure to radioactive iodine-131 for scintigraphy or therapy does not preclude pregnancy in thyroid cancer patients. J Nucl Med 1996;37(4):606–12.
77. Garsi JP, Schlumberger M, Rubino C, et al. Therapeutic administration of 131I for differentiated thyroid cancer: radiation dose to ovaries and outcome of pregnancies. J Nucl Med 2008;49(5):845–52.
78. Yeo CP, Khoo D, Eng P, et al. Prevalence of gestational thyrotoxicosis in Asian women evaluated in the 8th to 14th weeks of pregnancy: correlations with total and free beta human chorionic gonadotropin. Clin Endocrinol 2001;55:391–8.
79. Glinoer D. The regulation of thyroid function in pregnancy: pathways of endocrine adaptation from physiology to pathology. Endocr Rev 1997;18:404–33.
80. Tan JY, Loh KC, Yeo GS, et al. Transient hyperthyroidism of hyperemesis gravidarum. BJOG 2002;109(6):683–8.
81. Goodwin TM. Hyperemesis gravidarum. Obstet Gynecol Clin North Am 2008; 35(3):401–17, viii.
82. Brent GA. Clinical practice. Graves' disease. N Engl J Med 2008;358(24): 2594–605.
83. Marx H, Amin P, Lazarus J. Hyperthyroidism and pregnancy. BMJ 2008;336: 663–7.
84. Towers CV, Thomas S, Steiger RM. The fetal heart monitor tracing in pregnancies complicated by fetal thyrotoxicosis. Am J Perinatol 2009;26:373–7.
85. Nachum Z, Rakover Y, Weiner E, et al. Graves' disease in pregnancy: prospective evaluation of a selective invasive treatment protocol. Am J Obstet Gynecol 2003; 189:159–65.
86. Davies L, Welch HG. Increasing incidence of thyroid cancer in the United States, 1973–2002. JAMA 2006;295(18):2164–7.
87. Smith LH, Danielsen B, Allen ME, et al. Cancer associated with obstetric delivery: results of linkage with the California cancer registry. Am J Obstet Gynecol 2003; 189(4):1128–35.
88. Moosa M, Mazzaferri EL. Outcome of differentiated thyroid cancer diagnosed in pregnant women. J Clin Endocrinol Metab 1997;82(9):2862–6.

89. Yasmeen S, Cress R, Romano PS, et al. Thyroid cancer in pregnancy. Int J Gynaecol Obstet 2005;91(1):15–20.

90. Cooper DS, Specker B, Ho M, et al. Thyrotropin suppression and disease progression in patients with differentiated thyroid cancer: results from the National Thyroid Cancer Treatment Cooperative Registry. Thyroid 1998;8(9): 737–44.

91. Johnson NA, Tublin ME. Postoperative surveillance of differentiated thyroid carcinoma: rationale, techniques, and controversies. Radiology 2008;249(2):429–44.

92. Lebouef R, Emerick L, Martorella A, et al. Impact of pregnancy on serum thyroglobulin and detection of recurrent disease shortly after delivery in thyroid cancer survivors. Thyroid 2007;17(6):543–7.

93. Belfort MA. Obstetric intensive care manual. In: Foley M, Strong T, Garite T, editors. Thyroid and other endocrine emergencies. 2nd edition. New York: McGraw-Hill; 2004. p. 125–9.

94. Kaplan MM, Meier DA. Principles and practice of medical therapy in pregnancy. In: Gleicher N, editor. Thyroid diseases in pregnancy. 3rd edition. Connecticut: Appleton and Lange; 1998. p. 441.

95. Burrow GN. Medical complications of pregnancy. In: Burrow G, Duffy T, editors. Thyroid disorders. 5th edition. Philadelphia (PA): WB Saunders Company; 1999. p. 145.

96. US Preventive Services Task Force. Screening for thyroid disease, topic page. Rockville (MD): Agency for Healthcare Research and Quality; 2004. Available at: http://www.ahrq.gov/clinic/uspstf/uspsthyr.htm. Accessed December 28, 2009.

97. Gharib H, Cobin RH, Dickey RA. Subclinical hypothyroidism during pregnancy: position statement from the American association of clinical endocrinologists. Endocr Pract 1999;5(6).

98. American Association of Clinical Endocrinologists Medical Guidelines for Clinical Practice for the Evaluation and Treatment of Hyperthyroidism and Hypothyroidism. AACE thyroid task force. Endocr Pract 2002;8(6). 2006 Amended version. Available at: http://www.aace.com/pub/pdf/guidelines/hypo_hyper.pdf. Accessed December 31, 2009.

99. UK Guidelines for the Use of Thyroid Function Tests. The Association for Clinical Biochemistry, British Thyroid Association, and British Thyroid Foundation. Available at: http://www.british-thyroid-association.org/info-for-patients/Docs/TFT_guideline_final_version_July_2006.pdf; 2006. Accessed December 31, 2009.

Management of Renal Disease in Pregnancy

Tiina Podymow, MD[a], Phyllis August, MD, MPH[b],
Ayub Akbari, MD[c],*

KEYWORDS

- Pregnancy • Renal disease • Glomerulonephritis
- Dialysis • Renal function

In patients with renal disease who become pregnant, the possible harmful effects of pregnancy on kidney function and the impact of renal disease on pregnancy outcome should be considered. In this context, the nephrologist's role is to assess the risk for worsening renal function in pregnancy; ideally nephrologic opinion should be sought before conception. Assessment of maternal hypertension is also crucial, because it contributes significantly to the risk for deteriorating renal function and increases the risk for preeclampsia, preterm delivery, intrauterine growth restriction, and perinatal mortality.

Management of pregnant women with kidney disease may be complicated, and requires an understanding of the physiologic changes associated with pregnancy and close teamwork between obstetricians and nephrologists. Although some areas in obstetric medicine have been extensively studied in randomized controlled trials (eg, prevention of preeclampsia), renal disease in pregnancy has been so less commonly, and the quality of the evidence guiding clinical practice has not been of the highest level. Most evidence consists of case series with modest numbers of subjects. Based on population studies, the prevalence of chronic kidney disease in women of childbearing age is 0.03% to 0.2% of all pregnancies.

RENAL ANATOMY AND PHYSIOLOGY IN PREGNANCY
Anatomic and Functional Changes in Urinary Tract

Normally in pregnancy, increased renal blood flow and glomerular hypertrophy result in an increase in kidney length of approximately 1 cm during normal gestation, and overall kidney volume increases by up to 30%.[1] The major anatomic alterations of the urinary

[a] Division of Nephrology, McGill University, 687 Pine Avenue West Ross 2.38, Montreal, QC H3A 1A1, Canada
[b] Division of Nephrology and Hypertension, Weill Medical College of Cornell University, 525 East 68th Street, Starr 437, NY 10021, USA
[c] Division of Nephrology, University of Ottawa, Kidney Research Center, 1967 Riverside Drive, Ottawa, ON, K1H 7W9, Canada
* Corresponding author.
E-mail address: aakbari@ottawahospital.on.ca

Obstet Gynecol Clin N Am 37 (2010) 195–210
doi:10.1016/j.ogc.2010.02.012
0889-8545/10/$ – see front matter © 2010 Elsevier Inc. All rights reserved.

obgyn.theclinics.com

tract during pregnancy are seen in the collecting system, where calyces, renal pelvises, and ureters dilate, often giving the erroneous impression of obstructive uropathy.[2] The cause of the ureteral dilation has been attributed to hormonal mechanisms, such as increased progesterone, and mechanical obstruction by the enlarging uterus. These morphologic changes result in stasis in the urinary tract and a higher risk among pregnant women with asymptomatic bacteriuria for progression to pyelonephritis, particularly in those who have a history of prior urinary tract infections.[3] Rarely, "overdistension syndrome" may occur, which is a pregnancy-related syndrome characterized by severe hydronephrosis, abdominal pain, decline in renal function, and even hypertension, which may respond to lateral recumbency or require stent placement.

Renal Hemodynamics in Pregnancy

Marked vasodilation is a hallmark of pregnancy and occurs by 6 weeks gestation. Vasodilation is accompanied by a decrease in blood pressure, increase in cardiac output, and increases in renal plasma flow and glomerular filtration, all of which persist until late gestation. Increased progesterone, estrogen, nitric oxide, and relaxin have all been implicated as vasodilatory mediators. Because renal plasma flow increases slightly more than the glomerular filtration rate (GFR), filtration fraction remains constant or slightly lower in pregnancy. Increases in renal hemodynamics reach a maximum during the first trimester, and levels are approximately 50% greater than those of prepregnancy.[4] The increase in GFR (hyperfiltration) during normal pregnancy occurs without increase in intraglomerular pressure, and normal pregnancy is not injurious to the maternal kidney.

Acid–Base Regulation in Pregnancy

Because of the increased circulating level of progesterone, which directly stimulates the medullary respiratory center, tidal volume and alveolar ventilation are increased during pregnancy, resulting in respiratory alkalosis, with reduced arterial Pco_2. To compensate, the kidneys excrete more bicarbonate in pregnancy, which results in a 4- to 5-mEq/L decrease in serum bicarbonate to 20 to 22 mEq/L, changes that are apparent in the first trimester.[5] Compared with nonpregnant patients, the normal anion gap in pregnancy is lower at 8.5 ± 2.9, and normal strong ion difference ([Na+] + [K+] − [Cl-]) is 38.3 ± 2.9.[6] Finally, a Pco_2 of 40 mm Hg signifies considerable carbon dioxide retention in pregnancy.

Water Metabolism

Pregnancy is associated with a decrease in plasma osmolality of 5 to 10 mOsm/kg lower than that of nongravid women, reaching a nadir at 10 weeks gestation. The decrease in plasma osmolality is associated with appropriate responses to water loading and dehydration, and suggests a resetting of the osmoreceptor system, with thirst occurring at lower serum osmolality. Clinical studies showing decreased osmotic thresholds for thirst and arginine vasopressin (AVP) release in pregnant women support this hypothesis. The lower osmolality and serum sodium represent a new normal set-point. In addition to these changes, pregnant women metabolize AVP more rapidly because of increased production of placental vasopressinases.[7] Pregnant women may develop syndromes of transient diabetes insipidus from the increased metabolism of AVP. These syndromes may be treated with pharmaceutical desmopressin, which remains effective because of a different N-terminus that is resistant to the circulating vasopressinases.

Serum sodium is also lower in pregnancy, which may be caused partly by relaxin, a peptide hormone in the insulin family that is secreted by the corpus luteum and placenta during human gestation. Relaxin is associated with osmoregulatory changes and increases in GFR and vasodilation in early pregnancy.[8] Human chorionic gonadotropin seems to cause release of relaxin, which then stimulates the subfornical organ in the hypothalamus, resulting in thirst and AVP secretion. Chronic administration of relaxin to rats mimics several of the hemodynamic and osmotic changes of pregnancy, whereas antirelaxin antibodies reverse these changes.

Volume Regulation in Pregnancy

Total body water increases by 6 to 8 L during pregnancy, 4 to 6 L of which is extracellular. Plasma volume increases 50% during gestation, with the largest rate of increment occurring mid-pregnancy. Although serum sodium measurement decreases, a daily positive balance of 2 to 5 mEq and gradual accumulation of approximately 900 mEq of sodium is present during pregnancy (approximately 20 g of sodium chloride), which is distributed between the products of conception and the maternal extracellular space. Despite the increase in plasma volume during pregnancy, no evidence shows a hypervolemic (ie, overfilled circulation) state during pregnancy. Vasodilation, which is observed as early as the first trimester, may be the stimulus for increased sodium retention and increased plasma volume. The observations that blood pressure is significantly lower and the renin–angiotensin system is stimulated during normal pregnancy are consistent with primary vasodilation preceding and causing the increase in plasma volume.

Physiology of Renal Disease in Pregnancy

In patients with abnormal prepregnancy renal function, pregnancy may adversely affect maternal renal function, causing it to deteriorate irreversibly, both during gestation and after delivery. The causes are not altogether clear, although exacerbation of preexisting endothelial dysfunction, alterations in immune function, and increased inflammation associated with pregnancy may contribute. Platelet aggregation, formation of fibrin thrombi, and microvascular coagulation have also been implicated in renal and placental dysfunction. In general, the closer to normal the GFR and blood pressure, the greater the chance of successful pregnancy.

Assessment of Renal Function in Pregnancy

During pregnancy, GFR and creatinine clearance increase by 40% to 65% and creatinine production is unchanged; therefore, the increased clearance results in decreased serum levels. One study reported average values of 0.83 mg/dL (73 μmol/L) in nonpregnant women, and 0.74, 0.58, and 0.53 mg/dL (65, 51, and 46 μmol/L, respectively) in first, second, and third trimester of pregnancy, respectively, with values for the upper limit of normal of 0.96, 0.90, and 1.02 mg/dL (85, 80, and 90 μmol/L, respectively).[9]

In the nonpregnant population, the Cockroft-Gault and MDRD (Modification of Diet in Renal Disease) formulae are most commonly used to assess kidney function. Neither of these have been validated in pregnancy. The Cockroft-Gault formula uses body weight as a surrogate for muscle mass, but because the weight of a gravid women increases without affecting the muscle mass, using pregnancy weight in this formula yields inaccurate results. In one study using prepregnancy weight, the formula better approximated creatinine clearance. The MDRD formula yields results that are corrected for body surface area, but because the body surface area changes in pregnancy, this too yields inaccurate results. In one study, MDRD formula underestimated GFR by more than 40 mL/min.

Measurement of serum cystatin C had been proposed as a more sensitive marker for GFR because it was believed to be independent of age, weight, height, or muscle mass; however this has not been proven when studied in pregnancy.[10] Creatinine clearance measured with 24-hour urine collection remains the best approximate of the gold standard of inulin clearance, and is the most well-validated method for measuring renal function.

Because of the increased GFR in pregnancy, the tubular transport maximum is exceeded and reabsorption is decreased, causing increased excretion of glucose, amino acids, calcium, and urinary protein. The upper limit of normal for urinary protein excretion is 300 mg/d in pregnant patients versus 150 mg/d in nonpregnant patients. Abnormal proteinuria has been evaluated with 24-hour urine collection, urine dipstick, and protein/creatinine ratio, but the gold standard remains the 24-hour urine protein measurement. A 24-hour protein level greater than 300 mg is abnormal in pregnancy and correlates with a urine dipstick 1+ protein measurement. Although commonly used in an obstetrician's office to detect significant proteinuria, urine dipstick testing is susceptible to error because of variations in urine concentration, and may miss up to 1 of 11 hypertensive pregnant women with true proteinuria.[11] Therefore, if the level of suspicion is high, 24-hour urine testing should be performed. Total protein/creatinine ratio has been shown to accurately estimate 24-hour urine protein in nonpregnant patients and, according to a systematic review of 13 studies of pregnant patients, seems to be of value in ruling out proteinuria if less than 0.25 g per 24 hours. Misclassifications tend to occur when the proteinuria is borderline (250–400 mg/d), and therefore the 24-hour collection should be performed to diagnose preeclampsia if the results are equivocal. The protein/creatinine measurement also underestimates severe proteinuria in pregnancy, and therefore cannot be recommended as an alternative to 24-hour measurement.[12]

KIDNEY DISEASE IN PREGNANCY

Kidney disease during pregnancy may be caused by (1) preexisting renal disease that was diagnosed before conception, (2) chronic renal disease that was unappreciated before pregnancy and diagnosed for the first time during pregnancy, or (3) renal disease that develops for the first time during pregnancy. Some overlap exists with respect to the different diseases that are typical of the three categories. For example, lupus nephritis may be a chronic condition, or it may develop for the first time during pregnancy.

Chronic Renal Disease: General Principles

Fertility and ability to sustain an uncomplicated pregnancy are related to the degree of renal functional impairment rather than to the specific underlying disorder. The greater the functional impairment and higher the blood pressure, the less likely the pregnancy will be successful (**Table 1**). Patients with preserved renal function and normal or well-controlled blood pressure have favorable maternal and fetal outcomes. Those with mildly elevated creatinine, such as 1.2 to 1.4 mg/dL (106–124 μmol/L) seem to have some risk (16% in one study) for renal function decline. Those with moderate renal insufficiency (serum creatinine 1.4–2.5 mg/dL, or 124–220 μmol/L) are at increased risk for preeclampsia (20%–30%) and preterm delivery. Of these women, approximately 50% have a pregnancy-related decline in creatinine clearance (by 25%), and the renal function decline seems to persist or progress after delivery. Women with severe renal dysfunction, defined by a creatinine level greater than 2.5 mg/dL [220 μmol/L], should be discouraged from conceiving because 70% will experience

Table 1
Effect of pregnancy on renal disease

Author	No. Pregnant Patients	Renal Diagnosis	Clinical Status at Baseline	Outcome
Katz et al[52]	89	glomerulonephritis	Serum Cr $\leq$ 1.4 mg/dL	16% transient worsening of renal function
Abe et al[53]	72	glomerulonephritis	GFR >70 mL/min	No change
Jungers et al[54]	171	glomerulonephritis	Normal GFR	No change
Abe et al[55]	118	IgA nephropathy	GFR mean 70 mL/min	19% had renal function decline, 4% progressed to ESRD or dialysis 1–5 years after delivery
	166	Glomerular disease	GFR >70 mL/min GFR <50 mL/min	Good if GFR >70 and blood pressure <140/90 GFR <50: 33% had decrease in GFR
Jones and Hayslett[13]	67	glomerulonephritis	Cr >1.9 mg/dL	12% on dialysis within 1 year of delivery
Imbasciati et al[14]	49	Nondiabetic renal disease	CrCl 35 mL/min	31% on dialysis at 37 months postpartum
Chopra et al[56]	29	glomerulonephritis	Cr >1.5 mg/dL	29% had progression of disease

Abbreviations: Cr, creatinine; CrCl, creatinine clearance; ESRD, end stage renal disease; GFR, glomerular filtration rate.

preterm delivery, 40% will develop preeclampsia, and 40% will experience pregnancy or postpartum deterioration in renal function, leading to dialysis.[13]

Urine protein excretion may increase markedly in pregnant women with underlying renal disease—perhaps tripling from baseline—which may also adversely affect outcome. In one study of pregnant women with stage 3 to 5 kidney disease, the rate of decline in GFR accelerated in the subgroup with both estimated GFR of less than 40 mL/min and proteinuria greater than 1 g/d before pregnancy.[14] The level of blood pressure at conception is an important variable in pregnancy outcome. In the absence of hypertension, there is significantly less chance of irreversible deterioration in renal function during pregnancy. When hypertension is present, pregnancy outcome is rarely uncomplicated. Preterm delivery and deterioration in renal function are expected. Finally, in patients with renal disease in whom eventual renal transplant is anticipated, pregnancy may result in immune sensitization, leading to difficulty locating a suitable matching donor.

Renal Diseases Associated with Systemic Illness

Diabetes is one of the most common medical disorders of pregnancy, with most cases caused by gestational diabetes. Preexisting diabetes poses significant risks to pregnancy, and many women have type 1 diabetes; if their disease has been present for 10 to 15 years, they may have diabetic nephropathy. Women with diabetes, microalbuminuria, well-preserved renal function, and normal blood pressure have a good prognosis for pregnancy, although they are at increased risk for preeclampsia and urinary infection.[15,16]

One prospective cohort study from Denmark followed-up 240 women who had type 1 diabetes during pregnancy, 11% of whom had microalbuminuria and 5% overt diabetic nephropathy. Of this cohort, 62% of women with microalbuminuria and normal renal function and 91% of women with overt diabetic nephropathy had preterm deliveries (compared with 35% of women with no albuminuria). Preeclampsia developed in 6% of women with no albuminuria compared with 42% and 64% of women with microalbuminuria and overt diabetic nephropathy, respectively.[16] In another study of 72 pregnancies in 58 women with diabetic nephropathy, an elevated serum creatinine at enrollment was associated with preterm delivery, very low birth weight, and neonatal hypoglycemia, and was independent of urinary protein excretion.

With respect to progression of maternal renal disease as a consequence of pregnancy, one study from Denmark reported that 26 women with type 1 diabetes who became pregnant had similar rates of deterioration in renal function over a 16-year follow-up compared with 67 control subjects with comparable disease who had never been pregnant.[17] Thus, when baseline renal function and blood pressure are still normal, pregnancy is not likely to accelerate the progression of early diabetic nephropathy,[17] although urinary protein excretion often increases significantly during pregnancy. Women with non–nephrotic range proteinuria preconception may develop nephrotic range proteinuria during pregnancy, which is usually reversible. Women with overt nephropathy preconception, particularly those with impaired renal function and hypertension, have a high incidence of preterm delivery, preeclampsia, and deterioration in maternal renal function.[15] However, women with type 1 diabetes with microalbuminuria and normal renal function and normotension should be encouraged not to postpone pregnancy, because of the worse prognosis once overt nephropathy develops.

Blood pressure control is important; however, because angiotensin-converting enzyme inhibitors (ACEIs) and angiotensin receptor blockers are contraindicated during all three trimesters of pregnancy, and in the 2nd and 3rd trimesters carry a neonatal mortality rate of 25%, women should be switched to other agents that are safe to use in pregnancy, such as methyldopa, labetolol, or nifedipine, before conception. After delivery, if ACEIs are to be restarted and the patient wishes to breast-feed, enalapril has been deemed safe by the American Pediatrics Association; it is likely a class effect, but safety data are lacking in other ACEIs. No studies of pregnancy and nephropathy associated with type 2 diabetes have been published; however, given the increasing prevalence of this condition, it is an important area for future study.

Lupus nephritis during pregnancy presents unique problems. Although similar considerations apply regarding level of renal function and blood pressure and their relationship to pregnancy outcome, generally lupus is a much more unpredictable illness because of the tendency of the disease to flare. Recent data suggest that pregnancy duration, total disease duration, and disease activity and damage before pregnancy are associated with increased organ damage after pregnancy in women with lupus.[18] Whether pregnancy per se is a risk factor for lupus flares has been disputed. Although some experts report no increase in flares attributable to pregnancy in patients in remission, prospective data suggest that pregnancy is in fact associated with a greater chance of disease exacerbation.[19] Women with lupus nephritis are advised not to conceive unless their disease has been inactive for the preceding

6 months, because active disease is associated with a higher incidence of fetal demise. Disease is considered inactive when the creatinine measurement is less than 0.7 mg/dL or 62 µmol/L, proteinuria is less than 0.5 g/d, and, on spun urine examination, fewer than five red blood cells are present per high-powered field. Fetal loss occurs in 25% to 50% of women who conceive when their disease is active with a creatinine of greater than 1.2 mg/dL, or 106 µmol/L.[20]

Additional complications associated with lupus and pregnancy include placental transfer of maternal autoantibodies, which can cause a neonatal lupus syndrome characterized by heart block, transient cutaneous lesions, or both. Women with lupus are also more likely to have clinically significant titers of antiphospholipid antibodies (anticardiolipin, lupus anticoagulant), which are associated with spontaneous fetal loss of 50% to 75%, hypertensive syndromes indistinguishable from preeclampsia, and thrombotic events, including deep vein thrombosis, pulmonary embolus, myocardial infarction, and strokes.[21] Thus, all women with systemic lupus erythematosus should be screened for antiphospholipid antibodies early in gestation. When titers are elevated (>40 GPL), daily aspirin (80–325 mg) is recommended. If the woman has a history of thrombotic events or pregnancy loss, then heparin in combination with aspirin is recommended.

One difficulty in managing lupus nephritis during pregnancy is that increased activity of lupus may be difficult to distinguish from preeclampsia. Both are characterized by an increase in proteinuria, a decrease in GFR, and hypertension. Thrombocytopenia may also be observed in both conditions. Hypocomplementemia is not a feature of preeclampsia, whereas increases in liver function tests may be observed in preeclampsia but are not characteristic of lupus activity. If disease activity is present before 20 weeks of gestation, then the diagnosis is more likely to be a lupus flare. Spun urine microscopy for red blood cell casts can also signal lupus nephritis activity.

In the latter half of pregnancy, a renal lupus flare may be impossible to distinguish from preeclampsia; frequently both are present simultaneously, and what starts as increased lupus activity seems to trigger preeclampsia. Unfortunately, delivery may be necessary if immunosuppressive therapy and supportive care fail to stabilize the condition.

The approach to treating lupus nephritis during pregnancy is based largely on anecdotal experience, principles of treatment used in nonpregnant patients, and knowledge of fetal toxicity of immunosuppressants. Steroids and azathioprine are the mainstays of treatment. Hydroxychloroquine during pregnancy seems to be associated with improved outcomes and does not seem to be toxic to the fetus.[22] Cyclophosphamide is generally not recommended during pregnancy because of potential fetal toxicity, and should only be used when the mother's life is in jeopardy. Mycophenolate mofetil should not be used during pregnancy to treat lupus nephritis because it is embryotoxic in animal studies, has been associated with fetal malformations in humans, and recent reports have characterized it as a teratogen.[23]

Chronic Glomerulonephritis

Childbearing women may be afflicted with any of the forms of chronic glomerulonephritis, including immunoglobulin A nephropathy, focal and segmental glomerulosclerosis, membranoproliferative glomerulonephritis, minimal change nephritis, and membranous nephropathy. The authors are unaware of data that would support the notion that histologic subtype confers a specific prognosis for pregnancy. Rather, the previously mentioned principles are applicable to women with chronic glomerulonephritis; baseline renal function and blood pressure are what dictate outcomes.

Polycystic Kidney Disease

Young women with autosomal dominant polycystic kidney disease (ADPKD) are frequently asymptomatic, with normal renal function and normal blood pressure, and may be unaware of their diagnosis. Little has been written about polycystic kidney disease and pregnancy because many patients with this condition have well-preserved renal function until after childbearing.

A series involving 235 women with autosomal dominant polycystic kidney disease and 108 unaffected family members evaluated pregnancy outcomes reported an increased incidence of maternal complications in affected compared with unaffected women.[24] Preexisting hypertension was the most common risk factor for maternal complications during pregnancy, because hypertension is a well-known risk factor for preeclampsia.[24]

Pregnant women with polycystic kidney disease should also be considered at increased risk for urinary tract infection. Estrogen is reported to cause liver cysts to enlarge, and repeated pregnancies may result in symptomatic enlargement of liver cysts. Given the association between cerebral aneurysms and ADPKD in some families, screening for these aneurysms should be considered before natural labor. All patients should undergo genetic counseling before pregnancy to ensure they are aware that their offspring have a 50% chance of being affected.

Chronic Pyelonephritis

Chronic pyelonephritis is defined as nephropathies associated with recurrent urinary tract infection, often in association with urinary tract abnormalities (eg, vesicoureteral reflux). Chronic pyelonephritis caused by dilation and stasis in the urinary tract may exacerbate in pregnancy. Women with reflux nephropathy have been reported to have an adverse prognosis during pregnancy.

A prospective study of 54 pregnancies in 46 women with reflux nephropathy found that preeclampsia was present in 24%, most commonly in women with preexisting hypertension.[25] Deterioration in renal function during pregnancy occurred in 18%, and those with preexisting reduced renal function were at greater risk. One third of the infants were delivered preterm, and 43% had vesicoureteral reflux. These women should have a high fluid intake and be screened with urine cultures at least monthly for bacteriuria, and should be treated promptly when infections are present. In some cases, after a first infection, suppressive antibiotic therapy for the duration of pregnancy may be warranted.

Chronic Renal Diseases That May be First Diagnosed During Pregnancy

The presence of chronic renal disease may first be appreciated during pregnancy partly because pregnant women are scrutinized more closely, and also because the renal hemodynamic alterations during pregnancy may cause proteinuria to increase and be clinically detectable for the first time. Frequent measurement of blood pressure may also lead to diagnosis of renal diseases accompanied by hypertension. Furthermore, the presence of even mild preexisting renal disease is associated with an increased risk for preeclampsia, and therefore underlying renal disease may first become apparent after preeclampsia has developed.

Renal diseases that may have been silent preconception and may "present" during pregnancy include IgA nephropathy, focal and segmental glomerulosclerosis, polycystic kidney disease, and reflux nephropathy. Renal diagnostic testing during pregnancy can include blood and urine testing and ultrasonography. Renal biopsy is usually deferred until after delivery unless acute deterioration in renal function occurs[26] or morbid nephrotic syndrome is present.

Although experienced operators have reported few complications of renal biopsy during pregnancy, increased renal blood flow, hypertension, and difficulty positioning the patient are concerns.[27–29] The timing of renal biopsy after delivery depends on the clinical circumstances. If renal function is normal, and only proteinuria is present, it is reasonable to delay biopsy up to 6 months postpartum, because proteinuria may improve once the pregnancy-associated hemodynamic alterations have resolved. However, if renal function is impaired, then biopsy may be considered within a few weeks of delivery.

Renal Diseases That Develop for the First Time During Pregnancy

Pregnant women are at risk for any of the renal diseases that occur in women of child-bearing age, including pyelonephritis, glomerulonephritis GN, interstitial nephritis, and acute renal failure. Pyelonephritis is more likely to be associated with significant azotemia in pregnant women than nonpregnant women, and should be treated aggressively. Glomerulonephritis and interstitial nephritis are not more likely to develop during pregnancy, although they do occur.

Acute kidney injury in association with pregnancy is a rare complication in developed countries, and is also decreasing in incidence in the developing world, with only 190 cases observed in a 20-year period in Eastern India.[30] Recent estimates suggest that the incidence of acute kidney injury from obstetric causes is less than 1 in 20,000 pregnancies.[31]

Treatment of acute glomerulonephritis presenting during pregnancy is challenging because immunosuppressants are toxic to the fetus, and high-dose steroids have not been studied during pregnancy. Acute glomerulonephritis presenting in pregnancy should be treated in close collaboration with the obstetrician and nephrologist. If acute renal deterioration is seen after 28 to 32 weeks gestation, the patient should probably be delivered and renal biopsy performed postpartum.

When acute kidney injury occurs early in pregnancy (12–18 weeks), it is usually associated with septic abortion or prerenal azotemia caused by hyperemesis gravidarium. Most cases of acute kidney injury in pregnancy occur between gestational week 35 and the puerperium, and are primarily caused by preeclampsia and bleeding complications. Preeclampsia, particularly the HELLP variant (hemolysis, elevated liver enzymes, low platelet count), is an important cause of acute kidney injury in pregnancy.[15] Although most cases of preeclampsia are not usually associated with renal failure, the HELLP syndrome may be associated with significant renal dysfunction, especially if not treated promptly with delivery. In rare instances, dialysis may be necessary, but most women without preexisting renal or hypertensive disease do not require long-term dialysis therapy. Additional important clinical entities causing acute kidney injury during pregnancy are discussed.

Thrombotic Microangiopathy

Although rare, thrombotic microangiopathies (thrombotic thrombocytopenic purpura [TTP] and hemolytic uremic syndrome [HUS]) are an important cause of pregnancy-associated acute renal failure because they are associated with considerable morbidity. They also share several clinical and laboratory features of pregnancy-specific disorders, such as the HELLP variant of preeclampsia and acute fatty liver of pregnancy. Therefore, distinction of these syndromes is important for therapeutic and prognostic reasons.

Features that may be helpful in making the correct diagnosis include timing of onset and the pattern of laboratory abnormalities. Preeclampsia typically develops in the third trimester, with only a few cases developing in the postpartum period, usually within a few days of delivery. TTP usually occurs antepartum, with many cases developing in the second and third trimesters. HUS is usually a postpartum disease; symptoms may begin antepartum, but most cases are diagnosed postpartum.

Preeclampsia is much more common than TTP/HUS and is usually preceded by hypertension and proteinuria. Renal failure is unusual in women with preeclampsia, even in severe cases, unless significant bleeding or hemodynamic instability or marked disseminated intravascular coagulation occurs. In some cases, preeclampsia develops in the immediate postpartum period and, when thrombocytopenia is severe, it may be indistinguishable from HUS. However, preeclampsia spontaneously recovers, whereas TTP/HUS is often associated with persistent renal insufficiency and hypertension, with many requiring dialysis or transplantation long-term.[32]

In contrast to TTP/HUS, preeclampsia may be associated with mild disseminated intravascular coagulation and prolongation of prothrombin and partial thromboplastin times. Another laboratory feature of preeclampsia/HELLP syndrome that is not usually associated with TTP/HUS is marked elevations in liver enzymes. The presence of fever is more consistent with a diagnosis of TTP than preeclampsia or HUS. The main distinctive features of HUS are its tendency to occur in the postpartum period and the severity of the associated renal failure.

Treatment of TTP/HUS includes plasma infusion/exchange and other modalities used in nonpregnant patients with these disorders. Treatment of preeclampsia/HELLP syndrome involves delivery and supportive care. More aggressive treatment is rarely indicated. Some centers have reported the use of steroids in cases of severe HELLP syndrome, although this therapy has not been rigorously evaluated in placebo-controlled clinical trials.[33]

Acute Tubular Necrosis

Acute tubular necrosis induced by volume depletion or exposure to nephrotoxins may occur during pregnancy, although the incidence is low. In the first trimester, acute tubular necrosis is usually associated with hyperemesis gravidarium, whereas later in pregnancy and in the peripartum period it is usually associated with abruptio placenta or other causes of obstetric hemorrhage. Occasionally, nonsteroidal anti-inflammatory agents, used for postpartum analgesia, may precipitate acute kidney injury in patients who are volume-depleted from hemorrhage, decreased fluid intake, or both. In severe cases of obstetric hemorrhage, acute cortical necrosis with associated disseminated intravascular coagulation may be present, and ultrasonography or computed tomography may demonstrate hyperechoic or hypodense areas in the renal cortex. These patients usually require dialysis, but 20% to 40% may have partial recovery of renal function.

Acute Fatty Liver of Pregnancy

Acute fatty liver of pregnancy (AFLP) is a rare complication of late pregnancy characterized by rapidly progressive liver failure. Women usually present with nausea, vomiting, and anorexia, and many have clinical and laboratory features that overlap with preeclampsia or HELLP syndrome.[34] Other laboratory abnormalities (in addition to marked elevations in alanine aminotransferase and aspartate aminotransferase) frequently observed include elevated bilirubin, hypofibrinogenemia, prolonged partial thromboplastin time, hypoglycemia, anemia, and low platelet count.[35] Many cases are associated with significant azotemia, and one series comparing AFLP with HELLP syndrome observed that acute renal failure was significantly more common with AFLP.[36]

Because AFLP is believed to be a disease of mitochondrial dysfunction,[37] the kidney dysfunction associated with AFLP may reflect inhibition of β-oxidation of fats in the kidney. This disease occurs in women heterozygous for long-chain 3-hydroxyacyl-coenzyme A dehydrogenase (LCHAD) deficiency and whose fetus has the disorder. Abnormal fatty-acid metabolites produced by the fetus seem to enter the maternal circulation and overwhelm the mitochondrial-oxidation machinery of the heterozygous mother. Autopsy data have shown microvesicular fat in the kidneys of women with AFLP. Delivery is urgently required, and most patients improve shortly afterwards.

This disorder was formerly associated with a more ominous outcome, which may have been a consequence of late diagnosis, although in a recent case series maternal mortality occurred in 2 of 6 women.[35] When diagnosed early, long-term morbidity is reduced.

Urinary Tract Obstruction

Pregnancy is associated with dilation of the collecting system, which is not usually accompanied by renal dysfunction. Rarely, complications such as large uterine fibroids that enlarge in the setting of pregnancy can lead to obstructive uropathy. Occasionally, acute urinary tract obstruction in pregnancy is caused by a kidney stone. Diagnosis can usually be made with ultrasonography. Often the stone will pass spontaneously, but occasionally cystoscopy is needed to insert a stent to remove a fragment of stone and relieve obstruction, particularly if sepsis or a solitary kidney is present. Extracorporeal shock wave lithotripsy is contraindicated during pregnancy because of the possibility of adverse effects on the fetus.

Treatment of Acute Kidney Injury

Treatment of acute kidney injury occurring in pregnancy or immediately postpartum is similar to that in nongravid subjects, although several important considerations are unique to pregnancy. Uterine hemorrhage near term may be concealed and blood loss underestimated; thus, any overt blood loss should be replaced early. When dialysis is required, peritoneal dialysis and hemodialysis have been used successfully in patients with obstetric acute kidney injury. Neither pelvic peritonitis nor the enlarged uterus is a contraindication to the former method. In fact, this treatment is more gradual than hemodialysis and may be less likely to precipitate labor.

Because urea, creatinine, and other metabolites that accumulate in uremia traverse the placenta, dialysis should be undertaken early, with the goal of maintaining the blood urea nitrogen at approximately 50 mg/dL (8 mmol/L). Excessive fluid removal should be avoided, because it may contribute to hemodynamic compromise, reduction of uteroplacental perfusion, and premature labor. However, polyhydramnios is a complication of a high maternal urea, leading to high urea and solute diuresis by the fetus, and is also believed to contribute to premature labor. When large volumes of ultrafiltration are required, continuous fetal monitoring during dialysis may be advisable, particularly after mid-pregnancy.

THERAPY FOR END-STAGE RENAL DISEASE DURING PREGNANCY
Dialysis

Fertility is reduced in patients undergoing dialysis because of abnormalities of pituitary luteinizing hormone release leading to anovulation. Pregnancy that occurs in women undergoing maintenance dialysis is extremely high risk for the fetus, and conception should not be encouraged because of very high fetal mortality. Large surveys have shown that only 42% to 60% of these pregnancies result in a live-born infant. Preterm birth, very low birth weight, and intrauterine growth restriction are common, and more than 85% of infants born to women who conceive after starting dialysis are born before 36 weeks gestation.

Management of pregnant patients on dialysis includes several considerations, but the single most important factor influencing fetal outcome is the maternal plasma urea level.[38] In patients undergoing hemodialysis, the number of dialysis sessions per week must be increased and the session duration prolonged to a minimum of 20 h/wk, aiming for a predialysis urea of 30 to 50 mg/dL (5–8 mmol/L).[38–40]

In small series, daily nocturnal hemodialysis has also been used with success to this end.[41] Heparinization should be minimal to prevent obstetric bleeding. Dialysate bicarbonate should be decreased to 25 mEq/L to target a predialysis bicarbonate level of approximately 22 mEq/L. If peritoneal dialysis is used, decreasing exchange volumes through increasing exchange frequency or cycler use is recommended.[42]

Adequate calorie and protein intake is required; 1 g per kilogram body weight per day of protein intake plus an additional 20 g/d has been suggested.[43] After the first trimester, maternal "dry" weight should be increased by approximately 1 lb/wk (400 g/wk) to adjust for the expected progressive weight increase in pregnancy.

Antihypertensive therapy should be adjusted for pregnancy by discontinuing ACEIs and angiotensin receptor blockers, and aiming to maintain maternal diastolic pressure at 80 to 90 mm Hg using methyldopa, labetolol, and sustained release nifedipine in standard doses to achieve target. Anemia should be treated with supplemental iron, folic acid, and erythropoietin. Erythropoietin is safe in pregnancy, and pregnancy-related erythropoietin resistance requires a dose increase of approximately 50% to maintain hemoglobin target levels of 10 to 11 g/dL.[39] Frequent monitoring of iron stores and treatment with intravenous iron should be prescribed as necessary.[43]

Because of placental 25-hydroxyvitamin D3 conversion, decreased supplemental vitamin D may be required and should be guided by levels of vitamin D, parathyroid hormone, calcium, and phosphorus. Sevelamer should not be used in pregnancy because animal studies have shown reduced or irregular ossification of fetal bones. Oral magnesium supplementation may be needed to maintain the serum magnesium level at 5 to 7 mg/dL (2–3 mmol/L), particularly because magnesium is a tocolytic, and low serum levels could theoretically promote uterine contractions. Based on a large meta-analysis, low-dose aspirin to prevent preeclampsia in women at risk for this complication may be advisable in those also on dialysis.[44] Babies born to mothers on dialysis may require monitoring for osmotic diuresis in the immediate postpartum period if maternal urea was high at delivery.

Anticonvulsant Therapy

The presence of dialysis or significant renal dysfunction, loading dose, and infusion rate of magnesium sulfate must be modified and monitored with serial magnesium levels, because doses will accumulate.

Renal Transplantation

Josephson and McKay provide a more detailed discussion of renal transplantation in pregnancy elsewhere in this issue. However, a brief summary follows.

Menstruation and fertility resumes in most women at 1 to 12 months post–renal transplant. Several thousand women have undergone pregnancy after renal transplantation, and pregnancy in this population seems to involve much lower risk to mother and baby than pregnancy in patients on dialysis. Although pregnancy has become common after transplantation, little other than case reports, series, and voluntary databases are available to guide practice. A Consensus Conference generated a report in 2005 summarizing the literature, produced practice guidelines, and identified gaps in knowledge.[45] Most pregnancies (>90%) succeed that proceed beyond the first trimester; however, immunosuppressant effects, preexisting hypertension, and renal dysfunction cause maternal and fetal complications. Maternal complications of steroid therapy include impaired glucose tolerance, hypertension (47%–73%), preeclampsia (30%), and increased infection. Fetal complications include a 45% to 60% incidence of premature delivery (mean gestational age is 36 weeks) and intra-uterine growth restriction with lower birth weight (average 2.3–2.6 kg). Best practice guidelines outline criteria for considering pregnancy in renal transplant recipients,[45–47] and suggest that those contemplating pregnancy should meet the following:

Good health and stable renal function for 1 to 2 years after transplantation with no recent acute or ongoing rejection or infections
Absent or minimal proteinuria (<0.5 g/d)
Normal blood pressure or easily managed hypertension
No evidence of pelvicalcyceal distention on ultrasonography before conception
Serum creatinine less than 1.5 mg/dL (133 μmol/L)
Drug therapy: prednisone 15 mg/d or less; azathioprine 2 mg/kg or less; cyclosporine less than 5 mg/kg per day.

Because of risk for intrauterine growth restriction and preeclampsia, all pregnant transplant recipients should be managed by a high-risk obstetrician.

Future studies are required to address optimal immunosuppression in pregnancy. Although cyclosporine levels tend to decrease during pregnancy, no information is available on whether drug dosage should be increased. Experience with tacrolimus is increasing; although it has not been used as widely in pregnancy as cyclosporine, growing experience suggests that it is safe and has a similar side effect profile to cyclosporine.[48] Considerations regarding hypertension and growth restriction are important; no established blood pressure target exists, although 130/80 mm Hg or less is suggested by the authors and Josephson and McKay in their article found elsewhere in this issue.

Antihypertensives should be switched to those safe in pregnancy.[49] Mycophenolate mofetil and sirolimus are not considered safe in pregnancy.[50] Mycophenolate mofetil has been reported to be embryotoxic in animals, is associated with ear and other deformities in humans, and was recently characterized as a teratogen.[23] This drug should be discontinued 6 weeks before conception, and women should be switched to azathioprine if indicated. Sirolimus causes delayed ossification in animal studies, and although successful live-born human outcomes have been reported, its use is contraindicated until more data are available.

Finally, data from the National Transplantation Pregnancy Registry and European Dialysis and Transplant Association suggest that pregnancy rarely negatively affects the graft, although minor increases in serum creatinine may be seen postpartum compared with prepregnancy levels.[46,50] A long-term analysis of parous compared with nulliparous women who underwent transplantation followed up for 20 years suggests that a live birth in women with a functioning graft does not have an adverse impact on graft and patient survival.[51] Rejection is difficult to diagnose in pregnancy, and renal biopsy may be required; the consensus opinion is that steroids are safe treatment as is intravenous immunoglobulin, but the safety of antilymphocyte globulins and rituximab in pregnancy are unknown.[45]

SUMMARY

Although kidney disease in pregnancy is uncommon, it poses considerable risk to maternal and fetal health. Based on case series published over the past several decades, pregnancy outcome seems to be directly related to level of baseline renal function and degree of hypertension. Because these disorders are uncommon, multicenter efforts are needed to better identify risks and determine optimal therapeutic strategies.

REFERENCES

1. Christensen T, Klebe JG, Bertelsen V, et al. Changes in renal volume during normal pregnancy. Acta Obstet Gynecol Scand 1989;68(6):541–3.
2. Ramin SM, Vidaeff AC, Yeomans ER, et al. Chronic renal disease in pregnancy. Obstet Gynecol 2006;108(6):1531–9.
3. Weissenbacher ER, Reisenberger K. Uncomplicated urinary tract infections in pregnant and non-pregnant women. Curr Opin Obstet Gynecol 1993;5(4): 513–6.
4. Sturgiss SN, Dunlop W, Davison JM. Renal haemodynamics and tubular function in human pregnancy. Baillieres Clin Obstet Gynaecol 1994;8(2):209–34.
5. Wolfe LA, Kemp JG, Heenan AP, et al. Acid-base regulation and control of ventilation in human pregnancy. Can J Physiol Pharmacol 1998;76(9):815–27.
6. Akbari A, Wilkes P, Lindheimer M, et al. Reference intervals for anion gap and strong ion difference in pregnancy: a pilot study. Hypertens Pregnancy 2007; 26(1):111–9.
7. Davison JM, Sheills EA, Philips PR, et al. Metabolic clearance of vasopressin and an analogue resistant to vasopressinase in human pregnancy. Am J Physiol 1993; 264(2 Pt 2):F348–53.
8. Danielson LA, Conrad KP. Time course and dose response of relaxin-mediated renal vasodilation, hyperfiltration, and changes in plasma osmolality in conscious rats. J Appl Physiol 2003;95(4):1509–14.
9. Girling JC. Re-evaluation of plasma creatinine concentration in normal pregnancy. J Obstet Gynaecol 2000;20(2):128–31.
10. Akbari A, Lepage N, Keely E, et al. Cystatin-C and beta trace protein as markers of renal function in pregnancy. BJOG 2005;112(5):575–8.
11. Phelan LK, Brown MA, Davis GK, et al. A prospective study of the impact of automated dipstick urinalysis on the diagnosis of preeclampsia. Hypertens Pregnancy 2004;23(2):135–42.
12. Cote AM, Brown MA, Lam E, et al. Diagnostic accuracy of urinary spot protein:-creatinine ratio for proteinuria in hypertensive pregnant women: systematic review. BMJ 2008;336(7651):1003–6.
13. Jones DC, Hayslett JP. Outcome of pregnancy in women with moderate or severe renal insufficiency. N Engl J Med 1996;335(4):226–32.
14. Imbasciati E, Gregorini G, Cabiddu G, et al. Pregnancy in CKD stages 3 to 5: fetal and maternal outcomes. Am J Kidney Dis 2007;49(6):753–62.
15. Khoury JC, Miodovnik M, LeMasters G, et al. Pregnancy outcome and progression of diabetic nephropathy. What's next? J Matern Fetal Neonatal Med 2002; 11(4):238–44.
16. Ekbom P, Damm P, Feldt-Rasmussen B, et al. Pregnancy outcome in type 1 diabetic women with microalbuminuria. Diabetes Care 2001;24(10):1739–44.
17. Rossing K, Jacobsen P, Hommel E, et al. Pregnancy and progression of diabetic nephropathy. Diabetologia 2002;45(1):36–41.
18. Andrade RM, McGwin G Jr, Alarcon GS, et al. Predictors of post-partum damage accrual in systemic lupus erythematosus: data from LUMINA, a multiethnic US cohort (XXXVIII). Rheumatology (Oxford) 2006;45(11):1380–4.

19. Ruiz-Irastorza G, Lima F, Alves J, et al. Increased rate of lupus flare during pregnancy and the puerperium: a prospective study of 78 pregnancies. Br J Rheumatol 1996;35(2):133–8.

20. Rahman FZ, Rahman J, Al-Suleiman SA, et al. Pregnancy outcome in lupus nephropathy. Arch Gynecol Obstet 2005;271(3):222–6.

21. Erkan D. The relation between antiphospholipid syndrome-related pregnancy morbidity and non-gravid vascular thrombosis: a review of the literature and management strategies. Curr Rheumatol Rep 2002;4(5):379–86.

22. Clowse ME, Magder L, Witter F, et al. Hydroxychloroquine in lupus pregnancy. Arthritis Rheum 2006;54(11):3640–7.

23. Anderka MT, Lin AE, Abuelo DN, et al. Reviewing the evidence for mycophenolate mofetil as a new teratogen: case report and review of the literature. Am J Med Genet A 2009;149A(6):1241–8.

24. Chapman AB, Johnson AM, Gabow PA. Pregnancy outcome and its relationship to progression of renal failure in autosomal dominant polycystic kidney disease. J Am Soc Nephrol 1994;5(5):1178–85.

25. North RA, Taylor RS, Gunn TR. Pregnancy outcome in women with reflux nephropathy and the inheritance of vesico-ureteric reflux. Aust N Z J Obstet Gynaecol 2000;40(3):280–5.

26. Day C, Hewins P, Hildebrand S, et al. The role of renal biopsy in women with kidney disease identified in pregnancy. Nephrol Dial Transplant 2008;23(1): 201–6.

27. Packham D, Fairley KF. Renal biopsy: indications and complications in pregnancy. Br J Obstet Gynaecol 1987;94(10):935–9.

28. Chen HH, Lin HC, Yeh JC, et al. Renal biopsy in pregnancies complicated by undetermined renal disease. Acta Obstet Gynecol Scand 2001;80(10):888–93.

29. Kuller JA, D'Andrea NM, McMahon MJ. Renal biopsy and pregnancy. Am J Obstet Gynecol 2001;184(6):1093–6.

30. Prakash J, Kumar H, Sinha DK, et al. Acute renal failure in pregnancy in a developing country: twenty years of experience. Ren Fail 2006;28(4):309–13.

31. Gammill HS, Jeyabalan A. Acute renal failure in pregnancy. Crit Care Med 2005; 33(10 Suppl):S372–84.

32. Dashe JS, Ramin SM, Cunningham FG. The long-term consequences of thrombotic microangiopathy (thrombotic thrombocytopenic purpura and hemolytic uremic syndrome) in pregnancy. Obstet Gynecol 1998;91(5 Pt 1):662–8.

33. van Runnard Heimel PJ, Franx A, Schobben AF, et al. Corticosteroids, pregnancy, and HELLP syndrome: a review. Obstet Gynecol Surv 2005;60(1):57–70 [quiz: 73–4].

34. Castro MA, Fassett MJ, Reynolds TB, et al. Reversible peripartum liver failure: a new perspective on the diagnosis, treatment, and cause of acute fatty liver of pregnancy, based on 28 consecutive cases. Am J Obstet Gynecol 1999; 181(2):389–95.

35. Fesenmeier MF, Coppage KH, Lambers DS, et al. Acute fatty liver of pregnancy in 3 tertiary care centers. Am J Obstet Gynecol 2005;192(5):1416–9.

36. Vigil-De Gracia P. Acute fatty liver and HELLP syndrome: two distinct pregnancy disorders. Int J Gynaecol Obstet 2001;73(3):215–20.

37. Ibdah JA, Bennett MJ, Rinaldo P, et al. A fetal fatty-acid oxidation disorder as a cause of liver disease in pregnant women. N Engl J Med 1999;340(22): 1723–31.

38. Haase M, Morgera S, Budde K. A systematic approach to managing pregnant dialysis patients–the importance of an intensified haemodiafiltration protocol. Nephrol Dial Transplant 2005;20:2537–42.

39. Asamiya Y, Otsubo S, Matsuda Y, et al. The importance of low blood urea nitrogen levels in pregnant patients undergoing hemodialysis to optimize birth weight and gestational age. Kidney Int 2009;75(11):1217–22.

40. Shemin D. Dialysis in pregnant women with chronic kidney disease. Semin Dial 2003;16(5):379–83.

41. Barua M, Hladunewich M, Keunen J, et al. Successful pregnancies on nocturnal home hemodialysis. Clin J Am Soc Nephrol 2008;3(2):392–6.

42. Smith WT, Darbari S, Kwan M, et al. Pregnancy in peritoneal dialysis: a case report and review of adequacy and outcomes. Int Urol Nephrol 2005;37(1):145–51.

43. Holley JL, Reddy SS. Pregnancy in dialysis patients: a review of outcomes, complications, and management. Semin Dial 2003;16(5):384–8.

44. Askie LM, Duley L, Henderson-Smart DJ, et al. Antiplatelet agents for prevention of pre-eclampsia: a meta-analysis of individual patient data. Lancet 2007;369(9575):1791–8.

45. McKay DB, Josephson MA, Armenti VT, et al. Reproduction and transplantation: report on the AST Consensus Conference on Reproductive Issues and Transplantation. Am J Transplant 2005;5(7):1592–9.

46. EBPG Expert Group on Renal Transplantation. European best practice guidelines for renal transplantation. Section IV: Long-term management of the transplant recipient. IV.10. Pregnancy in renal transplant recipients. Nephrol Dial Transplant 2002;17(Suppl 4):50–5.

47. McKay DB, Josephson MA. Pregnancy in recipients of solid organs–effects on mother and child. N Engl J Med 2006;354(12):1281–93.

48. Kainz A, Harabacz I, Cowlrick IS, et al. Review of the course and outcome of 100 pregnancies in 84 women treated with tacrolimus. Transplantation 2000;70(12):1718–21.

49. Podymow T, August P. Update on the use of antihypertensive drugs in pregnancy. Hypertension 2008;51(4):960–9.

50. Armenti VT, Radomski JS, Moritz MJ, et al. Report from the National Transplantation Pregnancy Registry (NTPR): outcomes of pregnancy after transplantation. Clin Transpl 2004;103–14.

51. Levidiotis V, Chang S, McDonald S. Pregnancy and maternal outcomes among kidney transplant recipients. J Am Soc Nephrol 2009;20(11):2433–40.

52. Katz AI, Davison JM, Hayslett JP, et al. Pregnancy in women with kidney disease. Kidney Int 1980;18(2):192–206.

53. Abe S, Amagasaki Y, Konishi K, et al. The influence of antecedent renal disease on pregnancy. Am J Obstet Gynecol 1985;153(5):508–14.

54. Jungers P, Houillier P, Forget D, et al. Influence of pregnancy on the course of primary chronic glomerulonephritis. Lancet 1995;346(8983):1122–4.

55. Abe S. Pregnancy in IgA nephropathy. Kidney Int 1991;40(6):1098–102.

56. Chopra S, Suri V, Aggarwal N, et al. Pregnancy in chronic renal insufficiency: single centre experience from North India. Arch Gynecol Obstet 2009;279(5):691–5.

Pregnancy in the Renal Transplant Recipient

Michelle A. Josephson, MD[a],*, Dianne B. McKay, MD[b,c]

KEYWORDS

• Pregnancy • Kidney transplantation • Immunosuppression

March 10th, 1958, marks the birthday of the first baby born to a kidney transplant recipient. The pregnancy went to term and the baby was delivered by cesarean section for fear that a vaginal birth could adversely affect the allograft kidney sitting in the iliac fossa. Undoubtedly, this pregnancy more than 50 years ago was considered high risk because of its pioneering nature. However, given that the transplant recipient had received her kidney from her identical twin sister approximately 2 years before and was not taking any immunosuppressive medications, the pregnancy was associated with far fewer risks than most pregnancies in transplant recipients of today. Not only are immunosuppressants now available that have potential adverse affects on the developing fetus but also many kidney transplant recipients have kidney function that is suboptimal. Although thousands of women with kidney transplants have successfully delivered healthy babies, many new issues must be considered during a transplant recipient's pregnancy compared with 50 years ago. These issues are discussed below.

FERTILITY

Women become pregnant after transplantation more easily than they do during end-stage kidney disease. However, despite the many births that have occurred since the first child was born to a transplant recipient in 1958, quantifying the likelihood of pregnancy after transplant has been difficult.

Gill and colleagues'[1] 2009 study sheds some light on this issue. His group examined 16,194 female kidney transplant recipients between ages 15 and 45 years who

[a] Department of Medicine, Section of Nephrology, University of Chicago, 5841 South Maryland Avenue, Chicago, IL 60637, USA
[b] Department of Immunology and Microbial Science, The Scripps Research Institute, 10550 North Torrey Pines Road, La Jolla, CA 92037, USA
[c] Balboa Institute of Transplantation, Sharp Memorial Hospital, 7920 Frost Street, San Diego, CA 92123, USA
* Corresponding author.
E-mail address: mjosephs@medicine.bsd.uchicago.edu

Obstet Gynecol Clin N Am 37 (2010) 211–222
doi:10.1016/j.ogc.2010.02.008
0889-8545/10/$ – see front matter © 2010 Elsevier Inc. All rights reserved.

underwent kidney transplantation in the United States between 1990 and 2003. Using Medicare claims data for the first 3 years posttransplant, his team identified the pregnancy and live birth rate. The pregnancy rate in women with kidney transplants was 59 per thousand in 1990, and declined to 20 per thousand in 2000. This rate is much lower than in the general public, in which the pregnancy rate was greater than 100 per thousand each year between 1990 and 2000. Pregnancy rates declined over the 10-year period for both transplant recipients and the general public, but the drop was steeper for the transplant recipients. During this period the overall live birth rate was 19 per thousand female transplant recipients (dropping from 28.5 per thousand in 1990 to 6.2 per thousand in 2000), compared with 70.9 per thousand in 1990 and 65.9 per thousand in 2000 in the general public. The period examined showed a drop in therapeutic abortions; however, the proportion of pregnancies that led to fetal loss (45.6%) remained constant, indicating an increase in spontaneous abortions. The decrease in live births between 1990 and 2000 was a consequence of the falling pregnancy rate.

Fertility in women is not the only consideration for kidney transplant recipients. Men with kidney transplants taking sirolimus also may experience infertility.[2,3] Sirolimus can play a central inhibitory role in a stem cell factor that regulates spermatogenesis, thus causing infertility.[4]

OPTIMAL TIMING

Historically, female transplant recipients have been counseled to wait 2 years after successful transplantation before becoming pregnant.[5] This recommendation was based on the assumption that after 2 years, the risk for rejection would be low and the allograft function would be stable. A more recent examination of this 2-year wait was undertaken at a consensus conference conducted by the American Society of Transplantation,[6] which reported that transplant patients now routinely experience a lower rate of rejection because of newer immunosuppressive strategies. It was also realized that, because of longer waiting list times for the allograft, women are waiting longer to receive a transplant (rendering some women nearer to the end of their reproductive years). Therefore, the conference experts agreed that the older recommendations were too restrictive, and the consensus opinion was that pregnancy was safe by 1 year after transplantation under the following conditions: the patient experienced no rejection in the past year; allograft function was adequate (similar to other recommendations arbitrarily defined for kidney allografts as a serum creatinine less than 1.5 mg/dL and with no or minimal proteinuria[7]); no infections were present that could impact the fetus (eg, cytomegalovirus); the patient was not taking teratogenic medications; and the immunosuppressive medication dosing was stable at maintenance levels.[6] The consensus recommendations cautioned, however, that pregnancy after only 1 year might be too risky if the creatinine is greater than 1.5 mg/dL, any recent acute rejection episodes occurred, the patient has hypertension or other comorbid factors, or evidence shows noncompliance with immunosuppressive medications.[6] It was also realized that strict recommendations for the optimal timing of pregnancy might need to be individualized, particularly in older transplant recipients who might have fewer reproductive years.

In 2008, a paper by Kim and colleagues[8] suggested that women could safely conceive within the first year of transplantation. They reported on 74 pregnancies in 48 women; 11 pregnancies conceived within the first year of transplantation had obstetric and graft outcomes comparable to those conceived after a longer posttransplant interval.

However, despite these observations, early conception posttransplant has not been proven optimal. Gill and colleagues[1] analyzed data from The United States Renal Data System on women between ages 15 and 45 years who underwent kidney transplantation between January 1, 1990, and December 31, 2003, and evaluated those insured only by Medicare at transplant. A borderline increase in the risk for fetal loss occurred with conception during the first transplant year compared with subsequent years.[1] Given these findings, the recommendation to wait at least a year after transplantation is reasonable.

HYPERTENSION AND ITS MANAGEMENT DURING PREGNANCY

In the general population, 1% to 5% of pregnant women have been reported to have chronic hypertension.[9] The frequency of hypertension is much higher in the kidney transplant population, in which 21% to 73% have hypertension during the pregnancy, depending on whether calcineurin inhibitors are used.[10–12] As with other pregnancies in the setting of kidney dysfunction, hypertension should be well controlled. The American Society of Transplantation consensus opinion was that blood pressure should be maintained close to normal.[6] Current recommendations are that blood pressure in the pregnant transplant patient should be maintained at levels recommended for nonpregnant patients with kidney dysfunction.[13] The current Seventh Report of the Joint National Committee on Prevention, Detection, Evaluation, and Treatment of High Blood Pressure and Kidney Disease Outcomes Quality Initiative guidelines suggest a goal of less than 130/80 mm Hg.[14,15]

Chronic hypertension in pregnancy is associated with abruptio placentae, acute renal failure, cardiac decompensation, and cerebral accidents in the mother.[9] It is also associated with an increased incidence of growth restriction and death of the fetus.[13] These adverse events usually occur in the setting of superimposed preeclampsia (approximately 20% incidence in chronic hypertensives without kidney transplants and 30% incidence in kidney transplant recipients). These adverse outcomes may occur even more frequently in female transplant recipients older than 30 years, and in those with end-organ damage.[9] Because all kidney transplant recipients have chronic kidney disease, they are at increased risk for complications associated with pregnancy, and thus should be managed as patients with chronic kidney disease.

The need to control hypertension is certainly another reason that pregnancies are best planned prospectively in this patient population, for instance to allow for discontinuation of potentially fetotoxic antihypertensive agents (eg, angiotensin converting enzyme inhibitors) before pregnancy.[13,16] Atenolol used early in pregnancy has been associated with fetal growth restriction.[17] Acceptable oral agents often used in pregnancy include methyldopa (considered first line), labetolol, and nifedipine. Hydralazine and thiazide diuretics have been safely used as adjunctive agents.[18–20]

IMMUNOSUPPRESSANTS

The transplant recipient must be adequately immunosuppressed during the pregnancy or she risks graft rejection and, potentially, fetal loss.[11] The pregnancy does not cause systemic immunosuppression of the mother, and immunosuppressive drug levels vary during the course of pregnancy; immunosuppressive medication levels must be closely followed. Pregnancy in transplant recipients should be considered a pregnancy in the setting of chronic kidney dysfunction, with the added dimension of immunosuppression, which is a major consideration in the management of the pregnant transplant recipient.[6,7]

The US Food and Drug Administration (FDA) considers the immunosuppressants prescribed to transplant recipients risky based on their categorization as more than FDA category A. **Table 1** lists the FDA categories of maintenance immunosuppressants commonly used to prevent rejection. The immunosuppressants commonly used to prevent rejection of the transplanted organ are described here.

Corticosteroids

Prednisone and prednisolone cross the placenta. Whether the patient takes prednisone or prednisolone, the latter is the major compound in the circulation.[21] The placenta metabolizes a significant amount (51%–67%) of the prednisolone and cortisol that cross it, exposing the fetus to a reduced amount.[22] Fetal concentrations of prednisolone have been found to be 8- to 10-fold lower than maternal prednisolone concentrations.[21] By contrast, little (1.8%) dexamethasone is converted by the placenta.[22] Methylprednisolone also transverses the placenta.[23] Case reports describe fetal adrenal insufficiency and thymic hypoplasia when corticosteroids are used in high doses,[22,24] but this rarely occurs with doses of 15 mg/d or less.[25]

Azathioprine

Azathioprine, an inhibitor of purine metabolism, is a prodrug rapidly converted to 6-mercaptopurine (6-MP) in adults. 6-MP is converted by the enzyme inosinate pyrophosphorylase to its active form thioinosinic acid that targets DNA in dividing cells. Radioactive labeling studies in humans have shown that most azathioprine administered to mothers appears in fetal blood as the inactive metabolite thiouric acid. The literature suggests that a fetal lack of the enzyme inosinate pyrophosphorylase needed for conversion of 6-MP protects the fetus from azathioprine's effects.[26] Several chromosome anomalies and transient lymphopenia have been reported in children exposed in utero to azathioprine, but these have been scattered reports.[27–31]

Given the comfort that most physicians have using azathioprine during pregnancy, many are surprised that it is rated FDA category D. However, this rating was based on observations of rodent fetus abnormalities and sporadic structural malformations in human fetuses.[30,31]

Table 1
Maintenance therapy: used on a daily basis to prevent rejection of the graft

Medication	FDA Category
Calcineurin inhibitors	
Cyclosporine (Neoral, Sandimmune, Gengraf)	C
Tacrolimus, FK506 (Prograf)	C
Antiproliferative Agents	
Mycophenolate mofetil (CellCept, Myofortic)	D
Azathioprine (Imuran)	D
Rapamycin, sirolimus (Rapamune)	C
Leflunomide (Arava)	X
Corticosteroids	
Prednisone (Deltazone)	B

Calcineurin Inhibitors: Cyclosporine and Tacrolimus

Calcineurin inhibitors are currently the most commonly used maintenance immuno-suppressive agents. Their use has decreased rejection and prolonged kidney graft survival. When cyclosporine was first introduced, its safety in pregnancy was of concern.[32] But with clinical use, no indication of congenital malformations has been noted,[33] although a risk for fetal growth restriction[34] exists that may exceed that seen with azathioprine and prednisone alone.[35] Mothers treated with cyclosporine are also more likely to have hypertension and creatinines greater than 1.5 mg/dL.[35] Compared with cyclosporine, pregnant women taking tacrolimus have a lower inci-dence of hypertension and hyperlipidemia.[34] A higher incidence of diabetes mellitus and transient hyperkalemia in the newborn has been described.[36]

Leflunomide

Leflunomide is primarily used in rheumatoid arthritis but also is prescribed in trans-plantation. It is an inhibitor of dihydroorotate dehydrogenase, an enzyme necessary for the de novo biosynthesis of pyrimidines. Studies in rats and rabbits showed tera-togenicity.[37] Growth restriction and embryo death was noted.[37] Although whether leflunomide is teratogenic in humans is unclear, it is worrisome that the drug level at which it is teratogenic in rats and rabbits is the same as that achieved in humans during clinical use.[37] Few data are available for human pregnancies, although in one survey rheumatologists reported no malformations in 10 women exposed to lefluno-mide during pregnancy.[38] However, this evidence is not sufficient to support the drug's use during pregnancy; leflunomide is rated category X (see **Table 1**) and should not be used during pregnancy. Leflunomide has a long half-life; it may take up to 2 years to achieve a nondetectable plasma level (<0.02 mg/L). Consequently, when stopping leflunomide, women who wish to become pregnant are advised to undergo a drug elimination procedure.[37]

Mycophenolate Mofetil and Rapamycin

Several case reports in humans have shown congenital abnormalities in fetuses exposed in utero to mycophenolate mofetil (MMF).[39,40] A characteristic phenotype seems to be emerging: cleft lip and palate, microtia, and absence of auditory canals, and possible coloboma, brachydactyly of the fifth fingers, and hypoplastic tone-nails.[41–43] Premarketing animal studies found that MMF is teratogenic in rats and rabbits.[44,45]

Initially MMF was labeled as FDA pregnancy category C; however, a case series of malformations published by the National Transplantation Pregnancy Registry (NTPR) and case reports caused the FDA to reclassify the drug as category D.

Fewer data are available on rapamycin (sirolimus). At least one case report docu-ments birth of a child without structural defects to a transplant recipient maintained on rapamycin for the first 2 trimesters of pregnancy.[46] Although classified as FDA category C, whether rapamycin is safe to use during pregnancy is unclear. The single case report of a healthy child born to a mother immunosuppressed during pregnancy with rapamycin should not indicate that it is necessarily safe.

The European Best Practice Guidelines[7] endorse switching immunosuppression to avoid MMF during pregnancy. Although risk for a rejection after switching from MMF to azathioprine may seem low in the setting of kidney-only allograft recipients on triple immunosuppression, the risks may increase in the setting of a simultaneous kidney–pancreas recipient. The latter point is particularly noteworthy if the patient is only taking two immunosuppressant agents and not prednisone, as is becoming common at many transplant centers. Aside from how to switch immunosuppressants, the issue of whether to start prednisone during pregnancy must also be considered.

In addition to deciding which immunosuppressants to continue during pregnancy, practitioners must also consider adjustment of immunosuppressant dosing. The dose of immunosuppressive medications, particularly calcineurin inhibitors, may need to be adjusted throughout gestation because of changing total body volumes during gestation[47] and changes in hepatic metabolism of the immunosuppressive medications throughout the pregnancy.[48] Whether other immunosuppressive medications require adjustment is unknown.

Although Jain and colleagues[49] found no rejection episodes in a retrospective analysis of 21 pregnancies among recipients of kidney and kidney–pancreas allografts in whom tacrolimus levels were not adjusted during gestation, despite lowered trough levels, this evidence cannot be taken as proof that decreasing immunosuppressive levels will be tolerated without rejection. NTPR data show that pregnant kidney transplant recipients who retained stable function during pregnancies took higher doses of cyclosporine than patients with kidney dysfunction.[50] As noted by Jain and colleagues,[49] some patients may tolerate decreasing immunosuppression levels. Unfortunately, predicting which patients will tolerate reduced levels is impossible.

Confounding the decision making is the fact that diagnosing kidney dysfunction is difficult during pregnancy, partly because serum creatinines normally decrease with the increased glomerular filtration rate seen during gestation.[51] Furthermore, because it is difficult to predict which patients will experience a rejection episode after changes to immunosuppressive drug dosing, the current recommendations are to maintain therapeutic drug levels at their prepregnancy levels.[6] Clinicians must realize that the fetus is also an allograft and that the mother is not systemically immunosuppressed by the pregnancy. The fetal allograft is not rejected because of local mechanisms acting at the site of the maternal–fetal interface and specific to the paternal antigens.[11] Therefore, decreasing immunosuppressive dosing based on hypothetical immunologic privilege of the state of pregnancy cannot be justified.[52,53]

RECOGNIZING KIDNEY DYSFUNCTION

In kidney transplant recipients, creatinine is used as a marker for transplant graft health. Unfortunately, it is not a perfect surrogate because creatinine is insensitive and nonspecific. In clinically stable circumstances, creatinine may not adequately reflect intrinsic kidney perturbations, especially in a transplanted kidney. In the setting of pregnancy, the expected increase in intravascular volume and hyperfiltration should lead to an increase in glomerular filtration rate and a decrease in creatinine. Therefore, a "reassuringly" stable serum creatinine in a pregnant woman who underwent kidney transplantation may be just the opposite, and reflect an unstable process affecting the kidney parenchyma. Assessing the kidney transplant during pregnancy is important but can be complex.

SPECIAL CONSIDERATIONS
Urinary Tract Infections

Urinary tract infections are the most frequent complication found in otherwise normal pregnancies.[54] This condition is not benign; untreated bacteriuria is associated with acute pyelonephritis at the end of the second and in the third trimester in 20% to 30% of cases.[55] Acute pyelonephritis has been associated with prematurity. Treatment early in pregnancy results in a marked reduction in pyelonephritis and premature delivery.[55] Asymptomatic bacteriuria is common in kidney transplant recipients, especially in the early posttransplant period.[55]

Given the immunosuppressed state and likelihood for reflux in pregnant women with a kidney transplant, screening for pyuria and preventing pyelonephritis are important aspects of patient management. During gestation, asymptomatic bacteriuria may progress to acute pyelonephritis[54] and therefore most investigators recommend screening all pregnant women and treating any positive cultures.[56] Universal screening and treatment of patients who are culture-positive have reduced the incidence of pyelonephritis.[54] Current guidelines endorse screening on at least a monthly basis in kidney transplant recipients.[7]

Anemia

Anemia frequently complicates pregnancies in patients who have undergone kidney transplantation, even in the absence of kidney function deterioration. Compared with normal pregnancies, transplant recipients may have inappropriately low erythropoietin levels.[57] Given the increasing use of erythropoietin in the transplant population, some women with kidney transplants will already be taking an erythropoietin-stimulating agent (ESA) when they become pregnant. The safe use of ESAs has been reported during pregnancy in transplant recipients, although concern has been raised over the possibility of it playing a role in maternal hypertension.[58] No contraindication exists to using ESAs during pregnancy.

Management of anemia in women with kidney transplants is similar to that for women with preexisting kidney disease. ESA initiation and chronic dosing recommendations have changed because of cardiovascular complications associated with maintaining higher hemoglobin levels with ESAs. At this point, patients should not be started on an ESA until their hemoglobin is less than 10. Chronic administration should be performed to keep the hemoglobin less than 11.

Preeclampsia

Preeclampsia develops in approximately one third of pregnant women who have undergone a kidney or kidney–pancreas transplantation.[59] Diagnosis of preeclampsia is challenging because blood pressure often increases after the 20th week of gestation and many transplant patients have preexisting proteinuria.[60] In addition, calcineurin inhibitors raise uric acid levels, making uric acid an inaccurate marker for preeclampsia.[61]

The diagnosis of preeclampsia is subjective in the general population and, because of the ambiguity of potential clinical signs, even more subjective in transplant recipients. Observations that women with a history of preeclampsia are at increased risk for developing cardiovascular disease is of particular concern in transplant recipients who carry other risks for cardiovascular disease.[62–64] The fact that cardiovascular disease is greatest in women with small or preterm babies is noteworthy given the propensity for transplant recipients to have small or preterm babies.[63] Similarly, that preeclampsia had been found to be a marker for increased risk for subsequent end-stage renal disease is noteworthy.[65] Unfortunately, large-scale trials have failed to identify prophylactic interventions that will significantly reduce the incidence of preeclampsia.[66–69] Whether preeclampsia is a marker for preexisting increased cardiovascular risk or causes the increased risk is unclear. What is clear, however, is that kidney transplant recipients have a much higher propensity for preeclampsia than the general public.

Although potential markers for preeclampsia, such as sFlt-1, have been identified, their use in the clinical setting is untested.[70] Nevertheless, at least one case report has been published indicating that assaying for serum angiogenic factors may be clinically useful in establishing a diagnosis of preeclampsia.[71]

Breast-feeding

Breast-feeding in the setting of renal transplant is controversial. A survey conducted by the American Society of Transplantation (AST) noted that most physicians advise against breast-feeding.[72] Nevertheless, mothers may want to pursue breast-feeding. Resulting data from studies of breast-feeding mothers on immunosuppression are inconsistent, because the calcineurin inhibitor levels in breast milk can vary from undetectable to concentrations equal to those in the maternal blood.[11,73] The American Academy of Pediatrics (AAP) supports breast-feeding for mothers taking prednisone but advises against it for mothers on cyclosporine.[74] The AAP provides no recommendation regarding either azathioprine or tacrolimus. No data exist on the levels of mycophenolate mofetil, sirolimus, or leflunomide in breast milk. The NTPR has received input from 2 women who breast-fed with resumption of mycophenolate mofetil postpartum (Lisa A. Coscia, RN, BSN, CCTC, personal communication, 2009). Whether the risks associated with immunosuppressive medication exposure from breast milk outweigh the benefits of breast-feeding is currently unknown. The AST consensus opinion is that breast-feeding need not be viewed as absolutely contraindicated.[6]

Long Term Prognosis

Whether pregnancy adversely affects kidney transplant recipients remains a longstanding and unresolved question. Davison[75] showed that renal allografts adapt to pregnancy normally. Most studies have indicated that serum creatinine may rise slightly after a pregnancy, but an adverse effect on long-term outcome has not be shown.[76–78] At least one study, however, indicated that pregnancy has a negative effect on transplant function.[79] More recently, an analysis of 40 years of pregnancy-related outcomes for transplant recipients was performed. This analysis matched 120 parous and 120 nulliparous women according to year of transplantation, duration of transplant, age and predelivery creatinine for parous women, and creatinine for nonparous women. This analysis failed to show that pregnancy negatively influenced either graft or patient survival.[80]

Donors

Two recent reports, one based on registry data and the other on survey data, indicate that kidney donors may be at increased risk for preeclampsia after donation compared with before. Although the preeclampsia risk for kidney donors is comparable to the general public, their individual risk after donation may rise from a particularly low to a more normalized one. In other words, these individuals may be at increased risk compared with their pre-donation risk level.[81–83]

REFERENCES

1. Gill JS, Zalunardo N, Rose C, et al. The pregnancy rate and live birth rate in kidney transplant recipients. Am J Transplant 2009;9(7):1541–9.
2. Fritsche L, Budde K, Dragun D, et al. Testosterone concentrations and sirolimus in male renal transplant patients. Am J Transplant 2004;4(1):130–1.
3. Kaczmarek I, Groetzner J, Adamidis I, et al. Sirolimus impairs gonadal function in heart transplant recipients. Am J Transplant 2004;4(7):1084–8.
4. Tondolo V, Citterio F, Panocchia N, et al. Sirolimus impairs improvement of the gonadal function after renal transplantation. Am J Transplant 2005;5(1):197.

5. Davison JM. Pregnancy in renal allograft recipients: prognosis and management. Baillieres Clin Obstet Gynaecol 1987;1(4):1027–45.

6. McKay DB, Josephson MA, Armenti VT, et al. Reproduction and transplantation: report on the AST Consensus Conference on Reproductive Issues and Transplantation. Am J Transplant 2005;5(7):1592–9.

7. European best practice guidelines for renal transplantation. Section IV: long-term management of the transplant recipient. Nephrol Dial Transplant 2002;17(Suppl 4): 1–67.

8. Kim HW, Seok HJ, Kim TH, et al. The experience of pregnancy after renal transplantation: pregnancies even within postoperative 1 year may be tolerable. Transplantation 2008;85(10):1412–9.

9. Sibai BM, Lindheimer M, Hauth J, et al. Risk factors for preeclampsia, abruptio placentae, and adverse neonatal outcomes among women with chronic hypertension. National Institute of Child Health and Human Development Network of Maternal-Fetal Medicine Units. N Engl J Med 1998;339(10):667–71.

10. Armenti VT, Ahlswede KM, Ahlswede BA, et al. National transplantation Pregnancy Registry–outcomes of 154 pregnancies in cyclosporine-treated female kidney transplant recipients. Transplantation 1994;57(4):502–6.

11. McKay DB, Josephson MA. Pregnancy in recipients of solid organs–effects on mother and child. N Engl J Med 2006;354(12):1281–93.

12. Radomski JS, Ahlswede BA, Jarrell BE, et al. Outcomes of 500 pregnancies in 335 female kidney, liver, and heart transplant recipients. Transplant Proc 1995; 27(1):1089–90.

13. National High Blood Pressure Education Program Working Group Report on high blood pressure in pregnancy. Am J Obstet Gynecol 1990;163(5 Pt 1):1691–712.

14. K/DOQI clinical practice guidelines on hypertension and antihypertensive agents in chronic kidney disease. Am J Kidney Dis 2004;43:S1–290.

15. Chobanian AV, Bakris GL, Black HR, et al. The Seventh Report of the Joint National Committee on prevention, detection, evaluation, and treatment of high blood pressure: the JNC 7 report. JAMA 2003;289(19):2560–72.

16. Pryde PG, Sedman AB, Nugent CE, et al. Angiotensin-converting enzyme inhibitor fetopathy. J Am Soc Nephrol 1993;3(9):1575–82.

17. Podymow T, August P. Hypertension in pregnancy. Adv Chronic Kidney Dis 2007; 14(2):178–90.

18. Magee LA, Abalos E, von DP, et al. Control of hypertension in pregnancy. Curr Hypertens Rep 2009;11(6):429–36.

19. Umans JG. Medications during pregnancy: antihypertensives and immunosuppressives. Adv Chronic Kidney Dis 2007;14(2):191–8.

20. Yoder SR, Thornburg LL, Bisognano JD. Hypertension in pregnancy and women of childbearing age. Am J Med 2009;122(10):890–5.

21. Beitins IZ, Bayard F, Ances IG, et al. The transplacental passage of prednisone and prednisolone in pregnancy near term. J Pediatr 1972;81(5):936–45.

22. Blanford AT, Murphy BE. In vitro metabolism of prednisolone, dexamethasone, betamethasone, and cortisol by the human placenta. Am J Obstet Gynecol 1977;127(3):264–7.

23. Anderson GG, Rotchell Y, Kaiser DG. Placental transfer of methylprednisolone following maternal intravenous administration. Am J Obstet Gynecol 1981; 140(6):699–701.

24. Muirhead N, Sabharwal AR, Rieder MJ, et al. The outcome of pregnancy following renal transplantation–the experience of a single center. Transplantation 1992; 54(3):429–32.

25. Penn I, Makowski EL, Harris P. Parenthood following renal transplantation. Kidney Int 1980;18(2):221–33.
26. Saarikoski S, Seppala M. Immunosuppression during pregnancy: transmission of azathioprine and its metabolites from the mother to the fetus. Am J Obstet Gynecol 1973;115(8):1100–6.
27. Davison JM, Dellagrammatikas H, Parkin JM. Maternal azathioprine therapy and depressed haemopoiesis in the babies of renal allograft patients. Br J Obstet Gynaecol 1985;92(3):233–9.
28. Githens JH, Rosenkrantz JG, Tunnock SM. Teratogenic effects of azathioprine (imuran). J Pediatr 1965;66:959–61.
29. Rosenkrantz JG, Githens JH, Cox SM, et al. Azathioprine (Imuran) and pregnancy. Am J Obstet Gynecol 1967;97(3):387–94.
30. Tallent MB, Simmons RL, Najarian JS. Birth defects in child of male recipient of kidney transplant. JAMA 1970;211(11):1854–5.
31. Williamson RA, Karp LE. Azathioprine teratogenicity: review of the literature and case report. Obstet Gynecol 1981;58(2):247–50.
32. Pickrell MD, Sawers R, Michael J. Pregnancy after renal transplantation: severe intrauterine growth retardation during treatment with cyclosporin A. Br Med J (Clin Res Ed) 1988;296(6625):825.
33. Kainz A, Harabacz I, Cowlrick IS, et al. Analysis of 100 pregnancy outcomes in women treated systemically with tacrolimus. Transpl Int 2000;13(Suppl 1): S299–300.
34. Armenti VT, Moritz MJ, Cardonick EH, et al. Immunosuppression in pregnancy: choices for infant and maternal health. Drugs 2002;62(16):2361–75.
35. Hou S. Pregnancy in renal transplant recipients. Adv Ren Replace Ther 2003; 10(1):40–7.
36. Jain A, Venkataramanan R, Fung JJ, et al. Pregnancy after liver transplantation under tacrolimus. Transplantation 1997;64(4):559–65.
37. Brent RL. Teratogen update: reproductive risks of leflunomide (Arava); a pyrimidine synthesis inhibitor: counseling women taking leflunomide before or during pregnancy and men taking leflunomide who are contemplating fathering a child. Teratology 2001;63(2):106–12.
38. Chakravarty EF, Sanchez-Yamamoto D, Bush TM. The use of disease modifying antirheumatic drugs in women with rheumatoid arthritis of childbearing age: a survey of practice patterns and pregnancy outcomes. J Rheumatol 2003; 30(2):241–6.
39. Pergola PE, Kancharla A, Riley DJ. Kidney transplantation during the first trimester of pregnancy: immunosuppression with mycophenolate mofetil, tacrolimus, and prednisone. Transplantation 2001;71(7):994–7.
40. Sifontis NM, Coscia LA, Constantinescu S, et al. Pregnancy outcomes in solid organ transplant recipients with exposure to mycophenolate mofetil or sirolimus. Transplantation 2006;82(12):1698–702.
41. Anderka MT, Lin AE, Abuelo DN, et al. Reviewing the evidence for mycophenolate mofetil as a new teratogen: case report and review of the literature. Am J Med Genet A 2009;149(6):1241–8.
42. Dei Malatesta MF, Rocca B, Gentile T, et al. A case of coloboma in a newborn to a woman taking mycophenolate mofetil in pregnancy after kidney transplantation. Transplant Proc 2009;41(4):1407–9.
43. Merlob P, Stahl B, Klinger G. Tetrada of the possible mycophenolate mofetil embryopathy: a review. Reprod Toxicol 2009;28(1):105–8.
44. Mycophenolae mofetil [package insert]. Nutley (NJ): Roche Laboratories; 2007.

45. Tendron A, Gouyon JB, Decramer S. In utero exposure to immunosuppressive drugs: experimental and clinical studies. Pediatr Nephrol 2002;17(2):121–30.
46. Chu SH, Liu KL, Chiang YJ, et al. Sirolimus used during pregnancy in a living related renal transplant recipient: a case report. Transplant Proc 2008;40(7): 2446–8.
47. Thomas AG, Burrows L, Knight R, et al. The effect of pregnancy on cyclosporine levels in renal allograft patients. Obstet Gynecol 1997;90(6):916–9.
48. Harris RZ, Benet LZ, Schwartz JB. Gender effects in pharmacokinetics and pharmacodynamics. Drugs 1995;50(2):222–39.
49. Jain AB, Shapiro R, Scantlebury VP, et al. Pregnancy after kidney and kidney-pancreas transplantation under tacrolimus: a single center's experience. Transplantation 2004;77(6):897–902.
50. Armenti VT, Ahlswede KM, Ahlswede BA, et al. Variables affecting birthweight and graft survival in 197 pregnancies in cyclosporine-treated female kidney transplant recipients. Transplantation 1995;59(4):476–9.
51. Davison JM, Lindheimer MD. Pregnancy in renal transplant recipients. J Reprod Med 1982;27(10):613–21.
52. Aluvihare VR, Kallikourdis M, Betz AG. Tolerance, suppression and the fetal allograft. J Mol Med 2005;83(2):88–96.
53. Streilein JW. Peripheral tolerance induction: lessons from immune privileged sites and tissues. Transplant Proc 1996;28(4):2066–70.
54. Lindheimer MD, Katz AI. The normal and diseased kidney in pregnancy. In: Schrier R, editor. Diseases of the kidney. 7th edition. Philadelphia: Lippincott, Williams, Wilkins; 2001. p. 2129–65.
55. Nicolle LE. Asymptomatic bacteriuria: when to screen and when to treat. Infect Dis Clin North Am 2003;17(2):367–94.
56. Pedler SJ, Orr KE. Bacterial, fungal, and parasitic infections. In: Barron WM, Lindheimer MD, editors. Medical disorders during pregnancy. 3 edition. St. Louis (MO): Mosby; 2000. p. 411.
57. Magee LA, von DP, Darley J, et al. Erythropoiesis and renal transplant pregnancy. Clin Transplant 2000;14(2):127–35.
58. Goshorn J, Youell TD. Darbepoetin alfa treatment for post-renal transplantation anemia during pregnancy. Am J Kidney Dis 2005;46(5):e81–6.
59. Armenti VT, Radomski JS, Moritz MJ, et al. Report from the National Transplantation Pregnancy Registry (NTPR): outcomes of pregnancy after transplantation. Clin Transpl 2003131–41.
60. Stratta P, Canavese C, Giacchino F, et al. Pregnancy in kidney transplantation: satisfactory outcomes and harsh realities. J Nephrol 2003;16(6):792–806.
61. Morales JM, Hernandez PG, Andres A, et al. Uric acid handling, pregnancy and cyclosporin in renal transplant women. Nephron 1990;56(1):97–8.
62. Funai EF, Friedlander Y, Paltiel O, et al. Long-term mortality after preeclampsia. Epidemiology 2005;16(2):206–15.
63. Irgens HU, Reisaeter L, Irgens LM, et al. Long term mortality of mothers and fathers after pre-eclampsia: population based cohort study. BMJ 2001; 323(7323):1213–7.
64. Wolf M, Hubel CA, Lam C, et al. Preeclampsia and future cardiovascular disease: potential role of altered angiogenesis and insulin resistance. J Clin Endocrinol Metab 2004;89(12):6239–43.
65. Vikse BE, Irgens LM, Leivestad T, et al. Preeclampsia and the risk of end-stage renal disease. N Engl J Med 2008;359(8):800–9.

66. Villar J, Abalos E, Nardin JM, et al. Strategies to prevent and treat preeclampsia: evidence from randomized controlled trials. Semin Nephrol 2004;24(6):607–15.
67. Villar J, Abdel-Aleem H, Merialdi M, et al. World Health Organization randomized trial of calcium supplementation among low calcium intake pregnant women. Am J Obstet Gynecol 2006;194(3):639–49.
68. Poston L, Briley AL, Seed PT, et al. Vitamin C and vitamin E in pregnant women at risk for pre-eclampsia (VIP trial): randomised placebo-controlled trial. Lancet 2006;367(9517):1145–54.
69. Lindheimer MD, Sibai BM. Antioxidant supplementation in pre-eclampsia. Lancet 2006;367(9517):1119–20.
70. Levine RJ, Maynard SE, Qian C, et al. Circulating angiogenic factors and the risk of preeclampsia. N Engl J Med 2004;350(7):672–83.
71. Hladunewich MA, Steinberg G, Ananth KS, et al. Angiogenic factor abnormalities and fetal demise in a twin pregnancy. Nat Rev Nephrol 2009;5(11):658–62.
72. McKay DB, Adams PL, Bumgardner GL, et al. Reproduction and pregnancy in the transplanted patient: current practices. Prog Transplant 2006;16(2):127–32.
73. Grimer M. The CARI guidelines. Calcineurin inhibitors in renal transplantation: pregnancy, lactation and calcineurin inhibitors. Nephrology (Carlton) 2007; 12(Suppl 1):S98–105.
74. American Academy of Pediatrics Committee on Drugs. The transfer of drugs and other chemicals into human milk. Pediatrics 1994;93(1):137–50.
75. Davison JM. The effect of pregnancy on kidney function in renal allograft recipients. Kidney Int 1985;27(1):74–9.
76. First MR, Combs CA, Weiskittel P, et al. Lack of effect of pregnancy on renal allograft survival or function. Transplantation 1995;59(4):472–6.
77. Sturgiss SN, Davison JM. Effect of pregnancy on the long-term function of renal allografts: an update. Am J Kidney Dis 1995;26(1):54–6.
78. Tanabe K, Kobayashi C, Takahashi K, et al. Long-term renal function after pregnancy in renal transplant recipients. Transplant Proc 1997;29(1–2):1567–8.
79. Salmela KT, Kyllonen LE, Holmberg C, et al. Impaired renal function after pregnancy in renal transplant recipients. Transplantation 1993;56(6):1372–5.
80. Levidiotis V, Chang S, McDonald S. Pregnancy and maternal outcomes among kidney transplant recipients. J Am Soc Nephrol 2009;20(11):2433–40.
81. Ibrahim HN, Akkina SK, Leister E, et al. Pregnancy outcomes after kidney donation. Am J Transplant 2009;9(4):825–34.
82. Josephson MA. Transplantation: pregnancy after kidney donation: more questions than answers. Nat Rev Nephrol 2009;5(9):495–7.
83. Reisaeter AV, Roislien J, Henriksen T, et al. Pregnancy and birth after kidney donation: the Norwegian experience. Am J Transplant 2009;9(4):820–4.

Sickle Cell Disease in Pregnancy

Dennie T. Rogers, MD[a],*, Robert Molokie, MD[b,c,d]

KEYWORDS

- Sickle cell disease • Hemoglobinopathy • Anemia
- Pregnancy • Genetic disease

SICKLE CELL DISEASE: GENETICS, EPIDEMIOLOGY, AND PREGNANCY

The term sickle cell disease (SSD) encompasses several different sickle hemoglobinopathies, including homozygous hemoglobin S (sickle cell anemia Hb SS), the double heterozygote sickle hemoglobin C disease (Hb SC), sickle beta thalassemia plus (Hb $S\beta^+$), sickle beta thalassemia zero (Hb $S\beta^0$), the sickle cell anemias with alpha thalassemia (SS α-thalassemia), and sickle cell anemia with elevated fetal hemoglobin (Hb SS + F).

The sickle mutation is a point mutation in the β-globin gene (GAG to GTG) at the 6 amino acid position, causing valine to replace glutamic acid. The substitution of a hydrophilic amino acid with a hydrophobic one is the root cause of the disease, and allows for sickle hemoglobin to polymerize when it is deoxygenated, triggering a cascade of repeated injury to the red cell membrane, hemolysis, multiple organ dysfunctions, and frequently devastating effects for patients and their families. The mutation is believed to have 4 separate origins in Africa and another in the Indo-European area. The mutation is thought to have evolved, because those with one copy of the sickle gene (sickle cell trait Hb AS) have a survival advantage when infected with *Plasmodium falciparum*.

Approximately 5% of the world's population carries a genetic mutation for a hemoglobinopathy (sickle hemoglobinopathies and thalassemias).[1] The sickle hemoglobinopathies are more common among people whose ancestors are from sub-Saharan Africa, India, Saudi Arabia, and Mediterranean countries. In Africa it is estimated

The author has known disclosures and has not received any funding support for this article.

[a] Department of Obstetrics and Gynecology, University of Illinois at Chicago, 820 South Wood Street, M/C 808, Chicago, IL 60612, USA
[b] Department of Hematology/Medical Oncology, College of Medicine, University of Illinois at Chicago, 820 South Wood Street, M/C 808, Chicago, IL 60612, USA
[c] Department of Biopharmaceutical Sciences, College of Pharmacy, University of Illinois at Chicago, 820 South Wood Street, M/C 808, Chicago, IL 60612, USA
[d] Department of Internal Medicine, Jesse Brown VA Medical Center, Damen Avenue, Chicago, IL 60612, USA
* Corresponding author.
E-mail address: droger3@uic.edu

that more that 200,000 people are born each year with SSD,[1] while in the United States it is estimated that there are 70,000 to 100,000 cases and more than 2 million carriers, making it one of the most common lethal genetic diseases in this country. In the United States, people of all backgrounds have sickle hemoglobinopathies. Every organ system is affected by SSD, and because of its many complications it is probably best that patients are cared for in an interdisciplinary manner, with a hematologist or physician knowledgable in SSD as a member the team.[2]

Pregnancy in women with SSD has become more common as a direct result of improved survival from the advances in medical care and generalized interventions that begin at birth.[3] These interventions include early detection with newborn screening, institution of antibiotic prophylaxis with penicillin, immunization against encapsulated bacteria, and most recently the National Institutes of Health (NIH) consensus recommendation of administering hydroxyurea for its proven role in disease modification.[4] As survival improves, more women affected with SSD reach childbearing age and subsequently face the challenges associated with their fertility and desire for reproduction.

Prior to the last 3 decades maternal and fetal outcomes had been recognized as being associated with high mortality, which prompted many providers to suggest that pregnancy be contraindicated in this group of women.[1] However, many reported observations by investigators over the last 25 years have demonstrated significant improvement in outcomes, and women with SSD are no longer encouraged to avoid or discontinue pregnancy.[5,6]

Improved fetal and maternal outcomes may also be in part a result of advances in antenatal and obstetric care. Although the majority of women with SSD can achieve a successful uncomplicated birth, pregnancy is associated with an increased incidence of medical and pregnancy related complications, resulting in higher rates of morbidity and mortality when compared with their normal hemoglobin (AA) counterparts.[6]

Pregnancy in women with SSD is complicated not only by the maternal condition characterized by years of chronic organ damage, but by the physiologic changes and adaptations that are inherent to all child bearing women. Profound physiologic changes that involve virtually every organ system occur during pregnancy, which are typically well tolerated in healthy gravid woman. These changes are not always benign, particularly in women with underlying diseases, as reflected in the current maternal mortality rate of 8/100,000.[7] The adaptations required by the hematologic, cardiovascular, renal, and respiratory systems are by far the most concerning in women with SSD. Normally, plasma volume begins to expand between 6 and 8 weeks of gestation, ultimately achieving a 45% increase over nonpregnancy volume, 4700 to 5200 mL, at 32 weeks.[8] As a direct response to erythropoietin, red blood cell mass also increases throughout pregnancy, finally reaching 20% to 30% over the nonpregnant state.[8] The combination of increased plasma volume and slower increase in red blood cell mass produces a physiologic anemia of pregnancy (dilutional anemia), which is maximal in the third trimester. There are limited data on serial hematologic adaptation in women with SSD in pregnancy.

The 50% increase in blood volume triggers the cardiovascular system response of creating a hyperdynamic state characterized by a slightly increased resting pulse, increased cardiac output, and benign flow murmurs.[9] By the seventh week a progressive decrease in peripheral vascular resistance accounts for a marked decrease in blood pressure, reaching nadir at 24 to 32 weeks, followed by an increase toward nonpregnant values at term.[10] The glomerular filtration rate increases and remains elevated until after delivery.[11] There is increased minute ventilation as the respiratory system responds with a mild, compensated, respiratory alkalosis.[12] These routine physiologic changes of pregnancy often compound or can exacerbate underlying chronic organ damage initially created by SSD.

PREGNANCY-ASSOCIATED COMPLICATIONS IN SICKLE CELL DISEASE

Many investigators have focused on defining and quantifying the complications associated with SSD in pregnancy.[13–16] Although extremely valuable to our understanding, many of the reports are from single institutions, the majority is retrospective, some have small sample sizes, inclusion of different genotypes, lengthy time periods of data acquisition, as well as vast variability in definitions of stillbirth, acute anemia, and reporting incidences of morbidity and mortality. Due to the origin of the sickle cell gene, reports come from various parts of the world, but create questionable applicability to this condition, which has consistently been characterized by its variable course.[17] All of these factors lend to the difficultly in understanding how SSD and pregnancy affect one another.

Kobak and colleagues[13] published the first report outlining the effects and complications of SSD on pregnancy in 1941. Several additional reports soon followed, each highlighting experiences with this population, noting substantial maternal morbidity and maternal and perinatal mortality associated with pregnancy in women with SSD prior to 1972.[18,19]

Because of the poor perinatal outcomes experienced by sickle gravidas, Koshy and colleagues[15] undertook a landmark trial to determine the benefit of prophylactic blood transfusion at regular intervals compared with transfusion only for specific indications to improve fetal outcome. This prospective randomized, controlled, multicenter NIH-funded cooperative study was performed in pregnant women of greater than 20 weeks' gestation with hemoglobinopathies. Morbidity and mortality data were collected on 189 pregnancies (100 Hb SS, 66 Hb SC, 23 Hb Sβ) and 8981 pregnant, normal (Hb AA) African American controls.

The results failed to demonstrate a reduction in maternal or fetal morbidity and mortality in the sickle cell gravidas that received prophylactic blood transfusions. However, the comparisons clearly identified the obstetric, sickle cell related, and perinatal complications associated with SSD in pregnancy (**Tables 1–3**).

Women with SSD had higher rates of previous pregnancy loss, infection, preeclampsia, and their offspring had greater fetal and neonatal mortality, preterm

Table 1
Frequency of obstetric complications: outcomes from 189 pregnancies, 1979 to 1984

	Genotype			
	AA	**SS**	**SC**	**Sβ/Thal**
Number of subjects	8991	100	66	23
Mean EGA at delivery (weeks)	40	37.5	38.6	37.1
PTD	17%	26%	15%	22%
Previa	0.4%	1%	2%	4%
Preeclampsia	4%	18%	9%	13%
Endometritis	1%	3%	2%	4%

Abbreviations: EGA, estimated gestational age; PTD, preterm delivery.
Data from Koshy M, Burd L. Management of pregnancy in sickle cell syndrome. Hematol Oncol North Am 1991;5(3):585–96.

Table 2
Frequency of perinatal outcomes: outcomes from 189 pregnancies, 1979 to 1984

	Genotype		
	SS	SC	Sβ/Thal
Number of fetuses	104	66	23
IUGR	15.3%	6%	4%
Stillbirth	5.7%	2%	0
Neonatal death	1.9%	0	8%
Perinatal death	7.6%	2%	8%

Abbreviation: IUGR, intrauterine growth restriction.
Data from Koshy M, Burd L. Management of pregnancy in sickle cell syndrome. Hematol Oncol North Am 1991;5(3):585–96.

delivery, fetal distress, and fetal growth abnormalities compared with their normal hemoglobin controls. When hemoglobinopathy genotype comparisons were made, women with SSD overall had more complications compared with those with SC disease. Surprisingly, there were no maternal mortalities reported in this series.[15] Of note, this was the first attempt to manage sickle gravidas based on evidence of treatment effectiveness.

Sun and colleagues[20] reviewed 20 years of deliveries in women with SSD, not part of a prophylactic transfusion program, at Grady Hospital in Atlanta. The study group consisted of women with hemoglobin genotypes SS and SC and they were compared with normal controls. In regard to antepartum complications, women with SS and SC disease were more commonly hospitalized for pain crises, infections (antepartum, postpartum), and acute anemia requiring an average of 5 days of hospitalization. Women with Hb SS had increased risk for preterm labor or premature rupture of membranes, low birth weight, intrauterine growth restriction, and lower gestational age at delivery (mean 34.1 weeks). In contrast, those with Hb SC disease were only at increased risk for intrauterine growth restriction. When women were compared by genotype, women with Hb SS had significantly lower baseline hemoglobin, required twice as many blood transfusions, twice the number of hospitalizations for crises, and had an increased trend in perinatal mortality.[20] Neither Sun and colleagues

Table 3
Frequency of sickle-related complications: outcomes from 189 pregnancies, 1979 to 1984

	Genotype		
	SS	SC	Sβ/Thal
Number of subjects	100	66	23
ACS	7.6%	3%	9%
PE	1%	0%	9%
CHF	3.8%	0%	4%
UTI	10.6%	9%	4%
CRF	2%	0%	0%

Abbreviations: ACS, acute chest syndrome; CHF, congestive heart failure; CRF, chronic renal failure; PE, pulmonary embolism; UTI, urinary tract infection.
Data from Koshy M, Burd L. Management of pregnancy in sickle cell syndrome. Hematol Oncol North Am 1991;5(3):585–96.

nor Koshy and colleagues reported any maternal mortality, and they did not quantitate risks before 20 weeks' gestation.[15,20]

In a unique 2004 investigation Serjeant and colleagues[16] reported a prospectively followed cohort of 94 women with SSD (Hb SS) from birth to 25 years of age, and compared their obstetric outcomes to normal controls obtained through an established newborn screening program. Unlike other investigations, this analysis provided vital gynecologic and obstetric information from the fist half of gestation as well as later pregnancy. Women with SSD had later onset of menarche and an increased rate of spontaneous abortions, 36% versus 10% when compared with controls, and a slight increase in retained placenta following delivery beyond 24 weeks' gestation.[16] The women with SSD also had fewer liveborn infants, and a greater proportion of prematurity, lower mean gestational age at delivery, and lower birth weights (41.7% <2500 g), all significantly affected by the number of sickle related events (eg, pain crisis, acute chest, urinary tract infection) the women experienced during pregnancy.[16] Though not statistically significant, the rate of stillbirth occurred more frequently in the SSD group, 7.1%, versus 0.7% in normal controls. Serjeant and colleagues[16] also ascertained detailed accounts of maternal mortality, reporting a rate of 2.1% in the sickle women.

A more detailed account of maternal mortality and the effect of organized prenatal care were provided by Powars and colleagues[6] between 1972 and 1982, after establishing a comprehensive sickle center and collecting data prospectively; they compared their prospective observations to a historic cohort of sickle cell women. The investigators noted several improvements in obstetric and fetal outcomes: significant 3-week increases in mean gestational age among SSD women, increased birth weights in women with Hb SC disease, and in comparison to only 60% liveborn infants before 1972, nearly 80% of post-1972 infants were born live. There was also a significant decrease in fetal death rate after 1972, declining from 52.7% to 22.7% in women with SSD, a decreased spontaneous abortion rate, and decreased maternal death rate per pregnancy, dropping from 4.1% to 1.7% in the later era.[6]

Powars and colleagues[6] also reported uncomplicated pregnancies in 21% of women with Hb SS genotype, similar to that reported by Serjeant and colleagues, and 43% of those with Hb SC genotype. Their data also suggested that women with Hb SC genotype may represent a subset, which have better survival after 28 weeks' gestation, and fewer obstetric complications when compared with other sickle diseases. These data have proved consistent with those of other investigators and have also provided information on prognosis based on disease variation.

More recently, Villers and colleagues[21] assessed the morbidity and mortality associated with SSD in pregnancy using a large United States database, Nationwide Inpatient Sample from the Healthcare Cost and Use Project of the Agency for Healthcare Research and Quality, and queried all pregnancy-related discharges with a diagnosis of SSD from 2000 to 2003. A total of 17,952 deliveries to women with SSD were compared with 6,756,944 pregnancy-related discharges for women without the disease. The investigators reported that pregnant women with SSD had a significantly higher rate of cesarean delivery, were slightly older, more likely to experience infection (pyelonephritis, postpartum infection, sepsis), thromboembolic events (cerebral vein thrombosis, deep venous thrombosis), pneumonia, and systemic inflammatory response syndrome.[21] Although women with SSD may be more likely to experience stroke and pulmonary embolus, these did not reach significance. Finally, women with SSD were less likely to smoke or have a postpartum hemorrhage and no more likely to have a diagnosis of obesity or substance abuse.[21] Women with SSD accounted for only 0.1% of the pregnancies, but for 1% of all maternal deaths, mortality rate 72.4 deaths per 100,000, compared with nonsickle women, mortality rate 12.7 deaths per 100,000 (with the current United States rate being 8/100,000).[21]

Villers and colleagues[21] also noted that all pregnancy-related complications, with the exception of intrauterine fetal death and gestational diabetes, were significantly more likely among women with SSD including hypertensive disorders of pregnancy (gestational hypertension, preeclampsia, eclampsia), antepartum bleeding, preterm labor, fetal growth restriction, asymptomatic bacteruria, and genitourinary tract infection. Although the associated risks of pregnancy in women with SSD have declined from previous eras, this recent report documents that they remain at great risk for a wider range of morbidities in pregnancy than previously reported, and are at a significantly increased risk of mortality compared with their normal hemoglobin counterparts.

The fetal complications reported in the aforementioned studies all consistently document an increased incidence of fetal growth abnormalities: intrauterine growth restriction or low birth weight.[14–16,20,21] A myriad of hypotheses set forth to explain this consistent observation have ranged from maternal hemoglobin levels, maternal weight, maternal genotype, nutritional deficiencies, hypertensive disorders of pregnancy, uteroplacental insufficiency, gestational age at delivery, or number of sickle-related events during pregnancy.

The Cooperative Study of SSD by Smith and colleagues,[14] including 19 centers, documented that birth weight was influenced by the presence of preeclampsia, acute anemic events, and maternal hemoglobin levels. The Jamaican Cohort noted that birth weight was influenced by maternal genotype (Hb SS compared with Hb AA), gestational age, prepregnancy weight, and the number of prepartum clinical events sustained.[16] In 2007 Thame and colleagues[22] extended the Jamaican Cohort study to further delineate factors that influenced birth weight. Consistent with previous investigators, those with SS disease had infants with lower gestational age, lower birth weight, and lower placental weight. A multivariate analysis revealed that only gestational age and placental weight significantly affected low birth weight.[22] The growth abnormalities were characterized as asymmetric, suggesting a cause occurring later in pregnancy. None of these investigators demonstrated an effect of maternal steady-state hemoglobin (all means >6 g/dL) or fetal hemoglobin on the presence of low birth weight.

The ability to predict the clinical course of SSD during pregnancy is difficult, but may be associated with the level of chronic anemia, considered to have predictive value for comorbidities and mortality in the nonpregnant population.[14] Despite the differences in study design, patient acquisition, management, and variable frequency of adverse outcomes in SSD in pregnancy from 1941 to 2008, several themes consistently emerge. Women with SSD who become pregnant are clearly at increased risk of obstetric, fetal, and sickle cell related complications across each trimester and during the postpartum period, compared with women void of hemoglobinopathies.[13–16,20,22] Those with more severe anemia are more likely to have baseline organ damage, develop more frequent pain crises, and have worsening organ dysfunction, preterm labor, low birth weight neonates, and increased maternal mortality. Albeit despite a myriad of challenges, the majority of these women can achieve a successful pregnancy, including 25% without pain crisis[14] and more than 50% without medically indicated blood transfusion or hospital admission,[15] and the majority tend to deliver beyond 28 weeks' gestation[16] with a greater than 80% live birth rate.[16] Moreover, the majority can undergo more than one successful pregnancy.[6]

PREGNANCY MANAGEMENT IN SICKLE CELL DISORDERS

The cardinal manifestations of SSD are chronic hemolytic anemia and pain crises. Pregnant women with SSD may experience a relatively normal course punctuated by variable frequencies of painful episodes.[23] It is important to realize that chronic organ damage and decreased survival occur despite the number of vaso-occlusive episodes, thus emphasizing the need for access to expert care by providers familiar with the disease process as well as the complexity of the psychological aspects of the illness.[24] Pregnant women with SSD should be managed using a multidisciplinary team approach, comprising a high-risk obstetrician, hematologist, and other specialists as necessary, based on the patient's condition and comorbidities (eg, anesthesia pain specialist, pulmonologist, cardiologist).[2] This type of approach may have a positive impact on associated morbidity and mortality in the mother and her fetus.

Although most women typically know their diagnosis of sickle cell disorder before their pregnancy, a definitive diagnosis or confirmation and characterization by hemoglobin electrophoresis is required. One should avoid solubility tests (eg, Sickledex) for diagnosis, as these are positive in both SSD and sickle trait, and results may be invalid due to the presence of large amounts of Hb F.[25] Also, characterization of adult hemoglobins other than Hb S (eg, Hb C) cannot be discerned with this method. Even though pregnancy outcomes may differ by genotype,[6,15] the management during pregnancy does not change. Women with SSD, Hb SS, and Hb Sβ^0 genotypes, typically experience a greater frequency of pain crises and adverse outcomes, followed by Hb Sβ^+.[14-16,20,21] Women with Hb SC genotype tend to have a relatively more benign nonpregnant course, but are at greater risk of experiencing their initial crisis in pregnancy, tend to be more noncompliant with prenatal care, and have increased risk later in pregnancy.[26] The degree of anemia is most severe in patients with the genotype Hb SS and Hb Sβ^0 thalassemia, milder in Hb Sβ^+, Hb SC disease, and Hb SS with coexistent A thalassemia.[27]

Preconception

Once a diagnosis of SSD is confirmed and characterized, ideally a preconception consultation should occur. The counseling should be tailored appropriately for each patient, providing the information needed to make informed decisions about pregnancy. One should review the effects of pregnancy on SSD, highlighting increased risk for hospital admissions, pain crises, infections, severe anemia, and increased risk of maternal mortality.[21] Likewise, a discussion of the effects of SSD on pregnancy should include increased risks of preterm delivery, placental abnormalities, preeclampsia, and retained placenta.[21,22] The discussion should also entail a review of the effects of SSD on the fetus: increased risk of early pregnancy loss,[16] fetal growth abnormalities, and perinatal mortality, as well as risk for inherited hemoglobinopathies. Knowledge of the father's hemoglobin is required and he therefore should undergo hemoglobin electrophoresis if this is unknown.[28] A genetics consultation to discuss prenatal diagnosis should be offered if the fetus is identified to be at increased risk for a hemoglobinopathy. The objective is not to discourage the patient from pregnancy, as many women with SSD can achieve a successful live birth,[6] but to inform and review the associated medical and pregnancy morbidity, to optimize care, and to minimize complications.

Women with SSD are anemic, and the preconception visit is also an opportunity to optimize the hemoglobin status with addition of 1 to 4 mg folic acid daily, and a multivitamin.[29] Most patients with sickle cell disorders have an abundance of iron secondary to chronic hemolysis and typically do not require iron replacement.

However, iron deficiency does occur in approximately 20% of this population.[30] The diagnosis of iron deficiency may be obscured by the elevated serum iron levels associated with chronic hemolysis or the presence of coexisting undiagnosed thalassemia. This situation necessitates the detection of a low serum ferritin or an elevated serum transferrin level to assure correct diagnosis.[31] If iron status is unknown, the sickle patient should begin prenatal vitamins void of elemental iron, with replacement based on laboratory evaluation to avoid iron overload.

Preconception consultation should optimize nutrition and dietary modifications. Williams and Wang[32] reported that patients with SSD tended to have increased mineral and vitamin deficiencies, perhaps secondary to socioeconomic status or their persistent hypermetabolic state. Supplementation with an appropriate high caloric diet and vitamins should be recommended. Review of appropriate lifestyle changes (eg, smoking cessation) and scheduling of any necessary laboratory or procedures prior to pregnancy should be done. The frequency of prenatal visits, required laboratory testing, and importance of compliance with prenatal visits should be reviewed. Necessary medication changes should be made, assuring that identified teratogenic agents are discontinued before conception. One example is the important disease modification agent hydroxyurea (5HU), which has been demonstrated to improve long-term outcomes in SSD,[4] so many women reaching childbearing age may be undergoing this treatment. 5HU has teratogenic potential as exhibited in mice, and has caused appropriate concern for human fetuses.[33] Although animal model data do not always equate to similar effects in humans, it may be reasonable to determine the need for medication cessation on an individual basis. Data from more than 45 pregnancies conceived on 5HU therapy failed to demonstrate an increase in fetal anomalies or intrauterine fetal death.[34–36] At present, no randomized controlled studies regarding the efficacy and safety in human pregnancies have addressed these concerns. Additional medications that should be discontinued include, but are not limited to, iron chelation therapy, decitabine, and antihypertensives such as angiotensin-converting enzyme inhibitors and teratogens. In the latter case a satisfactory substitute antihypertensive agent such as α-methyldopa or labetalol should be prescribed.

Lastly, immunization status should be reviewed and necessary vaccines given, avoiding those that contain live virus as they are contraindicated in pregnancy. It is recommended that pregnant women with SSD be vaccinated annually for influenza and every 5 years for *Streptococcus pneumoniae*.[37] At present, vaccination for H1N1 influenza is also recommended.[38] These vaccines have been proven safe to be administered during pregnancy.

Pregnancy outpatient management

The authors believe that management of SSD during pregnancy can be best accomplished by separating the goals based on the setting: outpatient versus inpatient management.

The outpatient antepartum clinic management should be directed at initiating measures to prevent pain crises, fetal complications, monitoring baseline organ function, initiating measures to prevent further organ deterioration, identifying early evidence of infection, and avoidance of maternal and fetal mortality.

First Trimester

At the initial high-risk obstetric visit, a detailed medical history should be obtained directed at eliciting factors that influence pregnancy outcome such as alloimmunization, renal disease, and neurologic, pulmonary, or cardiac abnormalities. Preexisting renal disease, pulmonary hypertension, and congestive heart failure all may worsen during the adaptation to pregnancy.[6,39] The comprehensive history should include transfusion history, iron chelation therapy, thrombotic events, cerebrovascular accidents, acute chest syndrome, or chronic ulcers. In-depth information regarding pain crises triggers, locations, and optimal pain management regimen should be obtained.[40]

Baseline hemoglobin/hematocrit with reticulocyte count, antibody screen, blood urea nitrogen, creatinine, 24-hour urine collection, urinalysis and culture, liver function tests (aspartate aminotransferase, alanine aminotransferase), and lactate dehydrogenase are directed at quantifying the chronic hemolytic anemia and organ-specific complications of the renal, cardiac, or pulmonary systems. Trends can be evaluated to suggest an appropriate response or lack thereof to the normal adaptations of pregnancy. Urinary tract infections and pyelonephritis occur more frequently, and persistent urinary tract infections may be secondary to renal papillary necrosis.[14–16,21] All urinary tract infections in this population should be considered complicated, and 10 to 21 days of appropriate antibiotic therapy is required.[41] Because of the chronic hemolytic anemia and increased frequency of urinary tract infections, monthly blood counts, urinalyses, and cultures should be obtained. If any evidence of mineral deficiency or infection is identified they should be treated appropriately.

The recognition of pulmonary hypertension as a cause of early mortality in SSD warrants cardiac evaluation by an echocardiogram and a brain natriuretic peptide level.[42] Ophthalmologic examination should be performed if not done recently, especially if retinopathy has previously been diagnosed.[43] A first trimester sonogram to confirm dating and viability is recommended; this may prove beneficial later in gestation, especially if the fetus develops growth abnormalities. All patients should be given the option of prenatal diagnosis.[44] A major ethical issue pertains to inability to predict the severity of SSD in the fetus, hence the difficulty in counseling patients on prognosis for their child. However, one large survey noted that parents at risk for having a child with SSD were interested in prenatal diagnosis and would consider termination of pregnancy for an affected fetus.[44] Prenatal diagnosis can be safely performed by chorionic villus sampling (CVS) at 10 to 13 weeks or amniocentesis beginning at 15 weeks' gestation.[45] Percutaneous umbilical blood sampling is also available but is associated with a greater fetal risk than CVS or amniocentesis, and is therefore reserved for diagnosis only in centers where DNA-based testing is unavailable.[46]

In the first trimester pregnant women with SSD should be educated on how to avoid pain triggers, analgesia safety in pregnancy, and a plan for a home medication regimen.[40] Patients should be advised on the importance of hydration and adequate fluid intake resulting from the inability to concentrate their urine, thus avoiding the risk of dehydration.[40] Patients should also be aggressively counseled to seek medical attention for any febrile events.[47] Consultation with appropriate subspecialists should be obtained to establish a multidisciplinary plan of management, the team usually including the availability of a maternal fetal medicine specialist, hematologist, nutritionist, social support services, and a tertiary obstetric center.

Second and Third Trimesters

There are no specific therapies or treatments to prevent fetal growth abnormalities or perinatal mortality; however, early detection of growth restriction by measurement of fundal heights and serial ultrasounds can be helpful after a 20-week anatomy survey. Growth scans beginning at 24 to 28 weeks, as well as weekly antepartum testing initiated at 32 weeks, may affect management and improve outcomes. In the case that the fetus is diagnosed with growth restriction, more intensified fetal surveillance should be initiated (eg, increased frequency, Doppler testing). All routine prenatal screening examinations should be performed at the appropriate time. Continuation of monthly blood counts and urine evaluation should also occur. In the third trimester it is important to rescreen all women with SSD for red cell alloantibodies regardless of transfusion history.[48] If alloimmunization is identified, appropriate antepartum management should be undertaken (ie, middle cerebral artery Dopplers, fetal blood typing, and so forth).

Lastly, early arrangements with the blood bank should be made to identify sources of compatible blood. Although prophylactic transfusions have not been demonstrated to improve obstetric and perinatal outcomes in patients with SSD,[15] transfusion therapy is indicated for patients with cardiac or respiratory compromise, acute chest syndrome, hemoglobin levels less than 20% of steady state or less than 5 to 6 g/dL, and pain crisis in the setting of anemia in preparation for cesarean delivery, and is most likely beneficial for those with a previous history of perinatal death or current twin pregnancy.[49] Blood product transfusion is associated with alloimmunization, delayed hemolytic transfusion reactions, iron overload, antibody sensitization, and increased risk for transmission of viral illnesses, and should therefore be reserved for specific medical indications.[49]

Inpatient acute management

The majority of women with SSD are young, relatively healthy, and will carry their fetus safely to term, but more than 70% will experience associated vaso-occlusive pain crises, which is the leading cause (>85%) of emergency evaluation and hospital admissions.[40] Even in pregnancy one of the greatest challenges of SSD remains the vaso-occlusive painful event, and good management is essential. It is unclear whether the number of pain crises experienced during pregnancy correlates with early maternal death or poor fetal outcome.

It is not uncommon for those with a history of few to infrequent pain crises to present for initial episodes that require hospital management, or have an increased frequency of episodes during their pregnancy.[50] Although general consideration of vaso-occlusive severity and genotype has been posited, there is a large amount of variability between and within the different genotypes. Pain crises have been reported to be more frequent with Hb SS, low levels of Hb F, and higher hemoglobin concentrations.[51]

Many patients are familiar with the unfortunate experience of a typical pain crisis, and are usually managed in the home. The main reasons for hospital evaluation typically are failure of their home oral analgesia regimen or symptoms suggesting serious complications.[40] Some present because of uncertainty of the impact of a home analgesia regimen on the fetus. Therefore, an important component of the prenatal management scheme should include compassionate, prompt, effective, and safe relief of acute or chronic pain, optimally by a rapid assessment protocol that is readily available.

Sickle cell pain may involve any part of the body, and typically has a predictable location in an individual patient, but with an onset and severity that is unpredictable.[52] Pain may be precipitated by an event such as cold temperature, dehydration, infection, stress, hemorrhage, and alcohol consumption, but the majority has no identifiable cause.[53] Pain crisis may be associated with prodromal symptoms.[52] The uncomplicated crisis episode typically has duration of a few days to as long as 4 to 10 days, and requires hospital admission.[53] There are no specific clinical or laboratory findings that are pathognomonic of pain crises.[54]

Objective signs of pain on physical examination are usually absent, often creating frustration for the obstetrician and other health care providers. The diagnosis is established by history and physical examination, but often patients can confirm if it is a typical pain crisis or something worse.[52] Although laboratory values are monitored for evidence of complicated crisis, the changes in steady-state hemoglobin values, sickled cells on smear, and white blood cell counts are not reliable indicators of acute vaso-occlusion.[53]

The rapid assessment protocol should be directed at effective and safe relief of pain, assessment for pregnancy-related emergencies, and evaluation for SSD comorbidities. The management of pain crises does not differ during pregnancy.[55] Narcotics are the mainstay of pain management, and can be used in conventional doses and titrated upward as appropriate as women with SSD tend to metabolize narcotics more rapidly. Adjuvant therapies are also critical: hydration, supplemental oxygen, warm temperature, psychological support, and management of narcotic side effects.[40] It should be kept in mind that although hydration is a critical part of management, fluid balance must be monitored carefully. Likewise, inhaled oxygen therapy initially assists with improvement of the vaso-occlusion, but can also cause transient red cell hypoproduction due to supraphysiologic oxygen tensions acutely inhibiting erythropoietin production, and promptly suppressing reticulocytosis within 2 days.[56] Although vaso-occlusive crises cause significant maternal morbidity, it is the associated life-threatening complications associated with SSD that often lead to maternal mortality. It is important to remember that these same comorbid conditions characteristic of the damage caused by SSD can be compounded with pregnancy and prove to be fatal. Therefore, patients who present in the antepartum period with complaints of sickle pain require complete assessment for etiologic factors to tailor management appropriately. The major complications of SSD include sepsis, acute chest syndrome, aplastic crisis, cerebrovascular accident, thrombosis, pulmonary hypertension, cardiomyopathy, and chronic renal failure. Any one or more of these complications can occur during pregnancy and result in maternal demise.[6,21,39]

There is sufficient evidence to suggest that several treatments should be considered for initiation or continued therapy in pregnant patients with SSD. These treatments have demonstrated a decrease in symptoms and complications while improving survival. However, regarding treatment with 5HU, there are insufficient clinical data and trials to make a firm recommendation on its use, efficacy, and teratogenicity during pregnancy.[4]

Inpatient labor and delivery

The type of delivery should be based on routine obstetric practice, as there is no contraindication to vaginal delivery in uncomplicated SSD. Induction of labor at term versus allowing spontaneous labor has not been studied in this population, and should be directed by the individual clinical scenario. Cesarean delivery should be reserved for obstetric indications, and acute pain crisis does not constitute an indication for such management. Prophylactic transfusion before a cesarean delivery to avoid precipitating a crisis due to blood loss is not only acceptable but encouraged in patients with hemoglobins 7 to 8 g/dL or less. Otherwise blood loss should be replaced according to usual obstetric practices.

Pain during labor can be relieved with narcotics, regional anesthesia (epidural, spinal), or local infiltration of anesthesia via a pudendal block.[55,57] Any combination of these may be required depending on whether the patient is in crisis at the onset of labor.

During the postpartum period, women with SSD are at increased risk of thrombo-embolism, infections, dehydration, and worsening anemia.[21] In addition to routine care, hydration with intravenous fluids should be maintained. The risk of thrombosis can be decreased by early ambulation and antiembolic stockings, sequential compression devices, or prophylactic heparin if on bed rest. Hematologic parameters should continue to be assessed and transfusion administered only when indicated. Evidence of infection such as fevers, fundal tenderness, and dysuria should be aggressively diagnosed and treated with antibiotics, as these women are more likely to progress to sepsis and overwhelming infection.[6,15,58]

Breast feeding should be encouraged; few medications are contraindicated in this setting.[59–61] Hydroxyurea is excreted into human milk and there is the potential for adverse effects in the infant, therefore nursing should be considered contraindicated during hydroxyurea therapy. All newborns should be screened for hemoglobinopa-thies as well as routine genetic disorders.

Good prenatal care as described here does not directly affect the sickling process or remove the risk of maternal and fetal complications, but is believed to minimize them, thereby improving overall outcome. When maternal death has been reported, it has been secondary to a preexisting medical complication, which pregnancy may have exacerbated in an already compromised woman.[6,16,22] Hence, the importance of continued medical surveillance from before conception to well after delivery must be emphasized.

SUMMARY

The ability to predict the clinical course of SSD during pregnancy is difficult. Outcomes have improved for pregnant women with SSD and nowadays the majority can achieve a successful live birth. However, pregnancy is associated with an increased incidence of morbidity and mortality. Optimal management during pregnancy should be directed at preventing pain crises, chronic organ damage, and early mortality using a multidis-ciplinary team approach and prompt, effective, and safe relief of acute pain episodes. Although these measures do not remove the risk of maternal and fetal complications, they are thought to minimize them, promoting a successful pregnancy outcome for women with SSD.

REFERENCES

1. World Health Organization. Sickle-cell anaemia: report by the secretariat. 59th World health Assembly; 2006.
2. Yu CK, Stasiowska E, Stephens A, et al. Outcome of pregnancy in sickle cell disease patients attending a combined obstetric and haematology clinic. J Obstet Gynaecol 2009;29(6):512–6.
3. Platt OS, Brambilla DJ, Rosse WF, et al. Mortality in sickle cell disease. Life expectancy and risk factors for early death. N Engl J Med 1994;330(23):1639–44.
4. National Institutes of Health Consensus Development Conference Proceedings. Hydroxyurea treatment for sickle cell disease, February 25–27, 2008.
5. Charche S, Scott J, Niebl J, et al. Management of SSD in pregnant patient. Obstet Gynecol 1980;55:407–10.
6. Powars DR, Sandhu M, Niland-Weiss J, et al. Pregnancy in SSD. Obstet Gynecol 1986;67:217–28.
7. Hoyert DL. Maternal mortality and related concepts. National Center for Health Statistics. Vital Health Stat 3 2007;33:1–13.

8. Samuels P. Hematologic complications of pregnancy. In: Gabbe SG, Niebyl JA, Simpson JL, editors. Obstetrics: normal and problem pregnancies. 4th edition. Philadelphia: Churchill Livingstone; 2002. p. 1169–93.

9. Gilson GJ, Samaan S, Crawford MH, et al. Changes in hemodynamics, ventricular remodeling, and ventricular contractility during normal pregnancy: a longitudinal study. Obstet Gynecol 1997;89:957–67.

10. Halligan A, O'Brien E, O'Malley K, et al. Twenty four hour ambulatory blood pressure measurement in a primigravid population. J Hypertens 1993;11: 869–75.

11. Blackburn ST, Loper DL. Maternal adaptation to pregnancy. In: Polin RA, Fox WW, Abman SH, editors. Maternal, fetal, and neonatal physiology: a clinical perspective. Philadelphia (PA): WB Saunders; 1992. p. 201–12.

12. Awe RJ, Nicotra MB, Newsom TD, et al. Arterial oxygenation and alveolar-arterial gradients in term pregnancy. Obstet Gynecol 1979;53:182–6.

13. Kobak AJ, Stien PJ, Daro AF. Sickle cell anemia in pregnancy. A review of the literature and report of six cases. Am J Obstet Gynecol 1941;41:811–21.

14. Smith J, Espeland M, Bellevue R, et al. Pregnancy in sickle cell disease: experience of the cooperative study of sickle cell disease. Obstet Gynecol 1996;87(2): 199–204.

15. Koshy M, Burd L, Wallace D, et al. Prophylactic red-cell transfusions in pregnant patients with SSD. A randomized cooperative study. N Engl J Med 1988;319(22): 1447–52.

16. Serjeant GR, Loy LL, Crowther M, et al. Outcome of pregnancy in homozygous SSD. Obstet Gynecol 2004;103(6):1278–85.

17. Taylor JG. Chronic hyper-hemolysis in sickle cell anemia: association of vascular complications and mortality with less frequent vasoocclusive pain. PLoS One 2008;3(5):e2095.

18. Adams JQ, Whitacre FE, Diggs LW. Pregnancy and sickle cell disease. Obstet Gynecol 1953;2:335–52.

19. Eisenstien MI, Posner AC, Friedman S. Sickle cell anemia in pregnancy: a review of the literature with additional case histories. Am J Obstet Gynecol 1956;72: 622–34.

20. Sun PM, Wilburn W, Raynor D, et al. SSD in pregnancy: twenty years of experience at Grady Memorial Hospital, Atlanta, Georgia. Am J Obstet Gynecol 2001;184:1127–30.

21. Villers MS, Jamison MG, DeCastro LM, et al. Morbidity associated with SSD in pregnancy. Am J Obstet Gynecol 2008;1:e1–5.

22. Thame M, Lewis J, Trotman H, et al. The mechanisms of low birthweight in infants of mothers with homozygous SSD. Pediatrics 2007;120:686–92.

23. Smith WR, Penberthy LT, Bovbjerg VE, et al. Daily assessment of pain in adults with sickle cell disease. Ann Intern Med 2008;148(2):94–101.

24. Wilkie D, Molokie R, Boyd-Seal D, et al. Patient reported outcomes: descriptors of nociceptive and neuropathic pain and barriers to effective pain management in adult outpatients with sickle cell disease. J Natl Med Assoc 2010;102(1):18–27.

25. Goldberg CA. The ferrohemoglobin solubility test; its accuracy and precision together with values found in the presence of some abnormal hemoglobins. Clin Chem 1958;4:146–9.

26. Rahimy M, Gangbo A, Adjou R, et al. Effect of active prenatal management on pregnancy outcome in sickle cell disease in an African setting. Blood 2000; 96(5):1685–9.

27. Bonds D. Three decades of innovation in the management of sickle cell disease: the road to understanding the sickle cell disease clinical phenotype. Blood Rev 2005;19:99–110.

28. Ingram VM. Gene mutations in human haemoglobin: the chemical difference between normal and sickle cell haemoglobin. Nature 1957;180(4581):326–8.

29. Claster S, Vichinsky EP. Managing sickle cell disease. BMJ 2003;327(7424): 1151–5.

30. Markham MJ, Lottenberg R, Zumberg M. Role of phlebotomy in the management of hemoglobin SC disease: case report and review of the literature. Am J Hematol 2003;73(2):121–5.

31. Thinkhamrop J, Apiwantanakul S, Lumbiganon P, et al. Iron status in anemic pregnant women. J Obstet Gynaecol 2003;29:160–3.

32. Williams R, Wang W. Children with sickle cell disease may benefit from improved nutrition practices. J Am Diet Assoc Oct 1985;94:739–43.

33. Yan J, Hales B. Depletion of glutathione induces 4-hydroxynonenal protein adducts and hydroxyurea teratogenicity in organogenesis stage mouse embryo. J Pharmacol Exp Ther 2006;319:613–21.

34. Thauvin-Robinet C, Maingueneau C, Robert E, et al. Exposure to hydroxyurea during pregnancy: a case series. Leukemia 2001;8:1309–11.

35. Diav-Citrin O, Hunnisett L, Sher G, et al. Hydroxyurea use during pregnancy: a case report in sickle cell disease and review of the literature. Am J Hematol 1999;60:148–50.

36. Hasley C, Roberts I. The role of hydroxyurea in sickle cell disease. Br J Haematol 2003;120:177–86.

37. Halasa NB, Shankar SM, Talbot TR, et al. Incidence of invasive pneumococcal disease among individuals with sickle cell disease before and after the introduction of the pneumococcal conjugate vaccine. Clin Infect Dis 2007;44(11): 1428–33.

38. Zaman K, Roy E, Arifeen S, et al. Effectiveness of maternal influenza immunization in mothers and infants. N Engl J Med 2008;359:1555–64.

39. Hassel K. Pregnancy and sickle cell disease. Hematol Oncol Clin North Am 2005; 19:903–16.

40. Rees D. Guidelines for the management of the acute painful crisis in sickle cell disease. Br J Haematol 2003;120:744–52.

41. Gilstrap LC III, Cunningham FG, Whaley PJ. Acute pyelonephritis in pregnancy, an anterospective study. Obstet Gynecol 1981;57:409–13.

42. Castro O, Gladwin MT. Pulmonary hypertension in sickle cell disease: mechanisms, diagnosis, and management. Hematol Oncol Clin North Am 2005;19(5): 881–96.

43. Emerson GG, Lutty GA. Effects of sickle cell disease on the eye: clinical features and treatment. Hematol Oncol Clin North Am 2005;19(5):957–73.

44. Kototey-Ahulu FID. The sickle cell disease patient: natural history from a clinicoepidemiological study of the first 1550 patients of Korle Bu Hospital Sickle Cell Clinic. J Med Genet 1996;76:302–5.

45. Chang J, Golbus M, Kan Y. Antenatal diagnosis of sickle cell anaemia by direct analysis of the sickle mutation. Lancet 1981;318(8256):1127–9.

46. Kan Y, Trecartin R, Golbus M, et al. Prenatal diagnosis of B thalassaemia and sickle-cell anaemia experience with 24 cases. Lancet 1977;8006:269–71.

47. Steiner CMJ. Sickle cell disease patients in U.S. Hospitals, 2004. HCUP statistical brief #21. Rockville (MD): Agency for Healthcare Research and Quality; December 2006. p. 200.

48. Mohomed K. Prophylactic versus selective blood transfusion for sickle cell anaemia during pregnancy. Cochrane Database Syst Rev 1996;(2): CD000040.

49. Josephson C, Su L, Hillyer C, et al. Transfusion in the patient with sickle cell disease: a critical review of the literature and transfusion guidelines. Transfus Med Rev 2007;21:118–33.

50. Faron G, Corbisier C, Tecco L, et al. First sickle cell crisis triggered by induction of labor in primigravida. Eur J Obstet Gynecol Reprod Biol 2001;94:304–6.

51. Platt O, Thorington BD, Brambilla DJ, et al. Pain in sickle cell disease: rates and risk factors. N Engl J Med 1991;325:11–6.

52. Ballas SK. Sickle cell anemia with few painful crises is characterized by decreased red cell deformability and increased number of dense cells. Am J Hematol 1991;36(2):122–30.

53. Adams S. Caring for the pregnant woman with sickle cell crisis. Prof Care Mother Child 1996;6:34–6.

54. Martin JJ, Moore GP. Pearls, pitfalls, and updates for pain management. Emerg Med Clin North Am 1997;15(2):399–415.

55. Firth PG, Alvin C. Sickle cell disease and anesthesia. J Am Anesthesiol 2004; 101(3):766–85.

56. Embury SH, Garcia JF, Mohandas N, et al. Effects of oxygen inhalation on endogenous erythropoietin kinetics, erythropoiesis, and properties of blood cells in sickle cell anemia. N Engl J Med 1984;311:291–5.

57. Finer P, Blair J, Rowe O. Epidural analgesia in the management of labor pain and sickle cell crisis—a case report. Anesthesiology 1988;68(5):799–800.

58. Rappaport VJ, Velazquez M, Williams K. Hemoglobinopathies in pregnancy. Obstet Gynecol Clin North Am 2004;31(2):287–317.

59. Fort AT, Morrison JC, Berreras L, et al. Counseling the patient with SSD about reproduction. Pregnancy outcome does not justify the maternal risk. Am J Obstet Gynecol 1971;111:324.

60. Gaston MH, Verter JL, Woods G, et al. Prophylaxis with oral penicillin in children with sickle cell anemia: a randomized trial. N Engl J Med 1986;314:1593–9.

61. Mansouri HA, Anfanan N. Sickle cell disease in pregnancy. Bahrain Medical Bulletin 2005;4:27–9.

Abnormal Placentation, Angiogenic Factors, and the Pathogenesis of Preeclampsia

Michelle Silasi, MD[a], Bruce Cohen, MD[a],
S. Ananth Karumanchi, MD[a,b,c], Sarosh Rana, MD[a,d],*

KEYWORDS

- Pregnancy • Preeclampsia • Hypertension
- Angiogenic factors

Preeclampsia (PE) is a disorder occurring after week 20 of pregnancy and marked by hypertension and proteinuria. It is the major cause of maternal and fetal morbidity worldwide, and a leading cause of maternal and fetal morbidity and mortality in the United States. It is believed that PE is mediated by toxic factors that induce widespread injury to the maternal vascular endothelium, leading to dysfunction of the kidneys, liver, brain, and blood coagulation system.[1] Furthermore, the placenta plays a key role in this pathogenesis; abnormal placentation occurs first, which is followed by secretion of placental toxic factors that in turn induce widespread endothelial dysfunction. The authors' laboratory recently characterized several angiogenic factors

S.A.K is listed as a coinventor on multiple patents filed by the Beth Israel Deaconess Medical Center for the use of angiogenic proteins for the diagnosis and therapy of preeclampsia. S.A.K. is a consultant to Abbott Diagnostics (Abbott Park, IL, USA), Beckman Coulter (Chaska, MN, USA), Roche diagnostics (Mannheim, Germany) and Johnson & Johnson (New Brunswick, NJ, USA). SR is funded by 5K12 HD001255-08 (National Institutes of Health/National Institute of Child Health and Human Development).

[a] Division of Maternal Fetal Medicine, Department of Obstetrics and Gynecology, Beth Israel Deaconess Medical Center, Harvard Medical School, 330 Brookline Avenue, Kirstein 3182, Boston, MA 02215, USA
[b] Division of Nephrology, Department of Medicine, Beth Israel Deaconess Medical Center, Harvard Medical School, 330 Brookline Avenue, Kirstein 3182, Boston, MA 02215, USA
[c] Howard Hughes Medical Institute, 25 Francis Avenue, Cambridge, MA 02138, USA
[d] Department of Obstetrics and Gynecology, Beth Israel Deaconess Medical Center, Harvard Medical School, 330 Brookline Avenue, Kirstein 3182, Boston, MA 02215, USA
* Corresponding author. Department of Obstetrics and Gynecology, Beth Israel Deaconess Medical Center, 330 Brookline Avenue, Kirstein 3182, Boston, MA 02215.
E-mail address: srana1@bidmc.harvard.edu

Obstet Gynecol Clin N Am 37 (2010) 239–253
doi:10.1016/j.ogc.2010.02.013
0889-8545/10/$ – see front matter

and demonstrated how they contribute to the maternal endothelial dysfunction and clinical features of PE. This article will include a review of information on the clinical aspects, management, and molecular pathogenesis of PE, specifically focusing on the role of these recently characterized angiogenic factors.

CLINICAL FEATURES, MANAGEMENT AND COMPLICATIONS OF PE
Clinical Features

Worldwide, PE affects 3% to 5% of all pregnancies, making it the most common medical complication of pregnancy.[2] It is associated with a perinatal and neonatal mortality rate of 10%.[3] Risk factors for PE include primiparity, multifetal gestation, extremes of age in the mother, and a previous history of PE. In addition, medical comorbidities such as obesity, hypercoagulable states, chronic hypertension, renal disease, lupus, and diabetes mellitus also increase the risk of PE.[3–6] Furthermore, evidence has suggested that if a woman's mother, mother-in-law, grandmother, or sister had PE, she herself is at higher risk of developing the disease, suggesting a possible genetic predisposition.[7,8] Long interpregnancy time interval also has been implicated as a risk factor for PE.[9] It was once thought that a new partner increased the risk, but this is confounded by increased time between pregnancies. After approximately 10 years, a multiparous woman's risk for PE approaches that of a primiparous woman.[10]

PE is first suspected when a patient presents with new-onset hypertension, with or without proteinuria in the second half of pregnancy. Hypertension is defined as two blood pressure readings of at least 140/90 occurring on two separate occasions (more than 6 hours apart) after 20 weeks of gestation in a patient without an antecedent history of hypertension. Proteinuria is defined as a 24-hour urine collection having greater than 300 mg/dl of protein. More recently, the urinary protein to creatinine (P:C) ratio has become the preferred method for quantification of proteinuria in the nonpregnant population. Its use to estimate 24-hour protein excretion for the diagnosis of PE, however, has been controversial. A meta-analysis showed a pooled sensitivity of 84% and specificity of 76% using P:C ratio cutoff of greater than 30 mg/mmol, as compared with the gold standard of 24-hour urine protein excretion greater than 300 mg/d.[11]

Other symptoms include evidence of central nervous system irritation such as unrelenting headache or scotomata, as well as right upper quadrant or midepigastric pain. Edema no longer is included in the diagnostic criteria, as it is too nonspecific a finding, occurring in most normal pregnancies. On the other hand, the sudden onset of severe nondependent edema (ie, in the hands and face) is often noticed by the patient or her family, and could be the only symptom of the disease. Laboratory values that support the diagnosis of PE include evidence of hemolysis (such as elevated lactate dehydrogenase [LDH]) or hemoconcentration, thrombocytopenia, elevated liver enzymes (in patients with hemolysis elevated liver enzymes and low platelets [HELLP] syndrome), elevated creatinine, and uric acid. None of these laboratory values, however, are specific for PE, and laboratory tests can be normal even in severe cases of PE.

Given this wide constellation of findings, the differential diagnosis is extensive, making the diagnosis of PE sometimes difficult. For example, gestational hypertension is elevated blood pressure (using the same criteria as in PE) with no proteinuria. Women with mild gestational hypertension at or after term have similar outcomes compared with women with normotensive pregnancies, with the exception of more induction of labor and cesarean delivery. On the contrary, women with severe gestational hypertension have rates of placental abruption, preterm delivery, and small-for-gestational age babies similar to women with severe PE.[12] In addition, gestational hypertension can be associated with features of PE, such as elevated liver enzymes, hemolysis, or seizures.[13] Elevated liver enzymes also are seen in acute fatty liver of pregnancy, further confusing the picture. Patients with underlying medical conditions that share some features of PE also complicate the diagnosis. For example, in patients with chronic hypertension, blood pressure can be elevated secondary to underlying hypertension. In chronic kidney diseases such as lupus, proteinuria may already be present because of renal manifestations of the disease. This makes accurate diagnosis of PE very challenging. Treatment of these patients also presents management dilemmas, as pregnancy prolongation and treatment of underlying disease will be an option in contrast to PE, where prompt delivery usually is indicated. Currently there are no clinically available biomarkers that are specific to PE. However there is increasing evidence that there is angiogenic imbalance in patients with true PE, particularly who are at risk for complications such as preterm delivery or fetal growth restriction. The authors discuss the use of these biomarkers in screening and diagnosis of PE later in this article.

Complications

PE is a complex disease that can lead to complications in multiple organ systems. Central nervous system complications include eclampsia (generalized tonic clonic seizures), which complicates approximately 2% of PE cases in the United States. Although most cases of eclampsia occur as a progression from PE, it can happen without evidence of hypertension or proteinuria. Up to one third of eclampsia cases occur postpartum, even days to weeks after delivery.[14] Acute renal failure, liver failure, pulmonary edema, and HELLP syndrome are additional complications. HELLP syndrome is characterized by hemolysis, elevated liver enzymes, and low platelets. It is considered a severe variant of PE, and is associated with a higher risk of maternal and neonatal adverse outcomes than PE alone.

Recently literature has accumulated about long-term consequences of PE including increased risk of cardiovascular disease, renal disease, and stroke. Approximately 20% of women with PE develop hypertension or microalbuminuria within 7 years, compared with only 2% of women with normotensive pregnancies.[15] The long-term risk of cardiovascular and cerebrovascular disease is doubled in women with PE and gestational hypertension compared with age-matched controls.[16,17] Severe PE, recurrent PE, PE with preterm birth, and PE with growth restriction are most strongly associated with adverse cardiovascular outcomes. This increased risk of long-term cardiovascular disease is independent of whether the woman had vascular risk factors before the development of PE.

Fetal complications secondary to PE include intrauterine growth restriction, prematurity, placental abruption, and increased risk of perinatal death. PE is a leading cause of iatrogenic premature delivery and contributes significantly to increasing health cost associated with prematurity.

Management and Treatment

Management of PE depends on the severity of the disease and the gestational age of the patient. Strategies focus on maintaining the health status of the mother, while attempting to reduce neonatal morbidity for the fetus. Preterm gestational ages (before 37 completed weeks) require individual patient assessment. Patients less than 32 weeks with mild PE are managed expectantly while administering antenatal steroids. Close observation and surveillance are warranted for signs of severity. Upon becoming diagnosed as severe, delivery is indicated. If severe PE does not develop, the patient is delivered at 37 weeks. Very preterm pregnancies (<32 weeks) with severe PE may be appropriate candidates for expectant management to administer antenatal steroids. This protocol, proposed by Sibai[18,19] involves giving magnesium sulfate for seizure prophylaxis, checking serial laboratory values, and close monitoring of blood pressures for 48 hours. After 48 hours, the magnesium can be discontinued, but close in-house observation must continue to monitor for declining clinical status or signs of severity. Once this happens, delivery is indicated. Otherwise, the patient may remain pregnant until 34 weeks. PE at term (at least 37 weeks) is managed by immediate delivery. A recent large multicenter randomized controlled trial (HYPITAT) in the Netherlands enrolled patients with a singleton pregnancy at 36 to 41 weeks' gestation with either gestational hypertension or mild PE and randomized them to undergo either induction of labor or expectant monitoring. This study found that women in the induction of labor group had a lower rate of development of poor maternal outcome (relative risk 0.71, 95% confidence interval [CI] 0.59 to 0.86, $P<.0001$).[20]

PATHOGENESIS OF PE
Placental Vascular Development in Health and in Disease

Evidence implicates the placenta is a major determinant in the development of PE. This evidence includes

Resolution of most signs and symptoms of PE within 48 hours following delivery of the placenta

PE has been reported in molar pregnancies where there is no fetus present

PE can occur postpartum in the presence of retained placental fragments.[19,21–26]

The recently proposed mechanism of the pathogenesis of PE involves abnormal placentation that leads to the release of vascular endothelial-damaging antiangiogenic factors. During normal placentation, cytotrophoblast cells aggregate and anchor the embryo to the uterine wall. They then invade the interstitium of the decidua and maternal uterine spiral arteries to provide the fetus a pathway for accessing nutrients and oxygen while excreting waste products. To accomplish this, the placenta must form new blood vessels and increase the number of already existing blood vessels. During the first few weeks of pregnancy, placentation begins with the differentiation of cytotrophoblast stem cells into primary villi, cores of cytotrophoblast cells surrounded by a layer of syncytiotrophoblast. As these cores of primary villi fill with mesenchymal cells, secondary villi form. These mesenchymal cells will differentiate into hemangiogenic precursor cells that later will form the lining of the first blood vessels in the placenta, and Hofbauer cells, which are macrophages that may play a role in vasculogenesis[27] and trophoblast differentiation.[28] The cytotrophoblast cells located within the villi also differentiate into extravillous trophoblast (EVT) cells. When the villi anchor to the maternal endometrium, the syncytiotrophoblast layer disappears, allowing EVT cells to migrate into the maternal tissue, where they gravitate toward the maternal spiral arteries. A complex physiologic remodeling of these vessels ensues, by which the normal muscular and elastic structures of the spiral arteries are partially replaced by EVT cells. These physiologic changes occur in the spiral arteries as far as the inner third of the myometrium. During this process, EVT cells change from an epithelial phenotype to a more endothelial phenotype as reflected by changes in the expression of cell surface adhesion molecules.[29] The EVT cells widen and strengthen the diameter of the vessel walls, resulting in large-bore, low-resistance spiral arteries that can provide the growing fetus an optimal blood supply of blood. Plugs of endovascular trophoblast cells form within the distal segments of the maternal arteries. These plugs serve as barriers, preventing maternal blood from flowing into the intervillous space. As vascular remodeling of the spiral arteries continues; the trophoblast plugs become loose, allowing blood flow, and subsequently, oxygen transport between the mother and the intervillous space. Oxygen tension measurements in the intervillous space up to 10 weeks of gestation are approximately 20 mm Hg.[30] This relatively hypoxic environment switches to a more normoxic environment as maternal blood supplies oxygen to the intervillous space. Oxygen tension levels rise threefold, with highest levels in the peripheral areas of the developing placenta and lowest levels toward the center. Peak pO_2 is about 60 mm Hg at 16 weeks of gestation. The rise in oxygen levels not only stimulates the growth of the fetus, but also causes an upregulation of a range of adhesion molecules by cytotrophoblast cells that facilitate trophoblast invasion. When there is a deficient blood supply from the mother, prolonged hypoxia occurs, with detrimental effects to the formation of the placental vasculature.

Abnormal placentation occurs in preeclamptic patients as evidenced by shallow or absent remodeling of the maternal spiral arteries.[31] Histologic studies show that the physiologic remodeling of the spiral arteries is incomplete.[32,33] The spiral arteries in the myometrium retain their endothelial linings and muscular walls, thereby retaining their high-resistance phenotype. This failure of vascular remodeling may be the initial insult in the pathogenesis of PE. In addition, defects in the phenotypic switching of cellular adhesion molecules have been characterized in preeclamptic patients. For example, trophoblast cells from preeclamptic pregnancies fail to switch the expression of epithelial cell-associated cell surface integrins to an endothelial phenotype, thereby limiting their invasive potential.[34] It also has been hypothesized that decidual natural killer (NK) cells or activated macrophages may play a role in the vascular remodeling noted during pregnancy, and this process may be altered in PE.[35]

Angiogenic Growth Factors

Although several molecules are involved in angiogenesis and vascular homeostasis, this discussion only will include factors such as vascular endothelial growth factor (VEGF), placental growth factor (PIGF), soluble fms like tyrosine kinase (sFlt1) and soluble endoglin (sEng), as these have been implicated in the pathogenesis of human PE.

VEGF is a homodimeric disulfide-linked glycoprotein involved in both angiogenesis (the growth of new blood vessels from existing ones) and vasculogenesis (de novo formation of blood vessels).[36,37] VEGF family members include VEGF-A, (PIGF, VEGF-B, VEGF-C, and VEGF-D), and two not expressed in mammals (viral VEGF-E and snake venom VEGF-F).[38,39] Increased production of VEGF has been implicated in cancer, where it is thought to help the cancer grow and metastasize.[40] VEGF acts on endothelial cells by binding to its receptors, VEGFR-1 and VEGFR-2. Expression of VEGF also is induced by low oxygen tension environments. VEGF-A affects endothelial cells, mediating increased vascular permeability, inducing angiogenesis and vasculogenesis and endothelial cell growth. Murine studies show that both homozygote and heterozygote knockout mice of the VEGF-A gene die in the embryonic period because of defects in angiogenesis.[41,42] VEGF-B does not appear to play such an important role in angiogenesis as VEGF-A. It functions more to maintain the newly formed blood vessels under pathologic conditions.[43] Pathologic overexpression of VEGF-C causes lymphedema. PIGF is expressed by the placental trophoblast

Further, overexpression of sFlt1 causes PE-like signs and symptoms in rats including hypertension, proteinuria, and glomerular endotheliosis.[64] sEng has been shown to amplify the vascular damage mediated by sFlt1 in pregnant rats, inducing a severe PE-like syndrome with features of HELLP syndrome and fetal growth restriction.[69] Neutralizing circulating sFlt1 by coadministration of VEGF results in a reduction of hypertension and proteinuria and reverses the damaging effects of sFlt1 on the kidneys in mice and in rats.[70,71]

Recently four different splice variants of sFlt1 have been described (sFlt1_v1 to v4). Three out of these four variants are up-regulated in the placentas of women with PE.[72] The sFlt14 variant is primate-specific.[73] It appears to be the predominant VEGF-inhibiting protein and is dramatically increased in preeclamptic placentas, specifically in syncytial knots.[74] More work is needed to understand the role of the various isoforms of sFlt1 during normal placentation and in diseased states such as PE.

The regulatory mechanism of sFlt1 is not well understood, but several pathways have been suggested. Hypoxia has been shown to increase the production of sFlt1 in vitro.[65–67] Angiotensin 2, a potent vasoconstrictor has been implicated in the regulation of sFlt1. Infusion of angiotensin 2 increases circulating levels of sFlt1 in pregnant mice and stimulates the production of sFlt1 from human villous explants and cultured trophoblasts.[75] Heme oxygenase and carbon monoxide have been shown to inhibit the production of sFlt1 from endothelial cells and placental explants.[76] Importantly, both decreased hemoxygenase and increased angiotensin signaling due to the presence of a circulating autoantibody against angiotensin receptor have been reported in people with PE.[70,77] Therefore, these pathways may be one of the proximal etiologies for the increased sFlt1 and sEng production noted in PE.

Despite these advances, there are several unanswered questions related to the role of sFlt1 and sEng in the pathogenesis of PE. Little is known about the role of sFlt1 and sEng in normal placental development and in placental pseudovasculogenesis. Although placental hypoxia has been implicated in the overproduction of sFlt1, the precise mechanisms of this process are poorly understood. It is noteworthy that sFlt1 is elevated in most, but not all patients with mild PE.[57] The relationship of sFlt1 with known risk factors for PE, such as obesity or pre-existing hypertension, is not clear. It is possible that a threshold level of sFlt1 is required to cause PE and that this threshold is lowered by the existence of concomitant risk factors.

CLINICAL IMPLICATIONS FOR ANGIOGENESIS RESEARCH

In light of the changes noted in angiogenic factors seen in women with PE, multiple studies have proposed using angiogenic factors for screening. Data from retrospective studies have shown significant elevations in both maternal sFlt1 and sEng from midgestation onward, and this rise seems to occur 5 to 8 weeks before PE onset.[52,53,59,78] Elevations in both sEng and the sFlt1:PIGF ratio seen in the late second and early third trimester are associated with a significantly high risk for the development of preterm PE.[59] Also, the sFlt1/PIGF ratio has been suggested as an index of antiangiogenic activity that reflects changes in both biomarkers[79] and is a better predictor of PE compared with either measure alone.[59] In a recent large prospective longitudinal cohort study for risk assessment for PE, midtrimester PLGF/sEng X sFlt1 had a sensitivity of 100%, specificity of 95.3%, negative predictive value (NPV) of 100%, and positive likelihood of 57.6.[80] In all the studies, levels of angiogenic proteins were measured by enzyme-lined immunosorbent assay (ELISA); however, recently automated assays for sFlt1 and PIGF have been reported that have coefficient of variation under 5%, and results are available in less than 30 minutes. Using automated assays on clinical laboratory platforms, two different studies have demonstrated the clinical utility of serum sFlt1/PLGF ratios as an aid in the diagnosis of PE with receiver operating characteristic (ROC) curves greater than 0.97.[81,82] Both sFlt1 and sEng have been shown to correlate with PE complications such as abruption, IUGR, or early onset disease.[83,84] Finally, measurement of urinary PlGF has been proposed as a low cost screening strategy that would be followed by confirmation of serum sFlt1/PlGF ratio.[79] Prospective studies to test this hypothesis are still ongoing.

In addition to measurement of angiogenic proteins alone, combination of different screening techniques such as abnormal uterine artery Doppler in early pregnancy could be used for screening in combination with angiogenic factors.[85–87] Several studies show that the combination of the measurement of uterine perfusion in the second trimester and analysis of angiogenic markers have a high detection rate for PE, especially early onset PE.[88–90] A recent study found that the combination of abnormal uterine artery Doppler and low serum PlGF in the second trimester was strongly associated with early onset and severe PE.[91]

The discovery of the changes in key angiogenic factors in women with PE is opening new doors to the development of accurate and reliable screening methods for the detection of PE. This would allow early diagnosis and management as well as proper intervention. Given that the management of PE is gestational age-dependent, a proper screening or diagnostic tool would need not only to predict that PE is going to develop, but would also require predicting the time interval for development. Previous methods targeting screening for PE have largely been inaccurate and have not been used for widespread implementation into the clinical setting.[92] The use of angiogenic factors for prediction of PE continues to be actively explored.

Besides using angiogenic proteins to predict PE, potential treatment of PE may include factors that can reverse the antiangiogenic imbalance seen in PE. VEGF-121, a novel variant of VEGF-A, has been used in an sFlt1 rat model of PE.[71] Treatment of the rats with VEGF121 alleviated preeclamptic symptoms and reversed 125 of 268 sFlt1-induced changes in gene expression. VEGF-121 also was found to reverse the hypertension and improve glomerular filtration rate and vascular reactivity in a rat model of reduced uterine artery perfusion.[93] Other strategies such as neutralizing antibodies against these antiangiogenic proteins or agents such as statins that block the production of these antiangiogenic proteins are being pursued by several laboratories.

Implications for Long-term Women's Health

Previously, PE was thought to be a condition confined to pregnancy that resolved with delivery of the placenta; however, recent large studies have demonstrated that PE has long-term associations with cardiovascular disease, renal disease, and increased mortality.[17,94] An increased serum concentration of sFlt1 during pregnancy also has been shown to be associated with subclinical hypothyroidism during pregnancy and reduced thyroid function later in life.[95]

SUMMARY

PE is a complex disorder affecting multiple organ systems resulting in serious maternal and fetal morbidity and mortality. Angiogenic factors have been shown to be important players in the development of this condition, by targeting the maternal systemic vascular endothelium and inducing the clinical signs and symptoms of the disease. As of now, there is no reliable or accurate means of predicting the development of PE, but future studies using the time sequence of the changes seen in these factors may lead to a much needed and valuable screening method to be used in routine clinical practice. Furthermore, strategies looking at restoring the balance of these dysregulated factors may pave the way toward variable treatment options for this devastating disease.

REFERENCES

1. Roberts JM, Taylor RN, Musci TJ, et al. Preeclampsia: an endothelial cell disorder. Am J Obstet Gynecol 1989;161(5):1200–4.
2. Wang A, Rana S, Karumanchi SA. Preeclampsia: the role of angiogenic factors in its pathogenesis. Physiology (Bethesda) 2009;24:147–58.
3. Sibai B, Dekker G, Kupferminc M. Preeclampsia. Lancet 2005;365(9461): 785–99.
4. Alderman BW, Sperling RS, Daling JR. An epidemiological study of the immuno-genetic aetiology of pre-eclampsia. Br Med J (Clin Res Ed) 1986;292(6517): 372–4.
5. Bhattacharya S, Campbell DM, Liston WA. Effect of body mass index on pregnancy outcomes in nulliparous women delivering singleton babies. BMC Public Health 2007;7:168.
6. Roman H, Robillard PY, Hulsey TC, et al. Obstetrical and neonatal outcomes in obese women. West Indian Med J 2007;56(5):421–6.
7. Carr DB, Epplein M, Johnson CO, et al. A sisters risk: family history as a predictor of preeclampsia. Am J Obstet Gynecol 2005;193:965–72.
8. Esplin MS, Fausett MB, Fraser A, et al. Paternal and maternal components of the predisposition to preeclampsia. N Engl J Med 2001;344(12):867–72.
9. Tuffnell DJ, Jankowicz D, Lindow SW, et al. Outcomes of severe preeclampsia/eclampsia in Yorkshire 1999/2003. BJOG 2005;112(7):875–80.
10. Skjaerven R, Wilcox AJ, Lie RT. The interval between pregnancies and the risk of preeclampsia. N Engl J Med 2002;346(1):33–8.
11. Cote AM, Brown MA, Lam E, et al. Diagnostic accuracy of urinary spot protein: creatinine ratio for proteinuria in hypertensive pregnant women: systematic review. BMJ 2008;336(7651):1003–6.
12. Sibai BM. Diagnosis and management of gestational hypertension and preeclampsia. Obstet Gynecol 2003;102(1):181–92.
13. Buchbinder A, Sibai BM, Caritis S, et al. Adverse perinatal outcomes are significantly higher in severe gestational hypertension than in mild preeclampsia. Am J Obstet Gynecol 2002;186(1):66–71.
14. Sibai BM. Diagnosis, prevention, and management of eclampsia. Obstet Gynecol 2005;105(2):402–10.
15. Nisell H, Lintu H, Lunell NO, et al. Blood pressure and renal function seven years after pregnancy complicated by hypertension. Br J Obstet Gynaecol 1995; 102(11):876–81.
16. Ray JG, Vermeulen MJ, Schull MJ, et al. Cardiovascular health after maternal placental syndromes (CHAMPS): population-based retrospective cohort study. Lancet 2005;366(9499):1797–803.
17. Irgens HU, Reisaeter L, Irgens LM, et al. Long-term mortality of mothers and fathers after preeclampsia: population-based cohort study. BMJ 2001; 323(7323):1213–7.

18. Sibai BM, Barton JR. Expectant management of severe preeclampsia remote from term: patient selection, treatment, and delivery indications. Am J Obstet Gynecol 2007;196(6):514, e1–9.

19. Bombrys AE, Barton JR, Nowacki EA, et al. Expectant management of severe preeclampsia at less than 27 weeks' gestation: maternal and perinatal outcomes according to gestational age by weeks at onset of expectant management. Am J Obstet Gynecol 2008;199(3):247, e1–6.

20. Koopmans CM, Bijlenga D, Groen H, et al. Induction of labour versus expectant monitoring for gestational hypertension or mild preeclampsia after 36 weeks' gestation (HYPITAT): a multicentre, open-label randomised controlled trial. Lancet 2009;374(9694):979–88.

21. Norwitz ER, Repke JT. Preeclampsia prevention and management. J Soc Gynecol Investig 2000;7(1):21–36.

22. Report of the National High Blood Pressure Education Program Working Group on high blood pressure in pregnancy. Am J Obstet Gynecol 2000;183(1):S1–22.

23. Newman RB, Eddy GL. Association of eclampsia and hydatidiform mole: case report and review of the literature. Obstet Gynecol Surv 1988;43(4):185–90.

24. Brittain PC, Bayliss P. Partial hydatidiform molar pregnancy presenting with severe preeclampsia prior to twenty weeks gestation: a case report and review of the literature. Mil Med 1995;160(1):42–4.

25. Shembrey MA, Noble AD. An instructive case of abdominal pregnancy. Aust N Z J Obstet Gynaecol 1995;35(2):220–1.

26. Matsuo K, Kooshesh S, Dinc M, et al. Late postpartum eclampsia: report of two cases managed by uterine curettage and review of the literature. Am J Perinatol 2007;24(4):257–66.

27. Seval Y, Korgun ET, Demir R. Hofbauer cells in early human placenta: possible implications in vasculogenesis and angiogenesis. Placenta 2007;28(8–9):841–5.

28. Khan S, Katabuchi H, Araki M, et al. Human villous macrophage-conditioned media enhance human trophoblast growth and differentiation in vitro. Biol Reprod 2000;62(4):1075–83.

29. Zhou Y, Fisher SJ, Janatpour M, et al. Human cytotrophoblasts adopt a vascular phenotype as they differentiate. A strategy for successful endovascular invasion? J Clin Invest 1997;99(9):2139–51.

30. Jauniaux E, Watson AL, Hempstock J, et al. Onset of maternal arterial blood flow and placental oxidative stress. A possible factor in human early pregnancy failure. Am J Pathol 2000;157(6):2111–22.

31. Brosens IA, Robertson WB, Dixon HG. The role of the spiral arteries in the pathogenesis of preeclampsia. Obstet Gynecol Annu 1972;1:177–91.

32. Gerretsen G, Huisjes HJ, Elema JD. Morphological changes of the spiral arteries in the placental bed in relation to pre-eclampsia and fetal growth retardation. Br J Obstet Gynaecol 1981;88(9):876–81.

33. Meekins JW, Pijnenborg R, Hanssens M, et al. A study of placental bed spiral arteries and trophoblast invasion in normal and severe pre-eclamptic pregnancies. Br J Obstet Gynaecol 1994;101(8):669–74.

34. Zhou Y, Damsky CH, Fisher SJ. Preeclampsia is associated with failure of human cytotrophoblasts to mimic a vascular adhesion phenotype. One cause of defective endovascular invasion in this syndrome? J Clin Invest 1997;99(9):2152–64.

35. Kopcow HD, Karumanchi SA. Angiogenic factors and natural killer (NK) cells in the pathogenesis of preeclampsia. J Reprod Immunol 2007;76:23–9.

36. Connolly DT. Vascular permeability factor: a unique regulator of blood vessel function. J Cell Biochem 1991;47(3):219–23.

37. Nagy JA, Dvorak AM, Dvorak HF. VEGF-A(164/165) and PlGF: roles in angiogenesis and arteriogenesis. Trends Cardiovasc Med 2003;13(5):169–75.
38. Shibuya M, Claesson-Welsh L. Signal transduction by VEGF receptors in regulation of angiogenesis and lymphangiogenesis. Exp Cell Res 2006; 312(5):549–60.
39. Takahashi H, Shibuya M. The vascular endothelial growth factor (VEGF)/VEGF receptor system and its role under physiological and pathological conditions. Clin Sci (Lond) 2005;109(3):227–41.
40. Dvorak HF. Vascular permeability factor/vascular endothelial growth factor: a critical cytokine in tumor angiogenesis and a potential target for diagnosis and therapy. J Clin Oncol 2002;20(21):4368–80.
41. Carmeliet P, Ferreira V, Breier G, et al. Abnormal blood vessel development and lethality in embryos lacking a single VEGF allele. Nature 1996; 380(6573):435–9.
42. Ferrara N, Carver-Moore K, Chen H, et al. Heterozygous embryonic lethality induced by targeted inactivation of the VEGF gene. Nature 1996;380(6573):439–42.
43. Zhang F, Tang Z, Hou X, et al. VEGF-B is dispensable for blood vessel growth but critical for their survival, and VEGF-B targeting inhibits pathological angiogenesis. Proc Natl Acad Sci U S A 2009;106(15):6152–7.
44. Yamazaki Y, Morita T. Molecular and functional diversity of vascular endothelial growth factors. Mol Divers 2006;10(4):515–27.
45. Olofsson B, Korpelainen E, Pepper MS, et al. Vascular endothelial growth factor B (VEGF-B) binds to VEGF receptor-1 and regulates plasminogen activator activity in endothelial cells. Proc Natl Acad Sci U S A 1998;95(20):11709–14.
46. Carmeliet P, Moons L, Luttun A, et al. Synergism between vascular endothelial growth factor and placental growth factor contributes to angiogenesis and plasma extravasation in pathological conditions. Nat Med 2001;7(5):575–83.
47. Hiratsuka S, Nakamura K, Iwai S, et al. MMP9 induction by vascular endothelial growth factor receptor-1 is involved in lung-specific metastasis. Cancer Cell 2002;2(4):289–300.
48. Murakami M, Zheng Y, Hirashima M, et al. VEGFR1 tyrosine kinase signaling promotes lymphangiogenesis as well as angiogenesis indirectly via macrophage recruitment. Arterioscler Thromb Vasc Biol 2008;28(4):658–64.
49. Kendall RL, Wang G, Thomas KA. Identification of a natural soluble form of the vascular endothelial growth factor receptor, FLT-1, and its heterodimerization with KDR. Biochem Biophys Res Commun 1996;226(2):324–8.
50. Shibuya M. Structure and function of VEGF/VEGF-receptor system involved in angiogenesis. Cell Struct Funct 2001;26(1):25–35.
51. Jones RL, Stoikos C, Findlay JK, et al. TGF-beta superfamily expression and actions in the endometrium and placenta. Reproduction 2006;132(2):217–32.
52. Levine RJ, Maynard SE, Qian C, et al. Circulating angiogenic factors and the risk of preeclampsia. N Engl J Med 2004;350(7):672–83.
53. Wathen KA, Tuutti E, Stenman UH, et al. Maternal serum-soluble vascular endothelial growth factor receptor-1 in early pregnancy ending in preeclampsia or intrauterine growth retardation. J Clin Endocrinol Metab 2006;91(1):180–4.
54. McKeeman GC, Ardill JE, Caldwell CM, et al. Soluble vascular endothelial growth factor receptor-1 (sFlt-1) is increased throughout gestation in patients who have preeclampsia develop. Am J Obstet Gynecol 2004;191(4):1240–6.
55. Hertig A, Berkane N, Lefevre G, et al. Maternal serum sFlt1 concentration is an early and reliable predictive marker of preeclampsia. Clin Chem 2004;50(9): 1702–3.

56. Chaiworapongsa T, Romero R, Espinoza J, et al. Evidence supporting a role for blockade of the vascular endothelial growth factor system in the pathophysiology of preeclampsia. Young Investigator Award. Am J Obstet Gynecol 2004;190(6): 1541–7 [discussion: 1547–50].

57. Powers RW, Roberts JM, Cooper KM, et al. Maternal serum soluble fms-like tyrosine kinase 1 concentrations are not increased in early pregnancy and decrease more slowly postpartum in women who develop preeclampsia. Am J Obstet Gynecol 2005;193(1):185–91.

58. Livingston JC, Chin R, Haddad B, et al. Reductions of vascular endothelial growth factor and placental growth factor concentrations in severe preeclampsia. Am J Obstet Gynecol 2000;183(6):1554–7.

59. Levine RJ, Lam C, Qian C, et al. Soluble endoglin and other circulating antiangiogenic factors in preeclampsia. N Engl J Med 2006;355(10):992–1005.

60. Bdolah Y, Lam C, Rajakumar A, et al. Twin pregnancy and the risk of preeclampsia: bigger placenta or relative ischemia? Am J Obstet Gynecol 2008;198(4):428 e421–6.

61. Kanter D, Lindheimer MD, Wang E, et al. Angiogenic dysfunction in molar pregnancy. Am J Obstet Gynecol 2010;202(2):184, e1–5.

62. Koga K, Osuga Y, Tajima T, et al. Elevated serum soluble fms-like tyrosine kinase 1 (sFlt1) level in women with hydatidiform mole. Fertil Steril 2009. [Epub ahead of print].

63. Bdolah Y, Palomaki GE, Yaron Y, et al. Circulating angiogenic proteins in trisomy 13. Am J Obstet Gynecol 2006;194(1):239–45.

64. Maynard SE, Min JY, Merchan J, et al. Excess placental soluble fms-like tyrosine kinase 1 (sFlt1) may contribute to endothelial dysfunction, hypertension, and proteinuria in preeclampsia. J Clin Invest 2003;111(5):649–58.

65. Nagamatsu T, Fujii T, Kusumi M, et al. Cytotrophoblasts up-regulate soluble fms-like tyrosine kinase-1 expression under reduced oxygen: an implication for the placental vascular development and the pathophysiology of preeclampsia. Endocrinology 2004;145(11):4838–45.

66. Shore VH, Wang TH, Wang CL, et al. Vascular endothelial growth factor, placenta growth factor and their receptors in isolated human trophoblast. Placenta 1997; 18(8):657–65.

67. Gu Y, Lewis DF, Wang Y. Placental productions and expressions of soluble endoglin, soluble fms-like tyrosine kinase receptor-1, and placental growth factor in normal and preeclamptic pregnancies. J Clin Endocrinol Metab 2008;93(1):260–6.

68. Ahmad S, Ahmed A. Elevated placental soluble vascular endothelial growth factor receptor-1 inhibits angiogenesis in preeclampsia. Circ Res 2004;95(9):884–91.

69. Venkatesha S, Toporsian M, Lam C, et al. Soluble endoglin contributes to the pathogenesis of preeclampsia. Nat Med 2006;12(6):642–9.

70. Bergmann A, Ahmad S, Cudmore M, et al. Reduction of circulating soluble Flt-1 alleviates preeclampsia-like symptoms in a mouse model. J Cell Mol Med 2009. [Epub ahead of print].

71. Li Z, Zhang Y, Ying Ma J, et al. Recombinant vascular endothelial growth factor 121 attenuates hypertension and improves kidney damage in a rat model of preeclampsia. Hypertension 2007;50(4):686–92.

72. Heydarian M, McCaffrey T, Florea L, et al. Novel splice variants of sFlt1 are up-regulated in preeclampsia. Placenta 2009;30(3):250–5.

73. Thomas CP, Andrews JI, Raikwar NS, et al. A recently evolved novel trophoblast-enriched secreted form of fms-like tyrosine kinase-1 variant is up-regulated in hypoxia and preeclampsia. J Clin Endocrinol Metab 2009;94(7):2524–30.

74. Sela S, Itin A, Natanson-Yaron S, et al. A novel human-specific soluble vascular endothelial growth factor receptor 1: cell-type-specific splicing and implications to vascular endothelial growth factor homeostasis and preeclampsia. Circ Res 2008;102(12):1566–74.

75. Zhou CC, Ahmad S, Mi T, et al. Angiotensin II induces soluble fms-like tyrosine kinase-1 release via calcineurin signaling pathway in pregnancy. Circ Res 2007;100(1):88–95.

76. Cudmore M, Ahmad S, Al-Ani B, et al. Negative regulation of soluble Flt-1 and soluble endoglin release by heme oxygenase-1. Circulation 2007;115(13): 1789–97.

77. Irani RA, Xia Y. The functional role of the renin–angiotensin system in pregnancy and preeclampsia. Placenta 2008;29(9):763–71.

78. Park CW, Park JS, Shim SS, et al. An elevated maternal plasma, but not amniotic fluid, soluble fms-like tyrosine kinase-1 (sFlt-1) at the time of midtrimester genetic amniocentesis is a risk factor for preeclampsia. Am J Obstet Gynecol 2005;193: 984–9.

79. Levine RJ, Thadhani R, Qian C, et al. Urinary placental growth factor and risk of preeclampsia. JAMA 2005;293(1):77–85.

80. Kusanovic JP, Romero R, Chaiworapongsa T, et al. A prospective cohort study of the value of maternal plasma concentrations of angiogenic and antiangiogenic factors in early pregnancy and midtrimester in the identification of patients destined to develop preeclampsia. J Matern Fetal Neonatal Med 2009;22(11): 1021–38.

81. Verlohren S, Galindo A, Schlembach D, et al. An automated method for the determination of the sFlt-1/PlGF ratio in the assessment of preeclampsia. Am J Obstet Gynecol 2010;202(2):161, e1–11.

82. Sunderji S, Gaziano E, Wothe D, et al. Automated assays for sVEGF R1 and PlGF as an aid in the diagnosis of preterm preeclampsia: a prospective clinical study. Am J Obstet Gynecol 2010;202(1):40, e1–7.

83. Signore C, Mills JL, Qian C, et al. Circulating angiogenic factors and placental abruption. Obstet Gynecol 2006;108(2):338–44.

84. Signore C, Mills JL, Qian C, et al. Circulating soluble endoglin and placental abruption. Prenat Diagn 2008;28(9):852–8.

85. Poon LC, Karagiannis G, Leal A, et al. Hypertensive disorders in pregnancy: screening by uterine artery Doppler imaging and blood pressure at 11-13 weeks. Ultrasound Obstet Gynecol 2009;34(5):497–502.

86. Poon LC, Staboulidou I, Maiz N, et al. Hypertensive disorders in pregnancy: screening by uterine artery Doppler at 11-13 weeks. Ultrasound Obstet Gynecol 2009;34(2):142–8.

87. Grill S, Rusterholz C, Zanetti-Dallenbach R, et al. Potential markers of preeclampsia—a review. Reprod Biol Endocrinol 2009;7:70.

88. Stepan H, Unversucht A, Wessel N, et al. Predictive value of maternal angiogenic factors in second trimester pregnancies with abnormal uterine perfusion. Hypertension 2007;49(4):818–24.

89. Stepan H, Geipel A, Schwarz F, et al. Circulatory soluble endoglin and its predictive value for preeclampsia in second-trimester pregnancies with abnormal uterine perfusion. Am J Obstet Gynecol 2008;198(2):175, e171–6.

90. Savvidou MD, Noori M, Anderson JM, et al. Maternal endothelial function and serum concentrations of placental growth factor and soluble endoglin in women with abnormal placentation. Ultrasound Obstet Gynecol 2008;32(7): 871–6.

91. Espinoza J, Romero R, Nien JK, et al. Identification of patients at risk for early onset and/or severe preeclampsia with the use of uterine artery Doppler velocimetry and placental growth factor. Am J Obstet Gynecol 2007;196(4):326, e1–13.

92. Conde-Agudelo A, Villar J, Lindheimer M. World Health Organization systematic review of screening tests for preeclampsia. Obstet Gynecol 2004;104(6): 1367–91.

93. Gilbert JS, Verzwyvelt J, Colson D, et al. Recombinant vascular endothelial growth factor 121 infusion lowers blood pressure and improves renal function in rats with placentalischemia-induced hypertension. Hypertension 2010;55(2): 380–5.

94. Vikse BE, Irgens LM, Leivestad T, et al. Preeclampsia and the risk of end-stage renal disease. N Engl J Med 2008;359(8):800–9.

95. Levine RJ, Vatten LJ, Horowitz GL, et al. Preeclampsia, soluble fms-like tyrosine kinase 1, and the risk of reduced thyroid function: nested case-control and population based study. BMJ 2009;339:b4336.

Update on Gestational Diabetes

Gabriella Pridjian, MD*, Tara D. Benjamin, MD

KEYWORDS

- Gestational diabetes • Pregnancy complications
- Glyburide • Insulin

Gestational diabetes mellitus (GDM), diabetes first diagnosed in pregnancy, complicates about 5% to 10% of pregnancies, which is an expected wide range of prevalence, given the variation in populations studied, the current variability in screening and diagnosis,[1] and a recent disproportionate increase in younger, obese women.[2]

GLUCOSE METABOLISM AND GESTATIONAL DIABETES

In normal pregnancy, directly or indirectly, the growth of the fetal-placental unit increases cortisol, growth hormone, human placental lactogen, estrogen, progesterone, and prolactin, which in concert lead to hyperinsulinemia, insulin resistance, fasting hypoglycemia, and postprandial hyperglycemia.[3–5] A progressive transition of fuel sources occurs so that by the third trimester, the metabolic fuel to meet the demands of the fetus changes from predominately maternal carbohydrate to fat.

Pregnancy is characterized by increased and adaptive pancreatic beta-cell function to compensate for decreased insulin sensitivity and increased requirements.[6] Morphologically, maternal pancreatic hypertrophy and hyperplasia occur.[7] In response to elevated insulin levels, peripheral muscle glucose use and tissue glycogen storage increase in an effort to maintain normal insulin sensitivity in the first trimester of pregnancy.[8–10] As gestation advances, these responses become inadequate to meet the energy requirements of the fetus, and insulin resistance develops.[11,12]

Insulin resistance in normal pregnancy is estimated to increase by 40% to 70%, predominantly in the third trimester. In a longitudinal study of healthy pregnant women using the hyperinsulinemic-euglycemic clamp, Catalano and colleagues[11] found a 56% decrease in insulin sensitivity in nonobese women by late pregnancy. Using the euglycemic-hyperinsulinemic clamp, Sivan and colleagues[13] demonstrated that healthy women developed insulin resistance mostly in the third trimester and showed a 40% reduction in peripheral glucose uptake by muscle in the third trimester compared with the nonpregnant state. Using a minimal model technique, Buchanan

Division of Maternal-Fetal Medicine, Department of Obstetrics and Gynecology, Tulane University Medical School, 1430 Tulane Avenue, SL11, New Orleans, LA 70112, USA
* Corresponding author.
E-mail address: Pridjian@Tulane.edu

Obstet Gynecol Clin N Am 37 (2010) 255–267
doi:10.1016/j.ogc.2010.02.017
0889-8545/10/$ – see front matter © 2010 Elsevier Inc. All rights reserved.

and colleagues[14] found that insulin sensitivity in normal pregnant women was reduced to about one-third of that of nonpregnant women of similar weight and age. Furthermore, the reduction in insulin sensitivity was compensated by reciprocal increase of the first and second phase insulin response.

There seems to be no significant change in insulin receptor binding in pregnancy[15]; thus insulin resistance in normal pregnancy is likely related to postreceptor handling of glucose. Postreceptor mechanisms contributing to insulin resistance include (1) impaired tyrosine kinase activity,[16] which is normally responsible for the phosphorylation of cellular substrates; (2) decreased expression of insulin receptor substrate-1, a cytosolic protein that binds phosphorylated intracellular substrates and transmits signals downstream[17]; and (3) decreased expression of the GLUT4 glucose transport protein in adipose tissue, which promotes glucose uptake.[18] The cytokine tumor necrosis factor α[19] and leptin may also be involved in insulin resistance seen in normal pregnancy.[20,21]

Compared with normal pregnant women, women with GDM have impaired beta-cell function and reduced beta-cell adaptation resulting in insufficient insulin secretion to maintain normal glycemia. Women with GDM, and more so obese women with GDM, have greater insulin resistance and less endogenous hepatic glucose production than non-GDM women.[22] Catalano and colleagues[23] used the hyperinsulinemic-euglycemic clamp in a longitudinal study to assess insulin sensitivity and endogenous glucose metabolism in obese and nonobese pregnant women with and without GDM. These investigators found that obese women who develop GDM have a decreased insulin sensitivity along with suppression of hepatic glucose production during insulin infusion. Shao and colleagues[16] noted a more profound drop in tyrosine kinase activity in women with gestational diabetes when compared with healthy normal women, suggesting a postreceptor mechanism abnormality as at least one cause of the increased insulin resistance in GDM.

Pregnancy-induced insulin resistance unmasks the beta-cell defects, which underlie GDM. These defects range from beta-cell dysfunction secondary to autoimmune factors or chronic insulin resistance or highly penetrant genetic abnormalities of insulin secretion.[1]

SCREENING AND DIAGNOSIS

There has been a question regarding the need to diagnose and treat mild hyperglycemia in pregnancy[24,25]; however, recent evidence has quieted the debate. Crowther and colleagues[26] showed that treatment of hyperglycemia in pregnancy improved neonatal outcomes. The long-awaited Hyperglycemia and Adverse Pregnancy Outcomes (HAPO) study made unambiguous the linear positive association between maternal glycemia and adverse pregnancy outcomes.[27,28] The study was a prospective, blinded, international, and multicentered 10-year study, with 25,505 pregnant women enrolled. The objective of the study was to clarify risks of adverse pregnancy outcomes associated with degrees of maternal glucose intolerance less severe than overt diabetes. Women were excluded from the study and their clinicians informed of test results if fasting plasma glucose was more than 105 mg/dL (5.8 mmol/L), or the 2-hour value greater than or equal to 200 mg/dL (11.2 mmol/L), or a random plasma glucose greater than or equal to 160 mg/dL (8.9 mmol/L). An additional random plasma glucose was collected between 34 and 37 weeks to identify possible late development of GDM; hypoglycemic women were also excluded. Routine prenatal and neonatal care was delivered in each of the 15 centers. The study investigators reported a significant association between maternal hyperglycemia and their primary outcomes, birth weight greater than the 90th percentile, cesarean section, and cord plasma C-peptide level, reflective of fetal hyperinsulinemia. The degree of association for each outcome was graded across the spectrum of maternal hyperglycemia, with even mild maternal hyperglycemia of one standard deviation more than the mean associated with their primary outcomes (**Table 1**). Landon and colleagues[29] recently reported for the Maternal-Fetal Medicine Network a multicenter study of 958 women, in which mild GDM was compared with normal glycemia. Women with mild GDM had more overgrown babies, shoulder dystocia, cesarean delivery, preeclampsia, and gestational hypertension. The network investigators concluded that treatment of mild GDM is beneficial.

There continues to be no resolution regarding the best method for screening or diagnosis of GDM. The current practice in the United States is 2-step testing, screening, and diagnosis. Universal screening (screening every pregnant woman) is practiced by most obstetricians in the United States[30] because this method is associated with fewer errors of omission that might occur in a busy obstetric practice. However, now the American College of Obstetricians and Gynecologists[31] and the American Diabetes Association [32] recognize that there are low-risk women who do not need screening. The US Preventive Services Task Force[33] suggests that physicians do not need to screen routinely for GDM but do need to discuss screening with each woman and make a case-by-case decision.

In the United States alone, an abnormal screening test has variability with the O'Sullivan 50-g glucose, 1-hour screening test cutoff ranging from 130 to 140 mg/dL (7.2–7.8 mmol/L). Even the next diagnostic step, the 3-hour, 100-g glucose tolerance test has at least 2 different glucose algorithms that are used for diagnosis of GDM: the National Diabetes Data Group[34] and Carpenter-Coustan criteria (**Table 2**).[35] Most clinicians outside the United States use a 1-step, 2-hour, 75-g glucose tolerance test for detection. A fasting plasma glucose level is obtained; then, after a 75-gm glucose load, 1-hour and 2-hour plasma glucose levels are measured. Variability in screening and detection has been difficult to resolve because of lack of consensus on the level of glycemia associated with adverse pregnancy outcomes[36] until the recent HAPO study.

Table 1
Mild Hyperglycemia and Pregnancy Outcome Study

| Risk Factor | Adjusted Odds Ratio[a] | | |
	Birth Weight (>90th Percentile)	Primary Cesarean	Cord C-Peptide Level (>90th Percentile)
Fasting Plasma Glucose>1 SD (6.9 mg/dL, 0.4 mmol/L)	1.38 (1.32–1.44)	1.11 (1.06–1.15)	1.55 (1.47–1.64)
1-h Plasma Glucose>1 SD (30.9 mg/dL, 1.7 mmol/L)	1.46 (1.39–1.53)	1.10 (1.06–1.15)	1.46 (1.38–1.54)
2-h Plasma Glucose>1 SD (23.5 mg/dL, 1.3 mmol/L)	1.28 (1.32–1.44)	1.08 (1.03–1.26)	1.37 (1.30–1.44)

Women with blood sugar levels in the gestational diabetes range were excluded from the study. All 3 primary outcomes were significantly increased.
Abbreviation: SD, standard deviation.
[a] Odds ratio (95% confidence interval).
Data from The HAPO Study Cooperative Research Group. Hyperglycemia and adverse pregnancy outcome. N Engl J Med 2008;358:1991–2.

Table 2
Diagnostic parameters for the 3-hour, 100-g glucose tolerance test

Time of Value	National Diabetes Data Group Criteria		Carpenter-Coustan Criteria	
	mg/dL	mmol/L	mg/dL	mmol/L
Fasting	105	5.8	95	5.3
1 h	190	10.6	180	10.0
2 h	165	9.2	155	8.6
3 h	145	8.0	140	7.8

Two or more values met or exceeded required to make diagnosis.
Data from National Diabetes Data Group. Classification and diagnosis of diabetes mellitus and categories of glucose intolerance. Diabetes 1979;28:1039–57 and Carpenter MR, Coustan DR. Criteria for screening tests for gestational diabetes. Am J Obstet Gynecol 1982;144:768–73.

In addition to providing definitive confirmation of the association of hyperglycemia with adverse pregnancy outcome, the HAPO study[27] showed a positive, near-linear correlation between hyperglycemia and adverse pregnancy outcome. The HAPO study information should allow experts and stakeholders to reach a consensus on glycemic levels for diagnosis of GDM, which should be forthcoming.

Risk factors for GDM provide the basis for targeted screening. GDM is most frequent in women with prior GDM, severe obesity, or a sibling with diabetes. Many other risk factors are described (**Table 3**).[37–46] More recently published associations with GDM include periodontal disease,[47,48] low maternal birth weight,[49] and high consumption of sugar-sweetened colas (see **Table 3**).[50]

Table 3
Risk factors for gestational diabetes

Risk Factor	Odds Ratio	References
Overweight	2	Torloni et al; Chu et al
Obesity	3.7	Torloni et al; Chu et al
Severe Obesity	7	Torloni et al; Chu et al
Prior Gestational Diabetes	23	McGuire et al
Prior Macrosomic Infant	3.3	McGuire et al
Maternal Age Greater than 25 y	1.4	Cypryk et al
Maternal Age Greater than 35 y	2.3	Xiong et al
Multiple Gestation	2.2[a]	Rauh-Hain et al
South East Asian	7.6[a]	Dornhorst et al
Hispanic	2.4[a]	Dooley et al
African American	1.8[a]	Dooley et al
Polycystic Ovarian Syndrome	2.9	Toulis et al
Parent with Diabetes	3.2	Kim et al
Sibling with Diabetes	7.1	Kim et al
Periodontal Disease	2.6	Xiong et al
Low Maternal Birth Weight	1.9	Seghieri et al

[a] Relative risk compared with white race.
Data from Refs. [47,49]

Women at very high risk of development of GDM, such as those with obesity or prior GDM, may benefit from early screening in the first trimester. If early screening is normal, screening is repeated at 24 to 26 weeks of gestation.

MATERNAL AND FETAL RISKS

Glucose travels freely from the mother to the fetus, but maternal insulin does not. Thus, untreated hyperglycemia exposes the fetus to higher concentrations of glucose than normal, forcing the fetus to increase its own insulin production. Unfortunately, excess insulin produced by the fetus results in macrosomia, either from excessive fat deposition or as a direct growth effect of insulin. Mean maternal plasma glucose levels[51] and fetal blood insulin levels[52] are strongly associated with neonatal birth weight. Maternal glycemia during third trimester and prepregnancy body mass index are independent predictors of birth weight in pregnancies complicated by GDM.[53]

The occurrence of GDM imparts significant and long-lasting health risks on mother and baby (**Table 4**). Fetal programming in utero increases the risk of obesity and obesity-related complications in children of mothers with diabetes.[54]

MONITORING

Close monitoring and treatment of GDM are important to the long-term health of a pregnant woman and her baby. The fifth International Workshop-Conference on Gestational Diabetes recommended the following blood glucose concentrations: fasting plasma glucose of 90 to 99 mg/dL (5.0–5.5 mmol/L), 1-hour postprandial plasma glucose less than 140 mg/dL (<7.8 mmol/L), and 2-hour postprandial plasma glucose less than 120 to 127 mg/dL (<6.7–7.1 mmol/L).[1] Baseline and interval hemoglobin A_{1c} levels during treatment are helpful, particularly in women who have fasting hyperglycemia.

Most women with GDM on diet treatment alone monitor capillary blood glucose levels 4 times a day (fasting blood glucose once a day and postprandial blood glucose thrice a day); women on pharmaceutical therapy often monitor 4 to 6 times a day and include preprandial values. Weekly in-office monitoring and daily self-monitoring seem

Table 4
Health risks of gestational diabetes

Mother	Fetus	Newborn	Child/Adult
Birth trauma	Hyperinsulinemia	Respiratory distress syndrome	Obesity
Increased cesarean delivery	Cardiomyopathy	Hypoglycemia	Type 2 diabetes
Preeclampsia/ Gestational hypertension	Stillbirth	Hypocalcemia	Metabolic syndrome
Type 2 diabetes	Large for gestational age/ macrosomia	Hypomagnesemia	
Metabolic syndrome	Birth trauma	Hyperviscosity	
		Polycythemia	
		Hyperbilirubinemia	
		Cardiomyopathy	

to have comparable outcomes in perinatal mortality and morbidity. However, Hawkins and colleagues[55] suggested that women with daily, more frequent monitoring may have less macrosomia.

Women on dietary and exercise therapy alone with normal self-monitored blood glucose levels can decrease the frequency of monitoring to twice a day. Our center prefers a fasting blood glucose and 1 other postprandial level per day, alternated throughout the week.

DIET AND EXERCISE

The initial treatment for GDM continues to be diet and exercise. Generally, a 1900- to 2400-kcal/d diet with carbohydrate restriction to 35% to 40% of calories is prescribed, calculated on ideal prepregnancy body weight and using complex and high-fiber carbohydrates.[56] The assistance of a trained dietician is ideal for tailoring dietary needs for each woman.

Dietary therapy delays pharmacologic therapy. Moses and colleagues[57] used a low-glycemic diet as treatment for GDM and in a prospective fashion showed that a low-glycemic diet decreased the need and timing for insulin. Most women lose weight during the initial weeks of dietary therapy but then resume modest weight gain. Insufficient dietary calories can be judged by excessive hunger, excessive weight loss, or persistent ketonuria.

If exercise is not contraindicated for other obstetric complications of pregnancy, it can improve glycemic control in any type of diabetes. Women with GDM should be asked to walk 1 to 2 miles at least 3 times a week, if possible.

PHARMACOLOGIC THERAPY

Pharmacologic therapy is most commonly instituted once diet and exercise have failed as evidenced by abnormality in more than half of self-monitored glucose values or an abnormal value in those women tested weekly. Traditionally, insulin has been the drug of choice because of its safety in pregnancy, lack of significant transplacental passage, and history of use. Most women can be treated as outpatients. The recommended initial insulin dose for pregnancy is based on maternal weight and can be calculated by the following guidelines to determine total daily insulin needs: 0.8 U/kg actual body weight in the first trimester, 1.0 U/kg actual body weight in the second trimester, and 1.2 U/kg actual body weight in the third trimester. However, because women with GDM have varying degrees of severity, in practice, insulin is started at 0.7 U/kg actual body weight to prevent hypoglycemia at home. Clinical judgment and experience assist in the selection of the starting dose of insulin. Once the total daily insulin dose is calculated, two-thirds of the daily dose is given before breakfast, divided into two-thirds neutral protamine hagedorn (NPH) insulin and one-third regular insulin, and the remaining one-third of the daily dose is divided into half regular insulin before dinner and half NPH insulin at bedtime. Very-short-acting insulin can also be used, but is best dosed with each meal in place of the twice-daily regular insulin. Further discussion of insulin types and regimens (see the article by Gabriella Pridjian elsewhere in this issue for further exploration of this topic) and in other published reviews.[57,58]

In the twenty-first century, oral hypoglycemic agents have been included in the armamentarium of treatment modalities for GDM (**Table 5**). Earlier concerns with use of these agents in pregnancy were the unknown risk of teratogenicity and neonatal hypoglycemia caused by transplacental passage. In 2000, Langer and colleagues[59] published a small but landmark study describing the use of glyburide for treatment of GDM. Women from 11 to 33 weeks of gestation with GDM were randomized to treatment

Table 5
Pharmacologic agents for gestational diabetes

	Insulin	Glyburide	Metformin[b]
Mechanism of Action	Receptor-mediated glucose uptake; other actions	Stimulates pancreatic beta-cell insulin release	Increases sensitivity to insulin; stimulates insulin-induced glucose uptake
Onset of Action	Varies	Approximately 1 h	Approximately 1 h
Peak	Varies	4 h	2–4 h
Dosing	Varies	2.5 mg in AM or every 12 h, increase weekly by 2.5 mg to a maximum of 10 mg every 12 h	500 mg in AM or every 12 h; maximum 1000 mg every 12 h
Placental Transport	Minimal (only antibody-bound fraction)	Minimal to none (some conflicting studies)	Yes
FDA Pregnancy Category	B[a]	C	B
Experience with Use in Pregnancy	Substantial	Modest[c]	Limited
Failure Rate Requiring Insulin		20%	35%

Abbreviation: FDA, Food and Drug Administration.
[a] Certain newer insulin analogs category C.
[b] Insufficient evidence at present to recommended use in pregnancy.
[c] Minimal experience with use at less than 11 weeks of gestation; insufficient number of large studies addressing neonatal risk.

with glyburide or insulin. There were no significant differences between the insulin treated group (201 women) and the glyburide group (203 women) in demographics and other characteristics, blood glucose concentrations, or neonatal outcomes. Glyburide was started at 2.5 mg in the morning and increased weekly to a maximum of 10 mg twice a day. The investigators concluded that glyburide is a clinically effective alternative to insulin therapy. In a retrospective study, Jacobson and colleagues[60] compared women with GDM treated with glyburide with those treated with insulin and noted that women in the glyburide group were more likely to achieve mean fasting and postprandial glucose goals and had newborns with similar weights and that the newborns were less likely to be admitted to the neonatal intensive care unit. The glyburide group had a higher rate of preeclampsia and need for phototherapy treatment of their newborns. In a different report, these investigators noted a somewhat higher risk of neonatal hypoglycemia with glyburide therapy,[61] but neonatal hypoglycemia may have been related to the higher rate of macrosomic infants in the group studied.

Glyburide does not seem to cross the placenta when studied in an in vitro isolated, perfused cotelydon model[62] and may actually be actively transported from fetal to maternal circulations. However, other investigators[63] have noted that the umbilical cord/maternal plasma ratio of glyburide is 0.7 ± 0.4, suggesting transfer across the placenta and no active transport back.

Failures of glyburide treatment can be predicted. Kahn and colleagues[64] reviewed 95 women with GDM in their diabetes clinic who were treated with glyburide. Of the 95 women, 19% failed glyburide treatment. Failures were more likely in women diagnosed early in pregnancy, of older age and higher parity, and with higher fasting glucose levels, reflecting reduced beta-cell function and reduced capacity to respond to insulin secretagogues. These factors should be considered with counseling or initiating glyburide therapy. Glyburide therapy alone is not likely to achieve optimal blood sugar control if the fasting glucose level is greater than 140 mg/dL and may not even achieve optimal control if fasting glucose level is between 120 to 140 mg/dL.

Use of glyburide is not without pitfalls. Some practitioners and women have begun to believe that diabetes is not a critical complication of pregnancy because it can be taken care of with a pill. Thus, laxity in diet and compliance may occur more often. Experience with glyburide use in the first trimester, during embryogenesis, is limited, and safety in later trimesters should not automatically be extended to the early first trimester. Furthermore, glyburide may not be the ideal oral hypoglycemic agent for pregnancy. Its absorption and steady state and associated insulin secretion do not mimic the in vivo state. The ideal oral hypoglycemic agent for use in pregnancy is one that is not teratogenic, does not cross the placenta, and exerts its peak effect quickly after ingestion, mimicking in vivo insulin secretion and designed to be taken before each meal.

Metformin has been studied recently for treatment of GDM, because women often present to the obstetrician already pregnant and on metformin for treatment of polycystic ovarian syndrome, infertility, or metabolic syndrome. Rowan and colleagues[65] performed a randomized controlled trial of metformin versus insulin for treatment of GDM. A total of 363 women were assigned to metformin; 92.6% continued metformin until delivery, but 46.3% required supplemental insulin to achieve euglycemia. Neonatal outcomes were similar in each group, and women preferred metformin treatment even if insulin was added. In a randomized, controlled study, Moore and colleagues[66] compared the use of metformin with that of glyburide for the treatment of women with GDM. If glycemic control was achieved, women treated with metformin were comparable with women treated with glyburide in outcomes studied. However, failure of metformin therapy was 2.1 times higher than failure of glyburide therapy. Of the metformin group, 34.7% of women eventually required insulin, but only 16% of the glyburide group required insulin. The investigators speculated that ethnic differences may influence success of metformin.

Until more information is obtained regarding safety and efficacy of metformin use in pregnancy, the best approach is to not use metformin for treatment of GDM. If a woman is already on metformin for other reasons, it is best to discontinue its use and perform diabetes screening at the appropriate time as indicated by risk factors or universal screening. Women on metformin for treatment of type 2 diabetes are best changed to insulin if unexpected pregnancy occurs.

ANTENATAL AND INTRAPARTUM MANAGEMENT

Once GDM is diagnosed, the pregnant woman should be seen at least every 1 to 2 weeks, more frequently if other complications ensue. Frequency and timing of antenatal testing in women with GDM is controversial. Generally, women on diet control who do not have macrosomic infants can wait until 40 weeks for antenatal testing; their risk of stillbirth is not substantially higher than the general population. It is prudent to manage women who are noncompliant, require pharmacologic therapy, have macrosomic or growth-restricted fetuses, or have other pregnancy complications similar to those women with preexisting diabetes and initiate antenatal testing.[31] Close assessment of symptoms, blood pressure, and proteinuria to diagnose preeclampsia is paramount.

The timing and mode of delivery of women with GDM is also controversial given the lack of sufficient data to support a specific recommendation. There is no evidence to support delivery before 40 weeks of gestation. However, some investigators have found a higher incidence of shoulder dystocia by waiting for delivery until after 40 gestational weeks.[67] Induction of labor at 39 gestational weeks in women with good metabolic control should not require documentation of fetal lung maturity by amniocentesis.[68] Documentation of fetal lung maturity is prudent if delivery is electively planned earlier without other obstetric indications.

Women with GDM requiring pharmacologic therapy are best managed with intravenous insulin drips and glucose monitoring protocols during labor similar to women with pregestational diabetes.[57] Women with very mild GDM may not require insulin therapy but should have blood glucose assessment during labor.

In light of the somewhat poor prediction of macrosomia by ultrasonography and the higher rate of shoulder dystocia in GDM infants when compared with non-GDM infants of comparable size,[69] a fetal weight cutoff for vaginal delivery has not been easy to establish. The current recommendation is to offer women with GDM whose estimated fetal weight is 4500 g or greater elective cesarean to prevent shoulder dystocia. In those women whose fetal weight ranges from 4000 to 4500 g, clinical pelvimetry and other obstetric factors should assist in the decision to offer cesarean section.[31]

POSTPARTUM MANAGEMENT

Many women who are diagnosed with type 2 diabetes are classified first as having GDM, even though they really have undiagnosed pregestational diabetes; these women continue to be diabetic in the postpartum period. Women with GDM should have a fasting or random blood sugar level test in the immediate postpartum period to identify undiagnosed type 2 diabetes. There is epidemiologic evidence that about 15% to 50% of women with GDM develop diabetes or impaired glucose tolerance well after pregnancy. A 75-g glucose, 2-hour glucose tolerance test should be performed at or around the time of the routine postpartum visit. The frequency of subsequent testing for detection of glucose intolerance or type 2 diabetes ranges from annually to triannually. The American Diabetes Association recommends glucose tolerance testing at least once every 3 years,[70] even though more frequent testing might be appropriate if further pregnancies are contemplated.

It is not surprising that there is marked variability in the proportion of women with GDM who are screened postpartum as well as in the type of screening used.[71–73] Ferrara and colleagues[73] showed that between 1995 and 2006, the proportion of women in their study who were screened postpartum increased from 20.7% (95% confidence interval [CI], 17.8–23.5) to 53.8% (95% CI, 51.3–56.3). Independent predictors of successful postpartum screening in their study were women who were older, of Asian or Hispanic ethnicity, better educated, and diagnosed with GDM earlier in gestation. Obese women and women of low parity were less likely to have postpartum screening.

There are considerable data to support that weight loss and use of metformin or thiazolidinediones can prevent or delay progression of glucose intolerance and type 2 diabetes.[74,75] Dietary modifications and treatment of periodontal disease may also prevent glucose intolerance.[47] Additional research and specific clinical guidelines for women with history of GDM will allow interventional strategies to prevent or delay the onset of type 2 diabetes.

REFERENCES

1. Metzger BE, Buchanan TA, Coustan DR, et al. Summary and recommendations of the Fifth International Workshop-Conference on Gestational Diabetes Mellitus. Diabetes Care 2007;30:S251–60.

2. Hedley AA, Ogden CL, Johnson CL, et al. Prevalence of overweight and obesity among U.S. children, adolescents, and adults, 1999–2002. JAMA 2004;291:2847–50.
3. Kuhl C. Etiology and pathogenesis of gestational diabetes. Diabetes Care 1998; 21:B19–26.
4. Phelps RL, Metzger BE, Freinkel N. Carbohydrate metabolism in pregnancy XVII. Diurnal profiles of plasma glucose, insulin, free fatty acids, triglycerides, cholesterol, and individual amino acids in late normal pregnancy. Am J Obstet Gynecol 1981;140:730–6.
5. Butte N. Carbohydrate and lipid metabolism in pregnancy: normal compared with gestational diabetes mellitus. Am J Clin Nutr 2000;71:1256S–61S.
6. Sorenson RL, Brelje TC. Adaptation of islets of Langerhans to pregnancy: beta-cell growth, enhanced insulin secretion and the role of lactogenic hormones. Horm Metab Res 1997;29(6):301–7.
7. Van Assche F, Aerts L, De Prins F. A morphological study of the endocrine pancreas in human pregnancy. Br J Obstet Gynaecol 1978;85:818–20.
8. Assel B, Rossi K, Kalhan S. Glucose metabolism during fasting through human pregnancy: comparison of tracer method with respiratory calorimetry. Am J Phys 1993;265:E351–6.
9. Catalano P, Tyzbir E, Wolfe R, et al. Longitudinal changes in basal hepatic glucose production and suppression during insulin infusion in normal pregnant women. Am J Obstet Gynecol 1992;167:913.
10. Kalhan SC, D'Angelo LJ, Savin SM, et al. Glucose production in pregnant women at term gestation. Sources of glucose for human fetus. J Clin Invest 1979;63:388–94.
11. Catalano PM, Tyzbir ED, Roman NM, et al. Longitudinal changes in insulin release and insulin resistance in non-obese pregnant women. Am J Obstet Gynecol 1991;165:1667–72.
12. Fisher P, Sutherland H, Bewsher P. The insulin response to glucose infusion in normal human pregnancy. Diabetologia 1980;19:15–20.
13. Sivan E, Chen X, Homko CJ, et al. Longitudinal study of carbohydrate metabolism in healthy obese pregnant women. Diabetes Care 1997;20:1470–5.
14. Buchanan TA, Metzger BE, Frienkel N, et al. Insulin sensitivity and B-cell responsiveness to glucose during late pregnancy in lean and moderately obese women with normal glucose tolerance or mild gestational diabetes. Am J Obstet Gynecol 1990;162:1008–14.
15. Damm P, Handber A, Kuhl C, et al. Insulin receptor binding and tryrosine kinase activity in skeletal muscle from normal pregnant women and women with gestational diabetes. Obstet Gynecol 1993;82:251–9.
16. Shao J, Catalano PM, Yamashita H, et al. Impaired insulin receptor tyrosine kinase activity and over expression of PC-1 in skeletal muscle from obese women with gestational diabetes. Diabetes 2000;49:603–10.
17. Friedman JE, Ishizuka T, Huston L, et al. Impaired glucose transport and insulin receptor tyrosine kinase phosphorylation in skeletal muscle from obese women with gestational diabetes. Diabetes 1999;48:1807–14.
18. Okuno S, Akazawa S, Yasuhi I, et al. Decreased expression of GLUT4 glucose transporter protein in adipose tissue during pregnancy. Horm Metab Res 1995; 27:231–4.
19. Kirwan JP, Hauguel-de Mouson S, Lepercq J, et al. TNF-alpha is a predictor of insulin resistance in human pregnancy. Diabetes 2002;51:2207–13.
20. Highman TJ, Friedman JE, Huston LP, et al. Longitudinal changes in maternal serum leptin concentrations, body composition, and resting metabolic rate in pregnancy. Am J Obstet Gynecol 1999;178:1010–5.

21. Henson MC, Swan KF, O'Neal JS. Expression of placental leptin and leptin receptor transcripts in early pregnancy and at term. Obstet Gynecol 1998;92:1020–8.
22. Devlieger R, Casteels K, van Assche FA. Reduced adaptation of the pancreatic B cells during pregnancy is the major causal factor for gestational diabetes: current knowledge and metabolic effects on the offspring. Acta Obstet Gynecol 2008;87:1266–70.
23. Catalano PM, Huston L, Amini SB, et al. Longitudinal changes in glucose metabolism during pregnancy in obese women with normal glucose tolerance and gestational diabetes. Am J Obstet Gynecol 1999;180:903–16.
24. Jarrett RJ. Gestational diabetes: a non-entity? BMJ 1993;306:37–8.
25. Langer O, Yogev Y, Most O, et al. Gestational diabetes: the consequences of not treating. Am J Obstet Gynecol 2005;192:989–97.
26. Crowther CA, Hiller JE, Moss JR, et al. Effect of treatment of gestational diabetes mellitus on pregnancy outcomes. N Engl J Med 2005;352:2477–86.
27. The Hyperglycemia and Adverse Pregnancy Outcome (HAPO) Study Cooperative Research Group. Hyperglycemia and adverse pregnancy outcomes. N Engl J Med 2008;358:1991–2.
28. The Hyperglycemia and Adverse Pregnancy Outcome (HAPO) Study Cooperative Research Group. Hyperglycemia and Adverse Pregnancy Outcome (HAPO) Study: associations with neonatal anthropometrics. Diabetes 2009;58:453–9.
29. Landon MB, Spong CY, Thom E, et al. A multicenter, randomized trial of treatment for mild gestational diabetes. N Engl J Med 2009;361:1339–48.
30. Gabbe SG, Gregory RP, Power ML, et al. Management of diabetes mellitus by obstetrician-gynecologists. Obstet Gynecol 2004;103:1229–34.
31. ACOG Practice Bulletin No. 30. American College of Obstetricians and Gynecologists. Gestational diabetes. Obstet Gynecol 2001;98:525–38.
32. American Diabetes Association. Gestational diabetes mellitus. Diabetes Care 2004;27:S88–90.
33. U.S.Preventive Services Task Force. Screening for gestational diabetes mellitus: U.S. Preventive Services Task Force recommendation statement. Ann Intern Med 2008;148:759–65.
34. National Diabetes Data Group. Classification and diagnosis of diabetes mellitus and categories of glucose intolerance. Diabetes 1979;28:1039–57.
35. Carpenter MR, Coustan DR. Criteria for screening tests for gestational diabetes. Am J Obstet Gynecol 1982;144:768–73.
36. Reece EA, Laguizamon G, Wiznitzer A. Gestational diabetes: the need for common ground. Lancet 2009;373:1789–97.
37. Torloni MR, Betran AP, Horta BL, et al. Prepregnancy BMI and the risk of gestational diabetes: a systematic review of the literature with meta-analysis. Obes Rev 2009;10:194–203.
38. Chu S, Kim SY, Lau J. Re: prepregnancy BMI and the risk of gestational diabetes: a systematic review of the literature with meta-analysis. Obes Rev 2009;10:489–90.
39. McGuire V, Rauh MJ, Mueller BA, et al. The risk of diabetes in a subsequent pregnancy associated with prior history of gestational diabetes or a macrosomic infant. Paediatr Perinat Epidemiol 1996;10:64–72.
40. Cypryk K, Szymczak W, Czupryniak L, et al. Gestational diabetes – an analysis of risk factors. Endokrynol Pol 2008;59:393–7.
41. Xiong X, Saunders LD, Wang FL, et al. Gestational diabetes mellitus: prevalence, risk factors, maternal and infant outcomes. Int J Gynecol Obstet 2001;75:221–8.

42. Rauh-Hain JA, Rana S, Tamez H, et al. Risk for developing gestational diabetes in women with twin pregnancies. J Matern Fetal Neonatal Med 2009;22:293–9.
43. Dornhorst A, Paterson CM, Nicholls JSD, et al. High prevalence of gestational diabetes in women for ethnic minority groups. Diabetic Medicine 1992;9:820–5.
44. Dooley S, Metzger B, Cho N, et al. Gestational diabetes mellitus: influence of race on disease prevalence and perinatal outcome in the US population. Diabetes 1991;20(Supple 2):25–9.
45. Toulis KA, Goulis DG, Kolibianakis EM, et al. Risk of gestational diabetes mellitus in women with polycystic ovarian syndrome: a systematic review and a meta-analysis. Fertil Steril 2009;92(2):667–77.
46. Kim C, Liu T, Valdez R, et al. Does frank diabetes in first degree relatives of a pregnant woman affect the likelihood of her developing gestational diabetes mellitus or nongestational diabetes? Am J Obstet Gynecol 2009;201:576, e1–6.
47. Xiong X, Ellkind-Hirsch KE, Vastardis S, et al. Periodontal disease is associated with gestational diabetes mellitus, a case-control study. J Periodontol 2009;80: 1742–9.
48. Dasanayake AP, Chhun N, Tanner AC, et al. Periodontal pathogens and gestational diabetes mellitus. J Dent Res 2008;87:328–33.
49. Seghieri G, Anichini R, de Bellis A, et al. Relationship between gestational diabetes mellitus and low maternal birth weight. Diabetes Care 2002;25:1761–5.
50. Chen L, Hu FB, Yeung E, et al. Prospective study of pre-gravid sugar-sweetened beverage consumption and the risk of gestational diabetes mellitus. Diabetes Care 2009;32(12):2236–41.
51. Langer O, Levy J, Brustman L, et al. Glycemic control in gestational diabetes – how tight is tight enough: small for gestational age versus large for gestational age? Am J Obstet Gynecol 1989;61:646–53.
52. Salvesen DR, Brudenell JM, Proudler AJ, et al. Fetal pancreatic beta-cell function in pregnancies complicated by maternal diabetes mellitus: relationship to fetal macrosomia. Am J Obstet Gynecol 1993;168:1363–9.
53. Sacks DA, Liu AI, Wolde-Tsadik G, et al. What proportion of birth weight is attributable to maternal glucose among infants of diabetic mothers? Am J Obstet Gynecol 2006;194:501–7.
54. Catalano PM, Presley MS, Minium J, et al. Fetuses of obese mothers develop insulin resistance in utero. Diabetes Care 2009;32:1076–80.
55. Hawkins JS, Casey BM, Lo JY, et al. Weekly compared with daily blood glucose monitoring in women with diet-treated gestational diabetes. Obstet Gynecol 2009;113:1307–12.
56. American Diabetes Association. Evidence-based nutrition principles and recommendations for the treatment and prevention of diabetes and related complications. Diabetes Care 2003;26:S51–61.
57. Moses RG, Barker M, Winter M, et al. Can a low-glycemic index diet reduce the need for insulin in gestational diabetes mellitus? A randomized trial. Diabetes Care 2009;32(6):996–1000.
58. Gabbe SG, Carpenter LB, Garrison EA. New strategies for glucose control in patients with type 1 and type 2 diabetes mellitus in pregnancy. Clin Obstet Gynecol 2007;50:1014–24.
59. Langer O, Conway DL, Berkus MD, et al. A comparison of glyburide and insulin in women with gestational diabetes mellitus. N Engl J Med 2000;343: 1134–8.

60. Jacobson GF, Ramos GA, Ching JY, et al. Comparison of glyburide and insulin for the management of gestational diabetes in a large managed care organization. Am J Obstet Gynecol 2005;193:118–24.
61. Ramos GA, Jaboson GF, Kirby RS, et al. Comparison of glyburide and insulin for the management of gestational diabetics with markedly elevated oral glucose challenge test and fasting hyperglycemia. J Perinatol 2007;27:257–8.
62. Kraemer J, Klein J, Lubetsky A, et al. Perfusion studies of glyburide transfer across the human placenta: implications for fetal safety. Am J Obstet Gynecol 2006;195:270–4.
63. Heber MF, Ma X, Nraharisetti SB, et al. Are we optimizing gestational diabetes treatment with glyburide? The pharmacologic basis for better clinical practice. Clin Pharmacol Ther 2009;85:607–14.
64. Kahn BF, Davies JK, Lynch AM, et al. Predictors of glyburide failure in treatment of gestational diabetes. Obstet Gynecol 2006;107:1303–9.
65. Rowan JA, Hague WM, Gao W, et al. Metformin versus insulin for the treatment of gestational diabetes. N Engl J Med 2008;358:2003–15.
66. Moore LE, Clokey D, Rappaport VJ, et al. Metformin compared with glyburide in gestational diabetes. A randomized controlled trial. Obstet Gynecol 2010;115:55–9.
67. Lurie S, Insler V, Hagay ZJ. Induction of labor at 38 to 39 weeks of gestation reduces the incidence of shoulder dystocia in gestational diabetic patients Class A2. Am J Perinatol 1996;13:293–6.
68. Kjos SL, Walther FJ, Montoro M, et al. Prevalence and etiology of respiratory distress in infants of diabetic mothers: predictive values of fetal lung maturity tests. Am J Obstet Gynecol 1990;163:898–903.
69. Lager O, Berkus MD, Huff RW, et al. Shoulder dystocia: should the fetus weighing greater than or equal to 4000 grams be delivered by cesarean section? Am J Obstet Gynecol 1991;165:831–7.
70. American Diabetes Association. Standards of medical care in diabetes—2008. Diabetes Care 2008;31:S12–54.
71. Almario CV, Ecker T, Moroz LA, et al. Obstetricians seldom provide postpartum diabetes screening for women with gestational diabetes. Am J Obstet Gynecol 2008;198:528 e1-5.
72. Kim C, Tabaei BP, Burke R, et al. Missed opportunities for type 2 diabetes mellitus screening among women with a history of gestational diabetes mellitus. Am J Public Health 2006;96:1643–8.
73. Ferrara A, Peng T, Kim C. Trends in postpartum diabetes screening and subsequent diabetes and impaired fasting glucose among women with histories of gestational diabetes mellitus. Diabetes Care 2009;32:269–74.
74. Buchanan TA, Xiang AH, Peters RK, et al. Preservation of pancreatic beta-cell function and prevention of type 2 diabetes by pharmacological treatment of insulin resistance in high-risk Hispanic women. Diabetes 2002;51(2796):803.
75. Berkowitz K, Peters R, Kyos SL, et al. Effect of troglitazone on insulin sensitivity and pancreatic beta-cell function in women at high risk for NIDDM. Diabetes 1996;45:1572–9.

Cholestasis of Pregnancy

Bhuvan Pathak, MD[a], Lili Sheibani, MD[b], Richard H. Lee, MD[c],*

KEYWORDS

- Cholestasis • Pregnancy • Fetal death
- Ursodeoxycholic acid

ETIOLOGY

The prevalence of intrahepatic cholestasis of pregnancy (ICP) differs by geographic location. The estimated prevalence of ICP in the United States is 0.001% to 0.32%, Chile 4.0%, United Kingdom 0.7%, and Scandinavia 1.0% to 2.0%.[1–4] However, over the latter half of the 20th century, some regions have witnessed a decrease in the prevalence of ICP. Between the 1960s and 1990s, Chile had a decline in prevalence from 14% to 4%.[5–7] During the same era, the prevalence of ICP in Scandinavia decreased from 2.0% to approximately 0.1 to 1.5%.[6] ICP is similar to other medical conditions where the prevalence of disease varies by ethnicity, and this was demonstrated in the United Kingdom (0.6% Caucasians, 1.5% Pakistanis, 1.2% South Asians).[8] Furthermore, despite the rarity of ICP in the United States, the authors demonstrated that the prevalence of ICP may be as high as 5.6% in the predominantly Hispanic population based in Los Angeles.[9]

Reported risk factors for ICP include ethnicity, family history of biliary disease, hepatitis C, prior ICP, multi-fetal gestation, and maternal age greater than 35 years.[10,11] Factors that may play a role in the pathogenesis of ICP include the environment, nutritional deficiencies, genetic variations, and hormonal changes.[5] The prevalence of ICP may have seasonal cycles and may be more prevalent in the winter.[12] Of the possible nutritional deficiencies contributing to ICP, selenium has been the most investigated.[13] Selenium levels were lower in Chilean patients with ICP. Apropos to the prior point, serum selenium levels in patients with ICP were lower in the winter, which was attributed to seasonal variations in diet.[14] Although the exact link between low concentrations of selenium and ICP needs further study, a deficiency in this mineral may lead to defective bile formation or secretion because of its role as a cofactor for several oxidative hepatic enzymes.[13,14]

---

[a] Division of Maternal Fetal Medicine, Department of Obstetrics and Gynecology, University of Southern California, 2020 Zonal Avenue, IRD, Room 203, Los Angeles, CA 90033, USA
[b] Division of Maternal Fetal Medicine, Department of Obstetrics and Gynecology, University of Southern California, 1200 North State Street, Inpatient Tower, Room C3F107, Los Angeles, CA 90033, USA
[c] Division of Maternal Fetal Medicine, Department of Obstetrics and Gynecology, University of Southern California, 2020 Zonal Avenue, IRD, Room 206, Los Angeles, CA 90033, USA
* Corresponding author.
E-mail address: richarhl@usc.edu

Obstet Gynecol Clin N Am 37 (2010) 269–282
doi:10.1016/j.ogc.2010.02.011
0889-8545/10/$ – see front matter © 2010 Elsevier Inc. All rights reserved.

Several investigators have studied potential genes associated with ICP. The primary genes of interest encode biliary transport proteins (ie, *ABCB4*, *ATP8B1*, and *ABCB11*). The gene most studied is *ABCB4*, which encodes for multidrug resistant protein 3 (MDR3) P-glycoprotein. MDR3 P-glycoprotein is a transporter of phospholipids across the canalicular membrane of the hepatocyte, and mutations in this may lead to altered bile acid trafficking and subsequent elevation in bile acids.[15,16] *ATP8B1* is another gene potentially linked to ICP. *ATP8B1* encodes a protein belonging to a subfamily of P-type ATPases. The biochemical and cellular functions of its product, FIC1, and the mechanisms by which its absence or dysfunction leads to cholestasis are currently unknown.[17] Others have concluded that *ATP8B1* is not a major gene in ICP.[18] Mutations in the *ABCB11* gene, which encodes for bile salt export pump (BSEP), may have a role in the etiology of ICP. Huang and colleagues[19] showed BSEP was decreased in placentas from patients with ICP. Finally, Wei and colleagues demonstrated upregulated expression of placental genes involved with apoptosis, suggesting that apoptosis of placental trophoblasts may contribute to ICP.[20]

There are lines of evidence that suggest ICP might be caused by abnormal hormone profiles, specifically steroid hormones (eg, estrogen and progesterone). Several clinical circumstances lend support to this as seen by the higher occurrence of ICP in the third trimester of pregnancy, a time when estrogen levels are at their highest, and in pregnancies with multiple gestations, which have higher estrogen levels than singleton pregnancies. In addition, there are reports of recurrence of cholestasis when estrogen- and progesterone-containing contraceptives are given to patients with a history of ICP. Furthermore, ICP resolves after delivery of the fetus and placenta, a time when hormone levels are normalized.[21,22] Finally, there appears to be altered progesterone metabolism and excretion in patients with ICP.[23] Large amounts of these hormones may result in saturation of hepatic enzymes and transporters normally used for biliary secretion.[23]

DIAGNOSIS

The diagnosis of ICP is based on the combination of pruritus and biochemical evidence of liver dysfunction. The chief complaint is usually pruritus, which is classically described as total-body itching, localizing to the palms of the hands and the soles of the feet, with a nocturnal predominance.[24–26] Often the pruritus will precede any other physical or lab abnormalities.[24] The pruritus generally improves shortly after delivery, but is reported to recur in 40% to 60% of subsequent pregnancies.[5,7] Pruritus is reported in as many as 20% of pregnancies; therefore, it is important to distinguish ICP from other conditions.[27] The pruritus of ICP is hypothesized to be caused by the accumulation of bile salts in the skin. Although less frequently seen, other reported symptoms include jaundice and steatorrhea.[28]

Elevation in the serum total bile acid (TBA) concentration is the most frequent lab abnormality associated with ICP and is the most sensitive marker for ICP. TBAs appear to increase toward the third trimester of pregnancy.[29] Unfortunately, the scientific literature has a wide range of values used to diagnosis ICP. This variability brings into question the validity of studies evaluating the population prevalence of ICP and its associated morbidity and mortality. Although most authors have used an elevated total serum bile concentration above the laboratory provided reference range, ranging anywhere from greater than or equal to 2 µmol/L to greater than or equal to 20 µmol/L. The authors believe these reference ranges may be inadequate for the diagnosis of ICP primarily because established reference ranges for the general population incorporate men and women and generally exclude pregnant subjects.[9,30] Therefore, there is a need to create method-specific, population-specific, and trimester-specific bile acid ranges to assist clinicians in making the diagnosis of ICP. Furthermore, there are differences in the methodologies used to measure total serum TBA concentration. Depending on methodology, the mean serum TBA concentrations in the third trimester of pregnancy appear to be approximately 1.8 ± 2.2 μmol/L (range 0.5–12.0) using direct spectrophotometry and 6.5 μmol/L (2 SD range 1.7–11.3) using enzymatic methods.[31,32] Other laboratory abnormalities observed in ICP include elevations in alanine aminotransferase (ALT), aspartate aminotransferase (AST), alkaline phosphatase (ALP), gamma glutamyl transferase, and bilirubin.[26,29]

Glutathione S-transferase (GST) is another possible diagnostic marker for ICP and deserves further evaluation. GST is thought be an indicator of hepatocellular damage and may be more sensitive and specific than some of the other traditional markers of liver function, including ALT, AST, and ALP.[29] Furthermore, there appears to be a positive correlation between serum GST and TBA concentrations. The rise in serum GST may occur earlier than the elevation of TBA concentration and may possibly be used to detect ICP earlier in gestation.[29]

Several investigators have examined the bile acid ratio in ICP. The primary bile acids, cholic acid (CA) and chenodeoxycholic acid (CDCA), are made in equal quantities. CA is converted to the secondary bile acid, deoxycholic acid (DCA), and chenodeoxycholic acid to its secondary bile acid, lithocholic acid . Studies demonstrate disparate results in the physiologic changes of the primary bile acid concentrations during pregnancy.[33–35] That said, in normal pregnancies the ratio of CA/CDCA is approximately less than 1.5.[34,35] Conversely, the ratio between CA/CDCA in pregnant patients with ICP appears to be more than 1.5:1.[33–35] The use of the bile acid ratio to diagnose ICP was recently evaluated, and it was found that the CA/CDCA ratio added little to the diagnosis of ICP and that the total bile acid concentration and transaminase levels were more useful.[36]

IMPACT ON THE FETUS

The most concerning aspect of ICP is its association with adverse perinatal outcome.[37,38] Although maternal complications from ICP are rare, there are several adverse fetal effects including preterm labor, meconium aspiration, and fetal death.[37–40] Rencoret and Aste[37] reviewed 32 cases of jaundice in pregnancy (31 out of 32 cases with intrahepatic cholestasis) and reported two fetal deaths and a preterm labor rate of 33.3%. Reid and colleagues[38] analyzed complications in 56 pregnancies with ICP and reported an astonishingly high rate of adverse outcomes (ie, perinatal mortality rate 11%, meconium staining 27%, abnormal antepartum fetal heart rate pattern 14%, and preterm delivery rate 36%). They also reported an increased risk for postpartum hemorrhage theorized to be caused by a depletion of vitamin K dependent clotting factors caused by ICP-induced liver dysfunction. Similarly, Fisk and Storey[40] reported a 45% incidence of meconium staining, 44% incidence of preterm labor, 22% incidence intrapartum fetal distress, and a 3.5% perinatal mortality rate. The most important observations noted by Fisk and colleagues were twofold. Firstly, given the absence of growth restriction in cases with fetal deaths, chronic uteroplacental insufficiency was thought to be less likely a cause for this complication in ICP. Secondly, the lower perinatal mortality rate compared with previous reports was attributed to closer surveillance during pregnancy with induction of labor by 37 weeks or earlier if there were any signs of fetal distress. Williamson and colleagues[41] reported an overall intrauterine death rate of 7% with 90% (18 out of 20) of the deaths occurring after 37 weeks gestation.

The mechanism of fetal death is currently unknown. There are several studies investigating possible mechanisms. In rats, cardiac myocyte exposure to taurocholate provoked arrhythmias and impaired contractility. It was therefore hypothesized that the fetal deaths in ICP may be caused by an acute cardiac event caused by raised fetal serum taurocholate concentrations.[42,43] A different study demonstrated human chorionic vein constriction with exposure to cholate, a bile acid. Chorionic vein constriction was hypothesized to lead to an abrupt decrease in blood flow to the fetus and impaired fetal oxygenation, ultimately resulting in fetal death via asphyxia.[44] Although the rate of meconium passage is high in ICP, there is not sufficient evidence at this time to suggest a role for meconium in fetal death.[45]

Whether or not there is a critical bile acid concentration threshold at which adverse perinatal outcomes are avoided is uncertain at this time. Recently, Glantz and colleagues[4] found no increased fetal risk with total bile acid levels less than 40 µmol/L; however, individual case reports have described fetal deaths with bile acids in this lower range.[46,47]

There are limited studies in humans to explain the high rate of meconium passage and staining in ICP. In ewes, the administration of cholic acid was found to stimulate colonic motility.[48] That said, there are conflicting data in humans correlating bile acid concentrations with meconium passage.[49,50] Exactly how ICP causes preterm birth is also uncertain. One study demonstrated increased contractile activity in myometrium biopsied from patients with ICP. It was hypothesized that cholic acid may stimulate oxytocin receptor expression.[51]

PHARMACOLOGY

Several medications have been studied in the treatment of intrahepatic cholestasis of pregnancy. The overarching goal of these therapies is to alter the enterohepatic circulation of bile acids in a manner that reduces their concentration in maternal serum. By doing so, it is hoped that such treatment would improve perinatal outcome. Some medications may, to some degree, improve maternal pruritus and liver function; however, currently no medications have been shown to decrease the risk for stillbirth caused by ICP. A brief synopsis of the clinical effect of the medications used to treat ICP follows this discussion.

Activated Charcoal

Activated charcoal is a porous substance that has been shown to adsorb bile salts, decrease bilirubin levels, and inhibit bile acid absorption in in-vitro, animal, and human studies respectively.[52–54] One randomized study has been performed comparing the use of activated charcoal with placebo in 19 women with ICP.[55] Although orally administered activated charcoal decreased total bile acids, there were no differences in other serum measures, such as aminotransferases, bilirubin concentrations, or cholesterol. Furthermore, there were no significant decreases in pruritus symptoms, birth weight, or gestational age at delivery. No adverse effects on either the mother or the fetus were reported. Finally, many women found the oral suspension unpleasant to ingest. Given the lack of data and the inconvenience in administration, oral activated charcoal has not gained widespread acceptance as a treatment for ICP.

Guar Gum

Guar gum is a dietary fiber that decreases the bile acid pool by binding to bile acids in the intestinal lumen thereby increasing their elimination. There is a paucity of data surrounding the use of guar gum in the treatment of ICP; however, one small, randomized controlled-trial has compared the use of guar gum in incremental dosages of 5 to 15 g/day with placebo in 39 women.[56] Despite the women receiving guar gum reporting more effective control of their pruritus, it was not better than placebo in decreasing pruritus scores when measured either subjectively by the women themselves via visual analog scales or when defined objectively by the investigators. Of importance, there was no difference between the two groups in gestational age at delivery or birth weight. The same group reported on the effects of guar gum on measures of cholesterol by examining its effects on cholesterol and cholestanol levels, the latter being a metabolite of the former.[57] They found that in comparison to placebo, serum cholesterol levels were unchanged with the use of guar gum and that in fact, cholestanol levels were increased suggesting an increase in cholesterol production. Furthermore, guar gum had no effect on bile acid or bilirubin levels. There were no serious maternal or neonatal side effects of guar gum reported in either study.

Although guar gum has shown no adverse effects thus far and may even alleviate some of the pruritus associated with ICP, the studies are few in number and contain small numbers of subjects. Furthermore, serum analytes are not improved with the use of guar gum treatment.

Cholestyramine

Cholestyramine is an anion exchange resin that binds to bile acids and therefore decreases their absorption in the ileum. Fecal elimination of bile acids is thereby increased with a resultant smaller total bile acid pool. Initial small studies examining the effect of cholestyramine on women with ICP did not show promising results as pruritus was not well or consistently controlled and serum bile acids did not decrease consistently.[58,59] Liver function tests also did not improve. In a larger randomized study of 84 women with ICP receiving either ursodeoxycholic acid (UDCA) or 8 g of cholestyramine daily, the latter did not perform well.[60] Cholestyramine was effective in attaining the endpoint of a greater than 50% reduction in pruritus in only 19% of subjects compared with 66.6% of subjects in the UDCA group. Cholestyramine did not significantly decrease transaminases, gamma-glutamyl transpeptidase, or bile acid levels and was conversely associated with a significant increase in alkaline phosphatase and bilirubin levels. Women in the cholestyramine group delivered somewhat earlier than women in the UDCA group (37.4 vs 38.7 days respectively), however, there was no difference in birth weights between the two groups. Although there were no cases of coagulopathy in this study, of concern is a single case report of a neonatal demise caused by a large subdural hematoma.[61] This hematoma was thought to be caused by fetal vitamin K deficiency following maternal vitamin K deficiency caused by a combination of severe ICP and the administration of cholestyramine.

Side effects of cholestyramine are primarily gastrointestinal in nature and occur in up to 29% of women.[60] These side effects include nausea, vomiting, constipation, and even diarrhea. A significant and important side effect of cholestyramine is a decrease in the intestinal absorption of fat-soluble vitamins. This side effect can be compounded by the risk for malabsorption of fat-soluble vitamins in ICP itself because of reduced enterohepatic circulation of bile acids with decreased uptake in the ileum. Therefore, some concern exists regarding the possibility of vitamin K deficiency in the mother and the fetus. Some supplement with vitamin K to avoid potential complications of deficiency, such as maternal or fetal bleeding; however, no studies have been performed and the authors do not support this practice.

Given the poor performance of cholestyramine in ameliorating maternal pruritus, biochemistries, or newborn outcomes, its use in the treatment of ICP has not gained widespread acceptance. The frequent side effects associated with cholestyramine have also been met with a lack of enthusiasm in its use as a treatment modality.

Dexamethasone

Dexamethasone has also been proposed as a treatment for ICP given its effect on reducing circulating estriol levels thought to increase intrahepatic cholestasis. Dexamethasone crosses the placenta and reduces dehydroepiandrosterone sulfate (DHEAS) production from the fetal adrenals. Because DHEAS is a precursor for placental production of estriol, dexamethasone effectively decreases estriol levels. A small observational study of 10 women with ICP treated with dexamethasone initially showed promising results as all subjects had either a reduction or a cessation in their pruritus and a reduction in total bile acid and ALT levels.[62] No maternal or fetal adverse side effects were reported in this small study. A second small observational study of 12 women who failed treatment with UDCA also showed some improvement with dexamethasone, clinically and biochemically, and also without maternal or fetal side effects.[63] However, the largest study to date randomized 130 women to dexamethasone, UDCA, or placebo and did not show improvement in pruritus with dexamethasone.[64] Furthermore, subjects receiving dexamethasone had no reduction in ALT and had less of a decrease in bile acid and bilirubin levels when compared with those receiving UDCA. Treatment with dexamethasone did not improve any of the perinatal outcomes examined. One case report has documented worsening of ICP following treatment with dexamethasone.[65]

Several concerns exist with the use of dexamethasone. In the rat model, antenatal administration of dexamethasone resulted in decreased insulin sensitivity in offspring.[66] In the African vervet monkey, antenatal dexamethasone exposure is associated with impaired glucose tolerance, hyperinsulinemia, decreased pancreatic beta cell number, and increased blood pressures in the offspring.[67] In humans, dexamethasone administration for fetal lung maturity has been associated with decreased birth weight.[68] Finally, dexamethasone causes widespread maternal effects on almost every organ system, but especially affects the central nervous system, the endocrine and metabolic systems, the gastrointestinal system, the musculature, and the skin.

Given the suboptimal results of dexamethasone as a treatment for ICP along with the adverse side-effect profile associated with its prolonged use, the authors do not favor the use of this drug.

Phenobarbital

Phenobarbital was once used to treat ICP but is currently not used in the treatment of ICP given the lack of significant or consistent data. Small trials examining phenobarbital in dosages ranging from 100 to 150 mg/day have shown inconsistent improvements in maternal pruritus and negligible or no effects on serum biochemistries.[58,59]

S-Adenosyl-L-Methionine

S-adenosyl-L-methionine (SAMe) is a methyl group donor involved in the production of several different phospholipids, including phosphatidylcholine, which is found in the hepatic cell membrane. By altering function at the level of the hepatic surface membrane, SAMe improves the impairment of bile flow caused by increased levels of ethinyl estradiol.[69] Studies of SAMe in rats have shown reversal of cholestasis in those treated with ethinyl estradiol.[70]

Several randomized studies examining SAMe have been performed in humans with ICP. An initial placebo-controlled study in 18 women examined the effects of varying dosages of SAMe (200 vs 800 mg IV/d) and found that the higher dosage was associated with a greater decline in transaminases, conjugated bilirubin, and total bile acids.[71] Pruritus was also significantly decreased in this group and no adverse side effects were noted in either group. Although these results were reproduced in another single-blinded, placebo-controlled study,[72] a double-blinded, placebo-controlled trial of an even higher dosage of SAMe (900 mg IV/d) failed to show any advantages over placebo.[73]

SAMe has also been compared with UDCA in several, small randomized studies, and in one recent, larger study that enrolled 78 women.[30,74-76] With regard to improvement in pruritus, the studies have shown mixed results ranging from no improvement at all to an equivalent improvement when compared with UDCA or placebo.[30,74,75] SAMe is not as effective as UDCA in decreasing serum transaminases, bilirubin, and bile acids levels[75,76] and may cause no improvement at all in some cases.[73] There were no significant differences in preterm delivery rates or gestational age at delivery in any of these studies. Finally, although no serious adverse maternal, fetal, or neonatal effects have been reported, some women have noted problems with peripheral veins during administration of the drug.[73]

Given the painful intravenous or intramuscular route of administration and the lack of a convincing therapeutic effect when compared with placebo or UDCA, SAMe has not become a prime medication in the treatment of ICP.

Ursodeoxycholic Acid

Ursodeoxycholic acid is a naturally occurring bile acid that comprises approximately 5% of the total bile acids found in humans. It is less toxic than other bile acids and is used in the treatment of cholestatic liver disease, exerting its effects via three main mechanisms.[77] Firstly, the decreased biliary secretion of endogenous and toxic bile acids seen in patients with ICP is enhanced by UDCA, thereby decreasing serum levels of endogenous bile acids and bilirubin. A second mechanism involves protection of cholangiocytes from cytotoxic hydrophobic bile acids, and a third mechanism involves protection of hepatocytes from apoptosis caused by bile acids.

An early pilot study of five subjects showed efficacy and safety of UDCA at a dosage of 1 g/day.[78] Pruritus and serum levels of total bile salts and ALT improved, and there were no adverse outcomes in the mothers or their babies. Following this study, several reviews and randomized-controlled trials have confirmed positive results when using UDCA as a treatment for ICP in dosages ranging from 450 mg daily to 2 g daily.[30,60,64,75,76,79-82] UDCA is more effective at decreasing pruritus when compared with either placebo, SAMe, cholestyramine, or dexamethasone,[30,60,64,79] and more effectively improves parameters of liver function including serum bile acids when compared with these drugs. In addition to these improvements in maternal serum, concentrations of bile acids, such as conjugated cholic acid and conjugated chenodeoxycholic acid, are decreased in amniotic fluid and in cord blood with the use of UDCA.[81]

With respect to perinatal outcomes, the effects of UDCA are less clear. Although some studies have shown no differences in gestational age at delivery or rates of preterm birth,[30,64] several other trials have found differences in these parameters with the use of UDCA.[60,81,82] One study comparing 32 women who received UDCA to historical controls who did not receive UDCA, showed a striking difference in preterm birth of 12.5% versus 65.7% respectively, with treated fetuses weighing on average 500 g more. Whether UDCA decreases rates of fetal asphyxia and meconium staining of the amniotic fluid is also unclear. UDCA is well tolerated by mothers, and thus far no adverse effects have been reported in either mothers or neonates.

UDCA is now considered the mainstay of therapy for the treatment of ICP. The dosage usually required to attain an effect on maternal pruritus and serum bile acids

closely followed after pregnancy. Furthermore, women with ICP have a greater risk for developing liver and biliary diseases including hepatitis C (relative risk [RR] = 3.5), nonalcoholic liver cirrhosis (RR = 8.2), gallstones and cholecystitis (RR 3.7), and nonalcoholic pancreatitis (RR = 3.2) when compared with patients without ICP.[92]

Other notable associations with ICP include 20% of such women having cyclic pruritus either at the time of ovulation or in the luteal phase of the menstrual cycle.[41] In women with a history of ICP, pruritus is also associated with oral contraceptive pill use, although recurrence of cholestasis is not of great concern.[91] Finally, 13% of women with ICP have a history of cholelithiasis.[41]

SUMMARY

Intrahepatic cholestasis of pregnancy is a disease that is likely multifactorial in etiology and has a prevalence that varies by geography and ethnicity. The diagnosis is made when patients have a combination of pruritus and abnormal liver function tests. It is associated with a high risk for adverse perinatal outcome, including preterm birth, meconium passage, and fetal death. As of yet, the cause for fetal death is unknown. Because fetal deaths caused by ICP appear to occur predominantly after 37 weeks, it is suggested to offer delivery at approximately 37 weeks. Ursodeoxycholic acid appears to be the most effective medication to improve maternal pruritus and liver function tests; however, there is no medication to date that has been shown to reduce the risk for fetal death.

REFERENCES

1. Wilson B, Haverkamp A. Cholestatic jaundice of pregnancy: new perspectives. Obstet Gynecol 1979;54(5):650–2.
2. Laifer SA, Stiller RJ, Siddiqui DS, et al. Ursodeoxycholic acid for the treatment of intrahepatic cholestasis of pregnancy. J Matern Fetal Med 2001;10(2):131–5.
3. Berg B, Helm G, Petersohn L, et al. Cholestasis of pregnancy. Clinical and laboratory studies. Acta Obstet Gynecol Scand 1986;65:107–13.
4. Glantz A, Marschall HU, Mattsson LA. Intrahepatic cholestasis of pregnancy: relationships between bile acid levels and fetal complication rates. Hepatology 2004;40(2):467–74.
5. Reyes H, Gonzalez MC, Ribalta J, et al. Prevalence of intrahepatic cholestasis of pregnancy in Chile. Ann Intern Med 1978;88:487–93.
6. Lammert F, Marschall HU, Glantz A, et al. Intrahepatic cholestasis of pregnancy: molecular pathogenesis, diagnosis and management. J Hepatol 2000;33(6): 1012–21.
7. Reyes H. Review: intrahepatic cholestasis. A puzzling disorder of pregnancy. J Gastroenterol Hepatol 1997;12(3):211–6.
8. Abedin P, Weaver JB, Egginton E. Intrahepatic cholestasis of pregnancy: prevalence and ethnic distribution. Ethn Health 1999;4(1–2):35–7.
9. Lee RH, Goodwin TM, Greenspoon J, et al. The prevalence of intrahepatic cholestasis of pregnancy in a primarily Latina Los Angeles population. J Perinatol 2006;26:527–32.
10. Gonzalez MC, Reyes H, Arrese M, et al. Intrahepatic cholestasis of pregnancy in twin pregnancies. J Hepatol 1989;9(1):84–90.
11. Heinonen S, Kirkinen P. Pregnancy outcome with intrahepatic cholestasis. Obstet Gynecol 1999;94(2):189–93.
12. Hay JE. Liver Disease in Pregnancy. Hepatology 2008;47(3):1067–76.

13. Reyes H, Baez M, Gonzalez MC, et al. Selenium, zinc, and copper plasma levels in intrahepatic cholestasis of pregnancy, in normal pregnancies and in healthy individuals, in Chile. J Hepatol 2000;32(4):542–9.

14. Kauppila A, Korpela H, Makila UM, et al. Low serum selenium concentration and glutathione peroxidase activity in intrahepatic cholestasis of pregnancy. Br Med J (Clin Res Ed) 1987;294(6565):150–2.

15. Oude Elferink RP, Paulusma CC. Function and pathophysiological importance of ABCB4 (MDR3 P-glycoprotein). Pflugers Arch 2007;453(5):601–10.

16. Dixon PH, Weerasekera N, Linton KJ, et al. Heterozygous MDR3 missense mutation associated with intrahepatic cholestasis of pregnancy: evidence for a defect in protein trafficking. Hum Mol Genet 2000;9(8):1209–17.

17. Mullenbach R, Bennett A, Tetlow N, et al. ATP8B1 mutations in British cases with intrahepatic cholestasis of pregnancy. Gut 2005;54(6):829–34.

18. Painter JN, Savander M, Ropponen A, et al. Sequence variation in the ATP8B1 gene and intrahepatic cholestasis of pregnancy. Eur J Hum Genet 2005;13: 435–9.

19. Huang L, Zhao A, Lew JL, et al. Farnesoid X receptor activates transcription of the phospholipid pump MDR3. J Biol Chem 2003;278:51085–90.

20. Wei J, Wang H, Yang X, et al. Altered gene profile of placenta from women with intrahepatic cholestasis of pregnancy. Arch Gynecol Obstet Jun 2009. [Epub ahead of print]. DOI:10.1007/s00404-009-1156-3.

21. Schreiber A, Simon F. Estrogen induced cholestasis: clues to pathogenesis and treatment. Hepatology 1983;3(4):607–13.

22. Reyes H, Simon FR. Intrahepatic cholestasis of pregnancy: an estrogen-related disease. Semin Liver Dis 1993;13(3):289–301.

23. Meng LJ, Reyes H, Palma J, et al. Profiles of bile acids and progesterone metabolites in the urine and serum of women with intrahepatic cholestasis of pregnancy. J Hepatol 1997;27(2):346–57.

24. Kenyon AP, Piercy CN, Girling J, et al. Pruritus may precede abnormal liver function tests in pregnant women with obstetric cholestasis: a longitudinal analysis. BJOG 2001;108(11):1190–2.

25. Germain A, Carvajal J, Glasinovic J, et al. Intrahepatic cholestasis of pregnancy: an intriguing pregnancy-specific disorder. J Soc Gynecol Investig 2002;9(1):10–4.

26. Reyes H. The spectrum of liver and gastrointestinal disease seen in cholestasis of pregnancy. Gastroenterol Clin North Am 1992;21(4):905–21.

27. Roger D, Vaillant L, Fignon A, et al. Specific pruritic diseases of pregnancy: a prospective study of 3192 pregnant women. Arch Dermatol 1994;130(6): 734–9.

28. Reyes H, Radrigan ME, Gonzalez MC, et al. Steatorrhea in patients with intrahepatic cholestasis of pregnancy. Gastroenterology 1987;93(3):584–90.

29. Dann AT, Kenyon AP, Seed PT, et al. Glutathione S-transferase and liver function in intrahepatic cholestasis of pregnancy and pruritus gravidarum. Hepatology 2004;40(6):1406–14.

30. Floreani A, Paternoster D, Melis A, et al. S-adenosyl methionine versus ursodeoxycholic acid in the treatment of intrahepatic cholestasis of pregnancy: preliminary results of a controlled trial. Eur J Obstet Gynecol Reprod Biol 1996;67(2):109–13.

31. Carter J. Serum bile acids in normal pregnancy. Br J Obstet Gynaecol 1991; 98(6):540–3.

32. Bacq Y, Myara A, Brechot MC, et al. Serum conjugated bile acid profile during intrahepatic cholestasis of pregnancy. J Hepatol 1995;22(1):66–70.

33. Sjovall K, Sjovall J. Serum bile acid levels in pregnancy with pruritus (bile acids and steroids 158). Clin Chim Acta 1966;13(2):207–11.
34. Heikkinen J, Maentausta O, Ylostalo P, et al. Changes in serum bile acid concentrations during normal pregnancy, in patients with intrahepatic cholestasis of pregnancy and in pregnant women with itching. Br J Obstet Gynaecol 1981; 88(3):240–5.
35. Heikkinen J. Serum bile acids in the early diagnosis of intrahepatic cholestasis of pregnancy. Obstet Gynecol 1983;61(5):581–7.
36. Huang WM, Gowda M, Donnelly JG. Bile acid ratio in diagnosis of intrahepatic cholestasis of pregnancy. Am J Perinatol 2009;26(4):291–4.
37. Rencoret R, Aste H. Jaundice during pregnancy. Med J Aust 1973;1(4):167–9.
38. Reid R, Ivey K, Rencoret R, et al. Fetal complications of obstetric cholestasis. Br Med J 1976;1(6014):870–2.
39. Alsulyman OM, Ouzounian JG, Ames-Castro M, et al. Intrahepatic cholestasis of pregnancy: perinatal outcome associated with expectant management. Am J Obstet Gynecol 1996;175(4 Pt 1):957–60.
40. Fisk NM, Storey GN. Fetal outcome in obstetric cholestasis. Br J Obstet Gynaecol 1988;95(11):1137–43.
41. Williamson C, Hems L, Goulis D, et al. Clinical outcome in a series of cases of obstetric cholestasis identified via a patient support group. BJOG 2004;111(7): 676–81.
42. Williamson C, Gorelik J, Eaton BM, et al. The bile acid taurocholate impairs rat cardiomyocyte function: a proposed mechanism for intra-uterine fetal death in obstetric cholestasis. Clin Sci (Lond) 2001;100(4):363–9.
43. Gorelik J, Harding SE, Shevchuk AI, et al. Taurocholate induces changes in rat cardiomyocyte contraction and calcium dynamics. Clin Sci (Lond) 2002;103(2): 191–200.
44. Sepulveda WH, Gonzalez C, Cruz MA, et al. Vasoconstrictive effect of bile acids on isolated human placental chorionic veins. Eur J Obstet Gynecol Reprod Biol 1991;42(3):211–5.
45. Kafkasli A, Belfort MA, Giannina G, et al. Histopathologic effects of meconium on human umbilical artery and vein: in vitro study. J Matern Fetal Med 1997;6(6): 356–61.
46. Lee RH, Incerpi MH, Miller DA, et al. Sudden fetal death in intrahepatic cholestasis of pregnancy. Obstet Gynecol 2009;113(2 Pt 2):528–31.
47. Sentilhes L, Verspyck E, Pia P, et al. Fetal death in a patient with intrahepatic cholestasis of pregnancy. Obstet Gynecol 2006;107(2 Pt 2):458–60.
48. Campos GA, Guerra FA, Israel EJ. Effects of cholic acid infusion in fetal lambs. Acta Obstet Gynecol Scand 1986;65(1):23–6.
49. Lee RH, Kwok KM, Ingles S, et al. Pregnancy outcomes during an era of aggressive management for intrahepatic cholestasis of pregnancy. Am J Perinatol 2008; 25(6):341–5.
50. Shaw D, Frohlich J, Wittmann BA, et al. A prospective study of 18 patients with cholestasis of pregnancy. Am J Obstet Gynecol 1982;142(6 Pt 1):621–5.
51. Israel EJ, Guzman ML, Campos GA. Maximal response to oxytocin of the myometrium from pregnant patients with intrahepatic cholestasis. Acta Obstet Gynecol Scand 1986;65(6):581–2.
52. Krasopoulos JC, De Bari VA, Needle MA. The adsorption of bile salts on activated carbon. Lipids 1980;15(5):365–70.
53. Davis DR, Yeary RA, Lee K. Activated charcoal decreases plasma levels in the hyperbilirubinemic rat. Pediatr Res 1983;17(3):208–9.

54. Kuusisto P, Vapaatalo H, Minninen V, et al. Effect of activated charcoal on hyper-cholesterolaemia. Lancet 1986;2(8503):366–7.
55. Kaaja RJ, Kontula KK, Raiha A, et al. Treatment of cholestasis of pregnancy with peroral activated charcoal. A preliminary study. Scand J Gastroenterol 1994; 29(2):178–81.
56. Riikonen S, Sanovius H, Gylling H, et al. Oral guar gum, a gel-forming dietary fiber relieve pruritus in intrahepatic cholestasis of pregnancy. Acta Obstet Gynecol Scand 2000;79(4):260–4.
57. Gylling H, Riikonen S, Nikkila K, et al. Oral guar gum treatment of intrahepatic cholestasis and pruritus in pregnant women: effects on serum cholestanol and other non-cholesterol sterols. Eur J Clin Invest 1998;28(5):359–63.
58. Laatikainen T. Effect of cholestyramine and phenobarbital on pruritus and serum bile acid levels in cholestasis of pregnancy. Am J Obstet Gynecol 1978;132(5):501–6.
59. Heikkinen J, Maentausta O, Ylostalo P, et al. Serum bile acid levels in intrahepatic cholestasis of pregnancy during treatment with phenobarbital or cholestyramine. Eur J Obstet Gynecol Reprod Biol 1982;14(3):153–62.
60. Kondrackiene J, Beuers U, Kupcinskas L. Efficacy and safety of ursodeoxycholic acid versus cholestyramine in intrahepatic cholestasis of pregnancy. Gastroenterology 2005;129(3):894–901.
61. Sadler LC, Lane M, North R. Severe fetal intracranial haemorrhage during treatment with cholestyramine for intrahepatic cholestasis of pregnancy. Br J Obstet Gynaecol 1995;102(2):169–70.
62. Hirvioja ML, Tuimala R, Vuori J. The treatment of intrahepatic cholestasis of pregnancy by dexamethasone. Br J Obstet Gynaecol 1992;99(2):109–11.
63. Diac M, Kenyon A, Nelson-Piercy C, et al. Dexamethasone in the treatment of obstetrics cholestasis: a case series. J Obstet Gynaecol 2006;26(2):110–4.
64. Glantz A, Marschall HU, Lammert F, et al. Intrahepatic cholestasis of pregnancy: a randomized controlled trial comparing dexamethasone and ursodeoxycholic acid. Hepatology 2005;42(6):1399–405.
65. Kretowicz E, McIntyre HD. Intrahepatic cholestasis of pregnancy, worsening after dexamethasone. Aust N Z J Obstet Gynaecol 1994;34(2):211–3.
66. O'Brien K, Sekimoto H, Boney C, et al. Effects of fetal dexamethasone exposure on the development of adult insulin sensitivity in a rat model. J Matern Fetal Neonatal Med 2008;21(9):623–8.
67. de Vries A, Holmes MC, Heijnis A, et al. Prenatal dexamethasone exposure induces changes in nonhuman primate offspring cardiometabolic and hypothalamic-pituitary-adrenal axis function. J Clin Invest 2007;117(4):1058–67.
68. Bloom SL, Sheffield JS, McIntire DD, et al. Antenatal dexamethasone and decreased birth weight. Obstet Gynecol 2001;97(4):485–90.
69. Boelsterli UA, Rakhit G, Balazs T. Modulation by S-adenosyl-L-methionine of hepatic Na+, K+-ATPase, membrane fluidity, and bile flow in rats with ethinyl estradiol-induced cholestasis. Hepatology 1983;3(1):12–7.
70. Stramentinoli G, Di Padova C, Gualano M, et al. Ethynylestradiol-induced impairment of bile secretion in the rat: protective effects of S-adenosyl-L-methionine and its implication in estrogen metabolism. Gastroenterol 1981;80(1):154–8.
71. Frezza M, Pozzaro G, Chiesa L, et al. Reversal of intrahepatic cholestasis of pregnancy in women after high dose S-adenosyl-L-methionine administration. Hepatology 1984;4(2):274–8.
72. Frezza M, Centini G, Cammareri G, et al. S-adenosylmethionine for the treatment of intrahepatic cholestasis of pregnancy. Results from a controlled clinical trial. Hepatogastroenterology 1990;37(Suppl 2):122–5.

73. Ribalta J, Reyes H, Gonzalez MC, et al. S-adenosyl-L-methionine in the treatment of patients with intrahepatic cholestasis of pregnancy: a randomized, double-blind, placebo-controlled study with negative results. Hepatology 1991;13(6):1084–9.

74. Nicastri PL, Diaferia A, Tartagni M, et al. A randomized placebo-controlled trial of ursodeoxycholic acid and S-adenosylmethionine in the treatment of intrahepatic cholestasis of pregnancy. Br J Obstet Gynaecol 1998;105(11):1205–7.

75. Roncaglia N, Locatelli A, Arreghini A, et al. A randomized controlled trial of urso-deoxycholic acid and S-adenosyl-l-methionine in the treatment of gestational cholestasis. Br J Obstet Gynaecol 2004;111(1):17–21.

76. Binder T, Salaj P, Zima T, et al. Randomized prospective comparative study of ur-sodeoxycholic acid and S-adenosyl-L-methionine in the treatment of intrahepatic cholestasis of pregnancy. J Perinat Med 2006;34(5):383–91.

77. Paumgartner G, Beuers U. Ursodeoxycholic acid in cholestatic liver disease: mechanism of action and therapeutic use revisited. Hepatology 2000;36(3):525–31.

78. Palma J, Reyes H, Ribalta J, et al. Effects of ursodeoxycholic acid in patients with intrahepatic cholestasis of pregnancy. Hepatology 1992;15(6):1043–7.

79. Diaferia A, Nicastri PL, Tartagni M, et al. Ursodeoxycholic acid therapy in pregnant women with cholestasis. Int J Gynaecol Obstet 1996;52(2):133–40.

80. Berkane N, Cocheton JJ, Brehier D, et al. Ursodeoxycholic acid in intrahepatic cholestasis of pregnancy. A retrospective study of 19 cases. Acta Obstet Gynecol Scand 2000;79(11):941–6.

81. Mazzella G, Rizzo N, Azzaroli F, et al. Ursodeoxycholic acid administration in patients with cholestasis of pregnancy: effects on primary bile acids in babies and mothers. Hepatology 2001;33(3):504–8.

82. Zapata R, Sandoval L, Palma J, et al. Ursodeoxycholic acid in the treatment of intra-hepatic cholestasis of pregnancy: a 12-year experience. Liver Int 2005;25(3):548–54.

83. Saleh MM, Abdo KR. Consensus on the management of obstetrics cholestasis: national UK survey. Br J Obstet Gynaecol 2007;114(1):99–103.

84. Laatikainen T, Tulenheimo A. Maternal serum bile acids and fetal distress in cholestasis of pregnancy. Int J Gynaecol Obstet 1984;22(2):91–4.

85. Matos A, Bernardes J, Ayres-de-Campos D, et al. Antepartum fetal cerebral hemorrhage not predicted by current surveillance methods in cholestasis of pregnancy. Obstet Gynecol 1997;89(5 Pt 2):803–4.

86. Rioseco AJ, Ivankovic MB, Manzur A, et al. Intrahepatic cholestasis of pregnancy: a retrospective case-control study of perinatal outcome. Am J Obstet Gynecol 1994;170(3):890–5.

87. Roncaglia N, Arreghini A, Locatelli A, et al. Obstetrics cholestasis: outcome with active management. Eur J Obstet Gynecol Reprod Biol 2002;100(2):167–70.

88. Kenyon AP, Piercy CN, Girling J, et al. Obstetric cholestasis, outcome with active management: a series of 70 cases. Br J Obstet Gynaecol 2002;109(3):282–8.

89. Gurung V, Williamson C, Chappell L, et al. Pilot study for a trial of ursodeoxycholic acid and/or early delivery for obstetric cholestasis. BMC Pregnancy Childbirth 2009;9:19.

90. Bacq Y, Sapey T, Brechot MC, et al. Intrahepatic cholestasis of pregnancy: a French prospective study. Hepatology 1997;26(2):358–64.

91. Leevy CB, Koneru B, Klein KM. Recurrent familial prolonged intrahepatic cholestasis of pregnancy associated with chronic liver disease. Gastroenterol 1997;113(3):966–72.

92. Ropponen A, Sund R, Ylikorkala O, et al. Intrahepatic cholestasis of pregnancy as an indicator of liver and biliary diseases: a population-based study. Hepatology 2006;43(4):723–8.

Update on Peripartum Cardiomyopathy

Meredith O. Cruz, MD, MPH, MBA[a],*, Joan Briller, MD[b,c],
Judith U. Hibbard, MD[a]

KEYWORDS
- Peripartum cardiomyopathy • Pregnancy
- Cardiac disease • Congestive heart failure

Peripartum cardiomyopathy (PPCM), or heart failure in association with pregnancy, was noted as early as the 1800s, but was first attributed to cardiomyopathy by Gouley and colleagues[1] in 1937. The incidence has been reported to vary by geographic location, with rates ranging from approximately 1:15,000 pregnancies in the United States to as frequent as 1:299 in a well-studied population in Haiti and 1:100 in a small region of sub-Saharan Africa.[2] Risk factors include hypertension, preeclampsia, multiparity, multiple gestations, African descent, and older maternal age. The prevalence of different risk factors in diverse populations may account for some of the wide range of reported prevalence estimates. Although rare, cardiomyopathy in pregnancy accounts for a significant proportion of maternal deaths, and in the United States may be increasing in frequency.[3,4] Reported mortalities have ranged as high as 18% to 56%. Even when the mother survives, she may not recover myocardial function and may require chronic therapy for heart failure or cardiac transplantation. Until recently, the cause has been poorly understood. Multiple mechanisms have been postulated as the inciting cause, including inflammation, myocarditis, autoimmune reactions, apoptosis, and oxidative stress.[5] This review addresses pathogenesis, risk factors, diagnosis, management, and prognosis.

CAUSE OF PROPOSED PATHOGENIC MECHANISMS

The investigation of the pathophysiology has been limited by the rare incidence of the disease, and the exact cause is unknown. It was previously believed that PPCM was

[a] Division of Maternal Fetal Medicine, Department of Obstetrics and Gynecology, University of Illinois at Chicago, 840 South Wood Street, M/C 808, Chicago, IL 60612, USA
[b] Department of Cardiology, University of Illinois at Chicago, 840 South Wood Street, M/C 715, Chicago, IL 60612, USA
[c] Department of Obstetrics and Gynecology, University of Illinois at Chicago, 840 South Wood Street, M/C 808, Chicago, IL 60612, USA
* Corresponding author.
E-mail address: mcruz9@uic.edu

Obstet Gynecol Clin N Am 37 (2010) 283–303
doi:10.1016/j.ogc.2010.02.003
0889-8545/10/$ – see front matter. Published by Elsevier Inc.

obgyn.theclinics.com

a result of an idiopathic dilated cardiomyopathy (IDCM) that was expressed in young, peripartal women, with a clinical and pathologic picture similar to that observed in older women or men.[6]

For many years it was believed that PPCM was a variant of IDCM that was unmasked by the hemodynamic stress of pregnancy.[7] If this were the case, then one would expect the incidence of PPCM to be the highest during the period when greatest hemodynamic stress is achieved, which is during the second trimester. However, PPCM usually occurs in the third trimester, and even more commonly in the puerperium.[8] Moreover, 30% of patients with PPCM experience complete recovery, with partial recovery in most cases, in contrast to rare recovery in IDCM.[9] Moreover, PPCM is diagnosed in young women during the peripartum period, whereas IDCM is more common in the older population.[10]

PPCM is likely its own distinct entity, and several hypotheses have been proposed regarding the pathophysiology, including viral myocarditis, abnormal immune response to pregnancy, increased myocyte apoptosis, stress-activated cytokines, maladaptive response to the hemodynamic stresses of pregnancy, excessive prolactin production, malnutrition, genetics, abnormal hormonal function, increased adrenergic tone, and myocardial ischemia (**Fig. 1**).[11] Several of these etiologic mechanisms seem plausible, but none is definite.

VIRAL MYOCARDITIS

Pregnancy results in an immunocompromised state.[12] The relationship between viral myocarditis and pregnancy was established as early as 1968 by Farber and Glasgow,[13] who showed that pregnant mice were more susceptible to viral infections than nonpregnant mice. They also found that viruses multiply to a greater level in

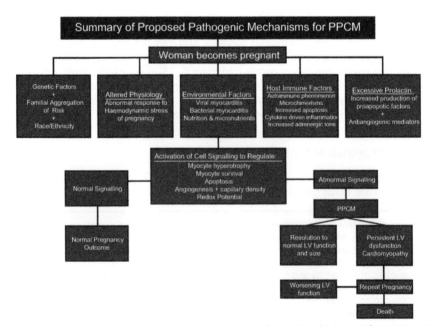

Fig. 1. Summary of proposed pathogenic mechanisms for PPCM. (*Adapted from* Ntusi NB, Mayosi BM. Etiology and risk factors of peripartum cardiomyopathy: a systematic review. Int J Cardiol 2009;131:168–79; with permission.)

the hearts of pregnant mice. The hemodynamic and physiologic changes of pregnancy may result in an increased susceptibility to viral myocarditis, higher viral loads (eg, Coxsackie and echoviruses), and worsening of myocardial viral lesions.[13,14]

PPCM secondary to myocarditis in humans was first shown by Gouley and colleagues,[1] who linked infection with enlarged hearts containing focal areas of necrosis and fibrosis in women dying of heart failure in the puerperium. Myocarditis has also been detected in endomyocardial biopsies in women with PPCM; however, there was a wide prevalence range among these studies (8.8%–76%).[15–20] Insufficient sample sizes prohibited achieving statistical significance in any of these studies. Multiple reasons have been suggested for this variability in prevalence, including challenge in defining PPCM clinically, inclusion of patients outside the accepted time frame, timing of biopsy in relation to the onset of symptoms, variability in inclusion of patients with borderline myocarditis along with those with clear histologic myocarditis as defined by the Dallas histologic criteria, and geographic variability of affected populations.[10]

Molecular studies within a German cohort of patients with PPCM found a high prevalence of virus-associated inflammatory changes and interstitial inflammation.[21] It is possible that there is a postviral immune response that is directed inappropriately toward the myocardium, resulting in decreased ventricular systolic function in the setting of increased circulating volume that is characteristic of pregnancy.[10] Further studies are needed to confirm the relationship between viral genomic particles and PPCM. In the future, newer technologies such as the polymerase chain reaction may be helpful in detecting viruses in the myocardium of PPCM patients.[11]

AUTOIMMUNE MECHANISMS

PPCM may be secondary to abnormal immunologic activity and inflammatory cytokines. Autoantibodies against select cardiac tissue proteins (eg, adenine nucleotide translocator, branched chain α-keto acid dehydrogenase) have been found in women with PPCM along with increased levels of inflammatory markers (eg, tumor necrosis factor-α, interleukin-6 [IL-6], and soluble Fas receptors).[22,23] These increased markers were significantly correlated with increased left ventricular (LV) dimensions and lower LV ejection fraction in patients who presented with PPCM.[23,24]

Other studies have suggested that PPCM is an acute, organ-specific, facultative autoimmune disease that is diagnosed in settings of altered immune and genetic environments.[25,26] In this setting, hematopoietic fetal cells may be introduced into maternal circulation during pregnancy without being rejected as a result of the immunosuppressive state of pregnancy. These cells are attracted to cardiac tissue and are later recognized as nonself during the post partum immune recovery, resulting in a pathologic autoimmune response.[10] Antibodies have also been suggested to form against proteins from the rapidly involuting uterus (eg, actin, myosin), which may cross-react with similar proteins found in the myocardium, resulting in PPCM.[10]

Warraich and colleagues[27] evaluated the effect of PPCM on humoral immunity and evaluated immunoglobulins (Ig; class G and subclasses G1, G2, G3) against cardiac myosin in 47 patients with PPCM from different global regions. Compared with healthy mothers and patients with IDCM, class G and all subclass Ig were nonselectively increased in PPCM, whereas there was a selective upregulation of IgG3s in IDCM.[27] Raised levels of G3-Ig in patients with chronic heart failure were found to correlate with poor clinical course at 6 month follow-up after conventional therapy.[28]

These multiple studies do not show with certainty that abnormal maternal autoimmune mechanisms account for the causation of PPCM. Moreover, it is not clear whether the autoantibodies may be secondary epiphenomena or whether they contribute directly to myocyte injury.[11]

CYTOKINE-MEDIATED INFLAMMATION

Investigations in molecular biology have shown that cytokines may contribute to the basic pathophysiology of cardiac failure.[29] Increased levels of cytokines have also been found in the serum of women with PPCM.[23] Cytokines are signaling molecules that are used extensively in cellular interaction. They are involved in a variety of biologic processes, and their effects on the cardiovascular system include promotion of inflammation, intravascular coagulation, oxidative stress, cardiac structural and functional abnormalities, endothelial injury, and cardiomyocyte apoptosis.[30] The proinflammatory cytokines include TNF-α, IL-1, IL-6, IFN-γ, which are involved in cardiac tissue repairs that result in immediate and delayed negative inotropic effects on myocardial contractility.[29,30] The inflammatory marker C-reactive protein (CRP) has been coexpressed with TNF-α in the myocardium of PPCM patients, as well as other human cardiomyopathies.[31] It is believed that in PPCM, as in other conditions that result in heart failure, the LV end-diastolic wall stress results in myocardial expression of a proinflammatory cytokine network, which influences cardiac contractile performance and promotes maladaptive ventricular remodeling, leading to heart failure.[29]

HEMODYNAMIC STRESS OF PREGNANCY

The cardiovascular changes in pregnancy are characterized by a high-volume, low-resistance state, with cardiac output increased up to 30% or 40% by the second and third trimester. These changes normally persist up to 2 or 3 weeks post partum, and may not resolve to normal physiology until 12 weeks post partum. It is believed that PPCM may be due to an exaggerated decrease in systolic function in the presence of the marked hemodynamic changes of pregnancy.

Echocardiographic and Doppler analysis of cardiac hemodynamics in normal pregnancy showed a 10% increase in preload (LV end-diastolic volume), a 45% increase in cardiac output, and a 28% decrease in afterload (end-systolic wall stress), with LV remodeling and transient LV hypertrophy.[32,33] Although LV anatomy may return to normal after pregnancy, contractile reserve in patients with PPCM was found to be decreased when assessed by dobutamine stress echocardiography.[34] There are not enough convincing data currently to support this hypothesis as the underlying cause for PPCM.

INCREASED MYOCYTE APOPTOSIS

Various animal models of heart failure have shown terminally differentiated cardiac myocytes undergoing apoptosis, or programmed cell death, as the final common pathway in cardiac disorders such as dilated and ischemic cardiomyopathy and acute myocardial infarction (MI).[35,36] It is believed that disruption of this homeostatic mechanism may lead to uncontrolled cellular proliferation and excessive cell death.[37] Studies have reported the G protein Gq to be responsible for coupling several cell surface receptors to intracellular signaling pathways involved in cardiac myocyte hypertrophy and cardiomyocyte apoptosis.[38,39] Apoptosis, which is mediated by proteases termed caspases, can be reduced by caspase inhibitors, which have been shown to improve LV function and survival in pregnant Gαq mice.[40] However, controversy still exists on the relevance of apoptosis to the development of PPCM.

EXCESSIVE PROLACTIN PRODUCTION

The involvement of prolactin in PPCM has been suggested, but recent studies have confirmed the potential role of excessive prolactin production in the pathogenesis of PPCM in mice and women.[41,42] Increased blood volume, decreased blood pressure, decreased angiotensin responsiveness, increased erythropoietin levels, reduced renal excretion of water, sodium, and potassium are all associated with prolactin.[43,44] A high incidence of PPCM has been noted in knockout mice for STAT-3, a cardiac tissue-specific DNA-binding protein. STAT-3 is involved in mediating cardiomyocyte hypertrophy and myocardial angiogenesis but also protects the heart from oxidative stress by upregulating antioxidative enzymes (eg, manganese superoxide dismutase [MnSOD]).[45] Reduced levels of STAT-3 lead to increased oxidative stress and activation of cathepsin D, resulting in cleavage of prolactin into an antiangiogenic and proapoptotic 16-kDa isoform.[41] Treatment of STAT-3–deficient pregnant mice with bromocriptine, an inhibitor of prolactin secretion, prevents the development of PPCM in these mice.[46]

NUTRITION

Nutrition was believed to play a role in the pathogenesis of PPCM. For example, selenium deficiency, which increases cardiovascular susceptibility to viral infection, hypertension and hypocalcemia, was detected in women with PPCM from the Sahel region of Africa.[47] Excessive salt consumption, leading to volume overload, may also be linked to PPCM.[48] However, malnutrition likely does not play a role in the cause of PPCM because many occurrences of the disease are documented in well-nourished patients.[17,48]

GENETICS

Some case reports suggest a possible familial clustering of PPCM. In each of these instances of women diagnosed with PPCM, at least 1 first-degree relative had also experienced PPCM.[49–53] There are also animal studies that suggest a genetic susceptibility to viral myocarditis in animals deficient in transforming growth factor-β (TGF-β); however, more studies are needed to investigate the role of TGF-β in PPCM.[54–58]

OTHER CAUSES

Abnormal hormonal regulation has been proposed as a potential cause of PPCM. The heart undergoes homeostatically regulated remodeling during pregnancy, including hypertrophy and growth of the capillary network to accommodate the increased pregnancy-related hemodynamic volume load and to maintain normal maternal-fetal health.[59] Estrogen is believed to promote cardioprotection during pregnancy, and the sudden drop noted after delivery of the placenta might explain why gravidas experience heart failure after delivery.[59] Relaxin, another ovarian hormone produced during pregnancy that promotes excessive relaxation of the cardiac muscle, may also play a role in PPCM.[60] There is a lack of convincing evidence that abnormal hormone levels result in PPCM.

Increased adrenergic tone secondary to emotional or physical stress has been implicated in the pathogenesis of PPCM, resulting in fluid overload, reduced colloid osmotic pressure, and transient LV dysfunction.[61] β1-adrenergic receptor antibodies may also play a role in PPCM, and, together with increased adrenergic tone, may contribute to cardiac muscle dysfunction.[62,63]

Vascular disease as a possible cause of PPCM has also been suggested, but coronary arteries were found to be normal when coronary angiography was performed.[64,65] Pathologic specimens also negate the possibility of vasculitis or intermittent coronary spasms.[66]

RISK FACTORS

Several risk factors are believed to be associated with the development of PPCM, including prolonged tocolysis, advanced maternal age, high gravidity/parity, multi-pregnancy, race, socioeconomic status, gestational hypertension, and cocaine abuse.[11] The use of prolonged tocolytics, such as terbutaline, ritodrine, salbutamol, isoxsuprine, and magnesium sulfate, has been known to cause pulmonary edema but has also been associated with LV dysfunction in the peripartum period.[67,68] The physiologic side effects of these drugs via interaction with β receptors include tachycardia, hyperglycemia, hypokalemia, and water retention. Cardiac failure and tocolysis seem to be unique in pregnancy, as these same medications, used for various other conditions, do not result in similar complications in nonpregnant women.[11] The underlying mechanisms by which these drugs might cause heart failure in pregnancy include (1) increased circulating blood volume resulting in overload; (2) prolonged β-sympathomimetic stimulation resulting in prolonged tachycardia as well as decreased serum albumin concentration and colloid oncotic pressure; (3) increased aldosterone and antidiuretic hormone secretion resulting in decreased excretion of sodium and water.[11,69]

Advanced maternal age was believed to be a risk factor for PPCM. In a review of several case series of patients with PPCM, their mean age was approximately 30 years.[9,23,70,71] However, the prevalence in all of the aforementioned studies was greatest in women at the upper and lower extremes of child-bearing age.[11] In terms of gravidity/parity as risk factors, PPCM has been documented to occur more often in women with high gravidity and parity.[9,23,71] Moreover, although most women with PPCM have a singleton pregnancy, the prevalence among women with multiple gestations is much higher.[72]

PPCM has been reported among a variety of races, including people of Caucasian, Hispanic, Asian, and African descent.[9,71,73] However, PPCM is generally believed to be more prevalent in women of African descent,[11] although it is not clear whether race is an independent risk factor or an association. Moreover, pregnancy-related hypertension and preeclampsia are also known risk factors for PPCM. However, some have debated whether to exclude pregnancy-related hypertensive disorders from the diagnosis of PPCM, although most investigators believe them to be separate entities. LV recovery at 6 months may be more frequent among women who suffered preeclampsia in contrast to those without this history.[11]

DIAGNOSIS

A thorough history and physical examination should be performed to identify cardiac and noncardiac disorders that may contribute to development or exacerbation of heart failure in pregnancy. This requirement includes attention to the presence of hypertension (chronic, gestational, preeclampsia), diabetes, dislipidemia, coronary, rheumatic or valvular heart disease, prior chemotherapy or mediastinal radiation, sleep disorders, current or past alcohol or drug use, collagen vascular disease, sexually transmitted diseases, thyroid disease, arrhythmias, and family history of cardiomyopathy or sudden death. Current use of alcohol, tobacco, illicit drugs or alternative therapy, diet, and sodium intake should also be assessed. Assessment should be made of the patient's ability to perform activities of daily living. Careful evaluation of volume status should be performed, including orthostatic blood pressure changes, weight, height, and body mass index. Initial laboratory assessment should include complete blood count, urinalysis, serum electrolytes including calcium and magnesium, fasting glucose and hemoglobin A1C, lipid profile, liver function tests, and thyroid-stimulating hormone. Measurement of natriuretic peptides (brain natriuretic peptide [BNP] and N-terminal pro-BNP [NT pro-BNP]) can be helpful in assessment of volume status and risk stratification, although criteria for abnormalities need to be adjusted in pregnancy. Increased BNP levels have been associated with reduced ejection fraction, LV hypertrophy, increased LV filling pressures, acute MI/ischemia, and preeclampsia, although they can occur in other settings such as pulmonary embolism or chronic obstructive pulmonary disease and may not be increased in the setting of morbid obesity.[74–78]

Twelve-lead electrocardiogram and posterior-anterior and lateral chest radiograph should be part of the initial assessment of all patients with clinical heart failure. Two-dimensional echocardiography with Doppler should also be performed to assess LV size, wall thickness, and valvular function, and can give clues to the presence of other precipitating causes such as rheumatic or congenital heart disease. Magnetic resonance imaging (MRI) may play an important role in the diagnosis of PPCM and assist in identifying the mechanism involved.[79] MRI can provide assessment of morphology and function, and has the ability to display myocardial fibrosis as a consequence of myocarditis through delayed contrast enhancement technique.[80] Radionuclide ventriculography or coronary arteriography in the nonpregnant patient may be considered for patients with symptoms or history suggestive of angina or underlying coronary disease without contraindication to revascularization. Noninvasive testing for myocardial ischemia may be substituted for some patients in this setting.

Additional screening for hemochromotosis, sleep disorders, human immunodeficiency virus (HIV), rheumatologic disease, amyloidosis, or pheochromocytoma should be based on clinical suspicion. Endomyocardial biopsy should not be performed routinely, although it is occasionally useful if there is suspected giant cell myocarditis as in autoimmune disorders, thymoma, drug hypersensitivity, anthracycline therapy, restrictive cardiomyopathy, sarcoid, or suspected arrhythmogenic right ventricular dysplasia.[81]

The diagnosis of PPCM is a diagnosis of exclusion (**Box 1**), but should be suspected whenever women present with symptoms of heart failure during the peripartum period. The diagnosis may be challenging because symptoms such as dizziness,

---

Box 1
Clinical criteria for the diagnosis of PPCM

- Development of cardiac failure in the last month of pregnancy or within 5 months post partum

- Absence of another identifiable cause for the cardiac failure

- Absence of recognizable heart disease before the last month of pregnancy

- LV systolic dysfunction shown by echocardiographic data such as depressed shortening fraction (eg, ejection fraction less than 45%, M-mode fractional shortening less than 30%, or both, and an LV end-diastolic dimension of more than 2.7 cm/m²)

Data from Demakis JG, Rahimtoola SH. Peripartum cardiomyopathy. Circulation 1971;44:964–8; Hibbard J, Lindheimer M, Lang R. A modified definition for peripartum cardiomyopathy and prognosis based on echocardiography. Obstet Gynecol 1999;94(2):311–6.

dyspnea, fatigue, or pedal edema of normal late pregnancy are similar to symptoms of early congestive heart failure.[82] Some would argue that the criteria for diagnosis in the last month of pregnancy are outdated and should be revised to include the entire span of pregnancy.[71,83]

There are currently no specific clinical criteria for differentiating between symptoms of normal late pregnancy and heart failure. One should have a high index of suspicion in any woman experiencing paroxysmal nocturnal dyspnea, chest pain, nocturnal cough, new regurgitant murmurs, pulmonary crackles, increased jugular venous pressure, or hepatomegaly.[82] Determining the presence of LV dysfunction is critical to the diagnosis.[84]

MANAGEMENT OF HEART FAILURE

Therapy is directed to improving symptoms, slowing progression of LV dysfunction, and improving survival, as summarized in **Box 2**.

Nonpharmacologic therapy, including fluid restriction and low-sodium diet for patients with evidence of volume overload, monitoring for pedal edema and measurement of daily weight are useful adjuncts. Control of blood pressure is a key component of therapy. Current guidelines for management of chronic heart failure include combinations of 3 types of drugs: diuretics, angiotensin-converting enzyme inhibitors

---

Box 2
Recommended therapy for PPCM

- Goals

  Treat hypertension

  Fluid restriction

  Dietary salt restriction

  Routine exercise post partum if stable

- Drugs for routine use

  Diuretics

  β-Blockers

  Vasodilators

  Digoxin[a]

- Therapies in selected patients

  Aldosterone antagonists

  Inotropes

  Anticoagulation

  Implantable defibrillators

  Biventricular pacing

  Cardiac transplantation

[a] See text for details.

Data from Hunt SA, Abraham WT, Chin MH, et al. Focused update incorporated into the ACC/AHA 2005 guidelines for the diagnosis and management of heart failure in adults: a report of the American College of Cardiology Foundation/American Heart Association Task Force on Practice Guidelines. Circulation 2009;119:e391–479.

(ACEIs) or angiotensin receptor blockers (ARBs), and β-blockers.[78] In women with PPCM, these recommendations need to be modified based on current gravid status and the woman's desire to lactate. Commonly used therapeutic agents with indications and precautions are summarized in **Table 1**. Management of PPCM should be performed in conjunction with a cardiologist versant in the use of these drugs in pregnancy.

Diuretics are indicated for most patients because they can improve pulmonary and peripheral edema within hours or days, but are usually inadequate to maintain clinical volume status in the absence of additional therapy. Furosemide, a loop diuretic, is most commonly used, but thiazides may be added if the loop diuretics are insufficient. Adverse effects are noted in **Table 1**. We typically use diuretics in the gravida with clear evidence of volume overload as well as early after delivery when volume shifts can be expected to increase intravascular volume. Aldosterone antagonists have been shown to improve survival in selected heart failure patients; these agents can be added post partum but we have not currently used these in pregnancy.

ACEIs improve survival in all severities of myocardial disease, but have multiple teratogenic risks and are typically avoided in pregnancy. When initiated post partum, we suggest that the patient should be counseled about the potential for teratogenicity or fetal demise with a recurrent pregnancy and appropriate steps for birth control be implemented. The risk/benefit ratio should be weighed for use in lactating mothers, although we have often prescribed these agents in this setting. For patients who are candidates for ACEIs, therapy is initiated at low dosages and titrated at intervals to a maximal tolerated dose.

ARBs are recommended because they improve mortality in patients with current or prior heart failure who do not tolerate ACEIs; it is not clear whether adding ARBs to ACEIs is beneficial. Teratogenic risks of ARBs are similar to those with ACEIs and we use similar precautions and counseling.

Hydralazine is an arterial vasodilator with little effect on venous tone and filling pressures. A large clinical experience with hydralazine in treating hypertension in pregnancy suggests that it is safe, and it is compatible with breast feeding. Nitrates decrease dyspnea and improve exercise tolerance. We currently use hydralazine and nitrates as the vasodilators of choice for women who are pregnant or if medications acting on the renin-angiotensin system are contraindicated, but ACEIs remain the first-line agent for nonpregnant patients. The combination of hydralazine and nitrates is considered to be a reasonable addition to standard therapy in symptomatic patients and some racial groups.[78,85] Amlodipine is an additional option for vasodilator therapy, especially if hydralazine is not tolerated or the patient has chronic hypertension. Goal systolic blood pressure is 100 to 110 mm Hg for most patients. We do not usually decrease doses of vasodilators for asymptomatic hypotension.

Three β-blockers (sustained-release metoprolol succinate, carvedilol, and bisoprolol), have been shown to reduce mortality with current or prior heart failure and reduced ejection fraction, and is therefore recommended for all stable patients unless contraindicated. Metoprolol is considered compatible with breast feeding, but we recommend monitoring of exposed neonates for signs and symptoms of β blockade, such as bradycardia, hypoglycemia, and growth restriction. Because transient worsening of heart failure symptoms has been reported with initiation of therapy, patients should have minimal evidence of fluid retention and not have required recent intravenous inotropic therapy. Initial therapy is started at a low dose, then doubled at 2-week intervals to achieve the target dose or until limited by symptoms. Improvement seems to be dose dependent; therefore target doses should be those noted in clinical heart failure trials.

Table 1
Common medications in the treatment of peripartum cardiomyopathy

Medication[a]	Indication	Drug Effect	Precautions	
			Maternal	**Fetal**
Diuretics Furosemide[C,L3] (first line) Thiazides[B,L3] (second line)	Evidence of volume overload or fluid retention	↓ Preload and afterload Improve cardiac function Decrease edema, improve exercise tolerance	Electrolyte abnormalities, fluid depletion, hypotension, azotemia	Decreased placental perfusion Thiazides: possible ↑ risk of birth defects or fetal thrombocytopenia
ACE inhibitors[D] Lisinopril[L3] Enalapril[L2] Captopril[L2]	History of LV dysfunction, stage B and C heart failure in the nonpregnant state	↓ preload and afterload Improves survival in all severities of myocardial disease	Electrolyte abnormalities Hypotension Cough Angioedema Worsening renal function	Skull hypoplasia, anuria, renal failure, limb contractures, craniofacial deformation, hypoplastic lungs, death
ARBs[D] Valsartan[L3] Candesartan[L3]	Intolerance to ACE inhibitors	↓ preload and afterload Improves mortality	Similar to ACE inhibitors	Similar to ACE inhibitors
Peripheral vasodilators[C] Hydralazine[L2] Nitrates[L3] Nesiritide[L3,b]	First-line vasodilator in pregnancy as ACE and ARBs are contraindicated	↓ preload and afterload	Hypotension Tolerance with long-term nitrate therapy Headache with nitrates Lupuslike reaction with hydralazine	

Medication	Blood pressure control	Peripheral vasodilation	Adverse effects
Calcium channel blocker[C] Amlodipine[L3]		Peripheral vasodilation	Peripheral edema Hypotension
β-Blockers[C] Metoprolol[L3] Carvedilol[L3] Bisoprolol[L3]	Always used with LV dysfunction unless contraindicated	Improves myocardial contractility by ↓ sympathetic tone Reduces mortality	Transient worsening of congestive heart failure symptoms Avoid initiation or increased dose in decompensated heart failure Bradycardia, hypoglycemia, growth retardation Animal fetal and teratogenicity with carvedilol at high human dose
Inotropes Digoxin[C,L2] Dopamine[C,L2,b] Dobutamine[B,L2,b]	Symptomatic heart failure in pregnancy	↑ myocontractility	Arrhythmias gastrointestinal symptoms Narrow therapeutic index
Aldosterone antagonists Spironolactone[C-D,L2] Eplerenone[B,L3]	May add post partum to ACEI and Arb in symptomatic patients	Improves survival in patients with class 3–4 symptoms	Hyperkalemia Feminization of male rat fetuses

Dr Hale's Lactation Risk Category: L1, controlled studies in breastfeeding women fail to show a risk to the infant and the possibility of harm to the breastfeeding infant is remote, or the product is not orally bioavailable in an infant; L2, drug that has been studied in a limited number of breastfeeding women without an increase in adverse effects in the infant. Or, the evidence of a demonstrated risk that is likely to follow is remote; L3, there are no controlled studies in breastfeeding women, but the risk of untoward effects to a breastfed infant is possible. Or, controlled studies show only minimal nonthreatening adverse effects. Give if potential benefits outweigh risks. Drugs in this category are essentially compatible with breastfeeding. (*Data from* Hale TW. Medications and mother's milk. 12th edition. Amarillo, TX: Hale Publishing; 2006.)

[a] Denotes US Food and Drug Administration class (A, B, C, D) and lactation safety.
[b] Reserved for refractory heart failure.

Digoxin improves symptoms, quality of life, and exercise tolerance in mild-to-moderate heart failure by attenuation of the neurohormonal system and inhibition of sodium potassium adenosine triphosphatase leading to increased myocontractility. Benefit with digoxin therapy has been shown regardless of underlying rhythm, cause of heart failure, or nature of concomitant therapy, but does not decrease mortality in class 2 or 3 heart failure.[86] Digoxin has a narrow therapeutic index and there have been concerns about increased morbidity and mortality when this agent is used[87]; therefore attention is required to avoid toxicity. We usually keep serum levels to between 1 and 1.2 ng/dL or less. However, we typically add digoxin early in the course of therapy in symptomatic women when ACEIs and ARBs are contraindicated.

For patients with ejection fraction of 35% or less on optimal therapy who have an expected survival of more than 1 year, implantable cardioverter defibrillator therapy may be warranted for primary prevention of sudden cardiac death.[78] Cardiac resynchronization therapy is recommended in patients with widened quantitative radioscintigraphy (QRS) by electrocardiograph (ECG) and class 3 or 4 symptoms despite optimal medical therapy.[78] LV-assist devices and transplantation are therapeutic options in the most critical patients.

LV dysfunction is associated with an increased risk of thromboembolic phenomena. In 3 large contemporary heart failure trials risk of embolic events ranged from 1 to 2.5 per 100 patient years.[88–90] Risk of embolic event correlated with severity of heart failure, presence of atrial fibrillation, and thrombus noted on transthoracic echocardiography. Furthermore, pregnancy and the puerperium are prothrombotic states. A recent review of 182 patients with PPCM documented thromboembolic complications in 4 patients (2.2%).[91] Choosing a specific antithrombotic agent during pregnancy is complicated by potential for teratogenicity with warfarin and dosing issues with heparin. In their practice, during pregnancy when warfarin is contraindicated, we have used low-molecular heparin in therapeutic doses when ejection fraction is 30% or less, atrial fibrillation is present, or there is documented thrombus/prior cardiac embolic event. Therapeutic dosing is typically based on weight to achieve an anti-Xa level of 0.6 to 1 IU/mL (enoxaparin) or 0.85 to 1.05 IU/mL (dalteparin). Warfarin can be used post partum in this setting to achieve an international normalization ratio (INR) of 2 to 3, and is safe with breastfeeding.

Drugs known to adversely affect clinical status in heart failure should be avoided whenever possible, including nonsteroidal antiinflammatories, many antiarrhythmic drugs, and nondihydropyridine calcium channel blockers. Exercise training can be an adjunct to improving status in stable post partum patients.[78]

Acute heart failure decompensation is usually manifested by signs of worsening pulmonary or peripheral congestion, particularly dyspnea, tachycardia, decreased oxygen saturation, large weight gain, and signs and symptoms of hypoperfusion such as hypotension or worsening mental status. The normal hemodynamic changes of pregnancy can make recognition of this syndrome difficult, but the presence of basilar rales, jugular venous distension, positive abdominal jugular reflex, increased heart rate, S3, and peripheral edema (all findings that can be normal in pregnancy) should raise the index of suspicion, particularly in those with a previous history of heart failure. Measurement of natriuretic peptides (BNP, NT pro-BNP) can be useful adjuncts to diagnosis.[75]

A search should be made for potentially confounding factors such as acute lung injury, embolus, pneumonia, preeclampsia, or MI. Therapy is directed at treatment of volume overload, afterload reduction, hypertension control, and treatment of confounding factors such as arrhythmias, anemia, and thyroid disease.[78]

Oxygen therapy should be administered to relieve symptoms related to hypoxemia. With significant volume overload we typically initiate loop diuretic therapy with furosemide, although caution must be used in the presence of preeclampsia because of concern for decreased placental perfusion. In pregnancy, hydralazine and nitrates are the vasodilators of choice because ACEIs and ARBs are contraindicated. Although evidence that digoxin is beneficial in acute decompensated heart failure is lacking, we have usually empirically added this drug. We use the same approach to β blockade in pregnant women as in nonpregnant women: initiation of β blockade once volume status has improved; in women already on this therapy it can often be continued, although occasionally dosage needs to be diminished. Intravenous nitroglycerine may be required in more severely decompensated patients, and inotropic therapy with dobutamine may be necessary in the setting of hypoperfusion with clearly increased filling pressures. Few human data are available, but, if blood pressure support is required, dopamine may have fewer potentially deleterious effects on placental blood flow than phenylephrine or norepinephrine.[92] Intravenous nitroprusside or nesiritide may be considered in certain circumstances for afterload reduction, although thiocyanate toxicity must be considered with the former and there are few human data in pregnancy with the latter. Invasive monitoring may be considered for patients with respiratory distress or impaired perfusion in which intracardiac filling pressures cannot be determined from clinical assessment.

OTHER NOVEL THERAPIES

In mouse models of PPCM, increased activity of cardiac cathepsin D promotes activity of a 16-kD proapoptotic form of prolactin, leading to myocardial injury. Bromocriptine as a specific therapy for PPCM is currently being evaluated. Several case reports documenting recovery of function in women with PPCM treated with bromocriptine have been published.[46,93] A series of 12 patients with previous PPCM at high risk for redevelopment were randomized to standard therapy with or without bromocriptine. In the 6 patients treated with bromocriptine there was no recurrence, whereas all patients treated with standard therapy alone developed worsening function.[41,59] MI has rarely been reported in women taking bromocriptine for suppression of lactation.[94] Hilfiker-Kleiner noted no complications in 18 PPCM women treated consecutively with bromocriptine (Denise Hilfiker-Kleiner, MD, Johannesburg, South Africa, personal communication, December 2009). Use of bromocriptine must be weighed against potential harm of decreased milk production, especially in Third World countries where risk of infant infection and malnutrition are high. Ongoing prospective trials should clarify the decision to treat with this agent.

In a study of 59 patients with PPCM, 30 were treated with pentoxifylline, which is known to decrease TNF-α, in addition to standard therapy with digoxin, ACEIs, and β blockade. They had lower mortality, greater decrease in LV end-diastolic and systolic chamber dimensions, and greater increase in functional status than the group treated with standard therapy alone.[95] Intravenous immune globulin has been associated with improved ejection fraction in several studies of cardiomyopathy associated with active inflammation[96,97]; however, treatment effect could not be proved because of a marked variability in outcome measures and the high rate of spontaneous recovery. Immunosuppressive therapy has been considered to be helpful in some patients with active myocarditis, although active viral infection must be excluded.[58,98] None of these novel agents are currently routinely recommended. A multicenter PPCM network is currently being established. Results of studies performed via this network should fuel development of prospective investigations with adequate power to address pathogenesis and new treatments for PPCM.

ANTEPARTUM MANAGEMENT

Serial clinical assessment should be performed at each return visit to assess the patient's ability to perform routine and desired activities of daily living, blood pressure, heart rate, weight, and volume status. Repeat assessment of ejection fraction and structural heart changes should be performed in patients who have had a change in clinical status, at intervals, and usually again before delivery. The value of serial measurements of BNP to guide therapy in pregnant patients with heart failure is not well established but in our practice we have found it a useful adjunct. Serum electrolytes and renal function should be monitored frequently. Potassium and magnesium concentrations are of particular importance because deficiency is a common adverse effect of diuretic therapy and a contributing factor to digoxin toxicity and fatal arrhythmias. Increased potassium levels are of potential concern in patients treated with ACEIs, ARBs, or aldosterone antagonists, although these are not routinely used in pregnancy.

We typically perform a sonogram at 20 weeks' gestation to assess fetal anatomy, and then serially to assess fetal growth, particularly for intrauterine growth restriction. In the third trimester, we routinely perform antenatal testing (eg, nonstress test and amniotic fluid index or biophysical profile) starting at 32 weeks and then weekly thereafter. If steroids for fetal lung maturity are indicated preterm, this medication can be administered safely with careful attention to the potential for fluid retention.

Fett[99] recently proposed a focused medical history test for PPCM patients during the latter portion of the pregnancy and post partum period, evaluating for orthopnea, dyspnea, unexplained cough, lower extremity swelling, excessive weight gain, and palpitations. Patients are assigned points based on symptomotology; tests for natriuretic peptide levels and high-sensitivity CRP (hs-CRP) are performed if the patient has 3to 4 points or more, with repeat echocardiography if these are increased. Fett[99] recommends performing all 3 tests if the patient reports symptoms resulting in 5 or more points. Prospective validation of this point scale in the future will be important in verifying risk.

MANAGEMENT OF DELIVERY

If medical management is successful in stabilizing a patient with PPCM, then early delivery is not required and spontaneous labor is not contraindicated. However, if the converse is true, then early delivery may be desirable. Labor induction can be conducted with minimal risk and, if cervical ripening is required, prostaglandins can be administered safely, as can oxytocin. One should consider administration of an early epidural to minimize sympathetic output; however, caution must be exercised in limiting fluid boluses and maintaining strict intake and output to avoid fluid overload. A predelivery anesthesia consultation is desirable in planning the anesthetic choice. Shortening the second stage of labor with the use of low forceps or a vacuum device is recommended to minimize ventricular work. Given the potential surgical risks encountered with cesarean delivery, including infection, blood loss, greater fluid shifts, and postoperative complications, we believe the cardiovascular benefits from vaginal delivery most often outweigh that of surgical delivery. We typically reserve cesarean delivery for obstetric indications; however, the need for prompt delivery may a play a role in the obstetrician's decision. Placement of invasive catheters for monitoring (eg, Swan-Ganz) have not been proven to achieve better outcomes in perioperative trials. We reserve invasive monitoring for individuals in whom volume status is problematic.[100] Thromboprophylaxis should be considered intrapartum (eg, sequential compression devices or prophylactic heparin). Strict monitoring of fluid status is critical, and we often administer diuretic therapy after delivery to prevent volume overload as fluids are resorbed into the intravascular space after delivery. The parturient should be seen 1 week after delivery to assess her cardiovascular status and make any necessary medication adjustments.

MATERNAL PROGNOSIS

Reports of long-term prognosis in women with PPCM vary, but outcome depends on LV function. Chapa and colleagues[83] reviewed 32 PPCM patients and noted that fractional shortening of less than 20% and LV end-diastolic dimension of 6 cm or more at diagnosis were associated with a threefold greater risk for persistent LV dysfunction. Amos and colleagues[101] reported 55 PPCM cases from 1990 to 2003, mean follow-up 43 months, and their mean initial ejection fraction was 20%. In this cohort, 62% of patients improved, 24% remained unchanged, and 4% died, whereas 10% required cardiac transplantation. Most who recovered significant LV function showed evidence of improvement by 2 months after diagnosis. Predictors of poor outcome included enlarged LV end-diastolic dimension (>5.6 cm), presence of LV thrombus, and African American race. Goland and colleagues[91] recently reviewed 182 PPCM patients for major adverse events (MAE) defined as death or life-threatening complications including heart transplantation, temporary circulatory support, cardiopulmonary arrest, pulmonary edema requiring intensive care unit therapy, thromboembolic complications, ventricular arrhythmias leading to placement of an implantable cardioverter defibrillator or bradyarrhythmias leading to pacemaker placement. Mean age was 29 (±7) years, follow-up 19 (±25) months (range 0–168 months) and ejection fraction 29% (±11%). MAE were noted in 25% of patients and 13 (7%) died: 5 of sudden cardiac death, 6 with progressive heart failure, and 2 from unknown causes. Eleven patients underwent heart transplantation (6%), whereas severe pulmonary edema was noted in 17 (9%) and thromboembolic complications in 4 (2.2%) women. All patients with MAE had severe LV dysfunction, were more commonly non-Caucasian, and more often had a delayed diagnosis. Greater complication rates in non-Caucasian women may reflect genetic or environmental status or disparities in access to health care. Similarly, Sliwa and colleagues[24] studied 100 women with newly diagnosed PPCM at a single center in South Africa for 6 months and noted normalization of LV function in only 23%. Fifteen patients died: 4 suddenly, the rest of progressive heart failure despite optimal medical therapy. Transplantation and placement of an LV-assist device were not available for financial reasons. Plasma markers of inflammation were significantly increased in PPCM patients, and correlated with lower ejection fraction and increased LV dimensions at presentation. Patients who died had a significantly lower mean ejection fraction and higher Fas/Apo-1 plasma levels.

Prognosis with Recurrent Pregnancies

Many women with PPCM desire another pregnancy. Information about risk of recurrent LV dysfunction is based predominantly on retrospective reviews of women who undertook subsequent pregnancies. Elkayam and colleagues[102] reviewed the risk of recurrent cardiomyopathy from a survey of 44 patients who underwent 60 subsequent pregnancies. Subjects were divided into those whose LV function normalized before recurrent pregnancy and those in whom LV function remained diminished. During subsequent pregnancy mean ejection fraction decreased in both groups, and heart failure symptoms were noted in 21% of gravidas with normal LV function and 44% of those with persistent dysfunction; mortality was 19% in those with persistent LV dysfunction. Prematurity was more frequent in the women with LV dysfunction. Fett and colleagues[103] documented 61 women with recurrent pregnancies identified from a Haitian PPCM registry or Internet support group and noted recurrent heart failure in 29% percent. As in the analysis by Elkayam and colleagues,[102] LV function at the start of pregnancy predicted recurrent heart failure at a rate of 46.2% when ejection fraction was less than 55%. Risk was inversely related to ejection fraction, with recurrent cardiomyopathy documented in only 17% of those with ejection fraction greater than 55%, compared with 66.7% recurrence in women with ejection fractions less than 45%.

There are no established protocols for following women with recurrent pregnancies who elect to continue pregnancy. Exercise stress echocardiography or dobutamine stress echocardiography may help define risk in women with recovered function.[34] Some patients with apparent improvement in LV function may still have decreased contractile reserve that becomes evident only with stress testing. Normal cardiac reserve does not preclude recurrent PPCM in any of the studies detailing recurrent pregnancy.[83,102,103] All patients, even those with recovered function, should be considered high risk, and close communication between the treating maternal-fetal medicine expert and cardiologist, and at time of delivery the obstetric anesthesiologist and perinatologist, is mandatory. Based on clinical experience with 61 recurrent gravidas, Fett[99] proposed baseline echocardiographic evaluation of LV function with follow-up evaluation in second and third trimesters, and in the first month post partum or if there is a change in symptoms suggestive of recurrent heart failure. Baseline BNP or pro-BNP and hs-CRP levels, with repeat values performed near term or with symptoms, can also provide useful clues to increased volume status suggestive of recurrent heart failure and increased inflammation associated with impending relapse, respectively. As the pathophysiology of PPCM becomes increasingly better defined, specific cytokine markers may prove useful adjuncts to predicting risk.

SUMMARY

Although multiple mechanisms have been postulated, PPCM continues to be a cardiomyopathy of unknown cause. Multiple risk factors exist and the clinical presentation does not allow differentiation among potential causes. Although specific diagnostic criteria exist, PPCM remains a diagnosis of exclusion. Treatment modalities are dictated by the clinical state of the patient, and prognosis is dependent on recovery of function. Randomized controlled trials of novel therapies, such as bromocriptine, are needed to establish better treatment regimens to decrease morbidity and mortality. The creation of an international registry will be an important step to better define and treat PPCM.

REFERENCES

1. Gouley BA, McMillan TM, Bellet S. Idiopathic myocardial degeneration associated with pregnancy and especially the puerperium. Am J Med Sci 1937;19: 185–99.
2. Mayosi B. Contemporary trends in the epidemiology and management of cardiomyopathy and pericarditis in sub-Saharan Africa. Heart 2007;93:1176–83.
3. Whitehead SJ, Berg CJ, Chang J. Pregnancy related mortality due to cardiomyopathy: United States, 1991–1997. Obstet Gynecol 2003;102(6):1326–31.

4. Kuklina VE, Callaghan WM. Cardiomyopathy and other myocardial disorders among hospitalizatons for pregnancy in the United States 2004–2006. Obstet Gynecol 2010;115:93–100.
5. Hilfiker-Kleiner D, Sliwa K, Drexler H. Peripartum cardiomyopathy: recent insights into its pathophysiology. Trends Cardiovasc Med 2008;18:173–9.
6. Ribner SH, Silverman RI. Peripartal cardiomyopathy. In: Elkayam U, Gleicher N, editors. Cardiac problems in pregnancy: diagnosis and management of maternal and fetal disease. 2nd edition. New York: Alan R Liss; 1990. p. 115–27.
7. Cunningham FG, Pritchard JA, Hankins GD, et al. Peripartum heart failure: idiopathic cardiomyopathy or compounding cardiovascular events? Obstet Gynecol 1986;67:157–68.
8. Robson SC, Hunter S, Boys RJ, et al. Serial study of factors influencing changes in cardiac output during human pregnancy. Am J Physiol 1989;256:1060–5.
9. Fett JD, Christie LG, Carraway RD, et al. Five-year prospective study of the incidence and prognosis of peripartum cardiomyopathy at a single institution. Mayo Clin Proc 2005;80:1602–6.
10. Pearson GD, Veille JC, Rahimtoola S, et al. Peripartum cardiomyopathy: National Heart, Lung, and Blood Institute and Office of Rare Diseases (National Institutes of Health) workshop recommendations and review. JAMA 2000;283:1183–8.
11. Ntusi NB, Mayosi BM. Aetiology and risk factors of peripartum cardiomyopathy: a systematic review [review]. Int J Cardiol 2009;131(2):168–79.
12. Krause PJ, Ingardia CJ, Pontius LT, et al. Host defense during pregnancy: neutrophil chemotaxis and adherence. Am J Obstet Gynecol 1987;157:274–80.
13. Farber PA, Glasgow LA. Viral myocarditis during pregnancy: encephalomyocarditis virus infection in mice. Am Heart J 1970;80:96–102.
14. Lyden DC, Huber SA. Aggravation of Coxsackie virus, group B, type-3-induced myocarditis and increase in cellular immunity to myocyte antigens in pregnant Balb/c mice and animal treated with progesterone. Cell Immunol 1984;87:462–72.
15. Rizeq MN, Rickenbacher PR, Fowler MB, et al. Incidence of myocarditis in peripartum cardiomyopathy. Am J Cardiol 1994;74:474–7.
16. O'Connell JB, Costanzo-Nordin MR, Subramanian R, et al. Peripartum cardiomyopathy: clinical, hemodynamic, histologic, and prognostic characteristics. J Am Coll Cardiol 1986;8:52–6.
17. Sanderson JE, Olsen EG, Gatei D. Peripartum heart disease: an endomyocardial biopsy study. Br Heart J 1986;56:285–91.
18. Midei MG, DeMent SH, Feldman AM, et al. Peripartum myocarditis and cardiomyopathy. Circulation 1990;81:922–8.
19. Melvin KR, Richardson PJ, Olsen EG, et al. Peripartum cardiomyopathy due to myocarditis. N Engl J Med 1982;307:731–4.
20. Felker GM, Jaeger CJ, Klodas E, et al. Myocarditis and long-term survival in peripartum cardiomyopathy. Am Heart J 2000;140:785–91.
21. Bultmann BD, Klingel K, Nabauer M, et al. High prevalence of viral genomes and inflammation in peripartum cardiomyopathy. Am J Obstet Gynecol 2005; 193:363–5.
22. Ansari AA, Neckelmann N, Wang YC, et al. Immunologic dialogue between cardiac myocytes, endothelial cells and mononuclear cells. Clin Immunol Immunopathol 1993;68:208–14.
23. Sliwa K, Skudicky D, Bergemann A, et al. Peripartum cardiomyopathy: analysis of clinical outcome, left ventricular function, plasma levels of cytokines and Fas/APO-1. J Am Coll Cardiol 2000;35:701–5.

24. Sliwa K, Forster O, Libhaber E, et al. Peripartum cardiomyopathy: inflammatory markers as predictors of outcome in 100 prospectively studied patients. Eur Heart J 2005;27:441–6.
25. Ansari AA, Fett JD, Carraway RE, et al. Autoimmune mechanisms as the basis for human peripartum cardiomyopathy. Clin Rev Allergy Immunol 2002;23: 301–24.
26. Sundstrom JB, Fett JD, Carraway RD, et al. Is peripartum cardiomyopathy an organ-specific autoimmune disease? Autoimmun Rev 2002;1:73–7.
27. Warraich RS, Sliwa K, Damasceno A, et al. Impact of pregnancy-related heart failure on humoral immunity: clinical relevance of G3-subclass immunoglobulins in peripartum cardiomyopathy. Am Heart J 2005;150:263–9.
28. Warraich RS, Young JB, Sestier F, et al. Clinical and prognostic relevance of Ig-G3 reactivity in heart failure: a substudy of vasogen's immune modulation therapy in patients with chronic heart failure. J Am Coll Cardiol 2004;43:226A.
29. Drexler H. Changes in the peripheral circulation in heart failure. Curr Opin Cardiol 1995;10:268–73.
30. Mann DL. Stress activated cytokines and the heart: from adaptation to maladaptation. Cytokine Growth Factor Rev 1996;7:341–54.
31. Satoh M, Nakamura M, Akatsu T, et al. C-reactive protein coexpresses with tumour necrosis factor-alpha in the myocardium in human dilated cardiomyopathy. Eur Heart J 2005;7:748–54.
32. Poppas A, Shroff SG, Korcarz CE, et al. Serial assessment of the cardiovascular system in normal pregnancy. Role of arterial compliance and pulsatile arterial load. Circulation 1997;95(10):2407–15.
33. Geva T, Mauer MB, Striker L, et al. Effects of physiologic load of pregnancy on left ventricular contractility and remodeling. Am Heart J 1997;133:53–9.
34. Lampert MB, Weinert L, Hibbard J, et al. Contractile reserve in patients with peripartum cardiomyopathy and recovered left ventricular function. Am J Obstet Gynecol 1997;176:189–95.
35. Wencker D, Chandra M, Nguyen K, et al. A mechanistic role for cardiac myocyte apoptosis in heart failure. J Clin Invest 2003;111:1497–504.
36. Narula J, Kolodgie FD, Virmani R. Apoptosis and cardiomyopathy. Curr Opin Cardiol 2000;15:183–8.
37. MacLellan WR, Schneider MD. Death by design: programmed cell death in cardiovascular biology and disease. Circ Res 1997;81:137–44.
38. Yussman MG, Toyokawa T, Odley A, et al. Mitochondrial death protein Nix is induced in cardiac hypertrophy and triggers apoptotic cardiomyopathy. Nat Med 2002;8:725–30.
39. Adams JW, Sakata Y, Davis MG, et al. Enhanced G alpha q signaling: a common pathway mediates cardiac hypertrophy and apoptotic heart failure. Proc Natl Acad Sci U S A 1998;95:10140–5.
40. Hayakawa Y, Chandra M, Miao W, et al. Inhibition of cardiac myocyte apoptosis improves cardiac function and abolishes mortality in the peripartum cardiomyopathy of G{alpha}q transgenic mice. Circulation 2003;108:3036–41.
41. Hilfiker-Kleiner D, Kaminski K, Podewski E, et al. A cathepsin D-cleaved 16 kDa form of prolactin mediates postpartum cardiomyopathy. Cell 2007;128:589–600.
42. Leinwand LA. Molecular events underlying pregnancy-induced cardiomyopathy. Cell 2007;128:437–8.
43. Corbacho AM, Martinez De La Escalera G, Clapp C. Roles of prolactin and related members of the prolactin/growth hormone/placental lactogen family in angiogenesis. J Endocrinol 2002;173:219–38.

44. Bryant EE, Douglas BH, Ashburn AD. Circulatory changes following prolactin administration. Am J Obstet Gynecol 1973;115:53–7.
45. Negoro S, Kunisada K, Fujio Y, et al. Activation of signal transducer and activator of transcription 3 protects cardiomyocytes from hypoxia/reoxygenation-induced oxidative stress through the upregulation of manganese superoxide dismutase. Circulation 2001;104:979–81.
46. Hilfiker-Kleiner D, Meyer GP, Schieffer E, et al. Recovery from postpartum cardiomyopathy in 2 patients by blocking prolactin release with bromocriptine. J Am Coll Cardiol 2007;50:2354–5.
47. Cenac A, Simonoff M, Moretto P, et al. A low plasma selenium is a risk factor for peripartum cardiomyopathy: a comparative study in Sahelian Africa. Int J Cardiol 1992;36:57–9.
48. Fillmore SJ, Parry EO. The evolution of peripartal heart failure in Zaria, Nigeria. Some etiologic factors. Circulation 1977;56:1058–61.
49. Pierce JA, Price BO, Joyce JW. Familial occurrence of postpartal heart failure. Arch Intern Med 1963;111:151–5.
50. Massad LS, Reiss CK, Mutch DG, et al. Familial peripartum cardiomyopathy after molar pregnancy. Obstet Gynecol 1993;81:886–8.
51. Pearl W. Familial occurrence of peripartum cardiomyopathy. Am Heart J 1995; 129:421–2.
52. Voss EG, Reddy CV, Detrano R, et al. Familial dilated cardiomyopathy. Am J Cardiol 1984;54:456–7.
53. Fett JD, Sundstrom BJ, Etta King M, et al. Mother-daughter peripartum cardiomyopathy. Int J Cardiol 2002;86:331–2.
54. Kuhl U, Pauschinger M, Michel Noutsias M, et al. High prevalence of viral genomes and multiple viral infections in the myocardium of adults with "idiopathic" left ventricular dysfunction. Circulation 2005;111:887–93.
55. Horwitz MS, Knudsen M, Fine C, et al. Transforming growth factor-beta inhibits Coxsackievirus-mediated autoimmune myocarditis. Viral Immunol 2006;19:722–33.
56. Lang C, Sauter M, Szalay G, et al. Connective tissue growth factor: a crucial cytokine-mediating cardiac fibrosis in ongoing enterovirus myocarditis. J Mol Med 2007;86:49–60.
57. Gluck B, Schmidtke M, Merkle I, et al. Persistent expression of cytokines in the chronic stage of CVB3-induced myocarditis in NMRI mice. J Mol Cell Cardiol 2001;33:1615–26.
58. Sliwa K, Fett J, Elkayam U. Peripartum cardiomyopathy. Lancet 2006;368:687–93.
59. Sliwa K, Forster O, Zhanje F, et al. Outcome of subsequent pregnancy in patients with documented peripartum cardiomyopathy. Am J Cardiol 2004;93: 1441–3, A10.
60. Coulson C, Thorp JM Jr, Mayer D, et al. Central hemodynamic effects of recombinant human relaxin in the isolated, perfused rat heart model. Obstet Gynecol 1996;87:610–2.
61. Wittstein IS, Thiemann DR, Lima JAC, et al. Neurohumoral features of myocardial stunning due to sudden emotional stress. N Engl J Med 2005;352:539–48.
62. Jahns R, Boivin V, Hein L, et al. Direct evidence for a β1-adrenergic receptor-directed autoimmune attack as a cause of idiopathic dilated cardiomyopathy. J Clin Invest 2004;113:1419–29.
63. Freedman NJ, Lefkowitz RJ. Anti-β1-adrenergic receptor antibodies and heart failure: causation, not just correlation. J Clin Invest 2004;113:1379–82.
64. Lampert MB, Lang RM. Peripartum cardiomyopathy. Am Heart J 1995;130: 860–70.

65. Homans DC. Peripartum cardiomyopathy. N Engl J Med 1985;312:1432–7.
66. Koide T, Saito Y, Sakemoto T, et al. Peripartal cardiomyopathy in Japan: a critical reappraisal of the concept. Jpn Heart J 1972;13:488–501.
67. Lampert MB, Hibbard J, Weinert L, et al. Peripartum heart failure associated with prolonged tocolytic therapy. Am J Obstet Gynecol 1993;168:493–5.
68. Hibbard JU. Case-control study of long-term terbutaline therapy and peripartum cardiomyopathy. Hypertens Pregnancy 1996;15:183–91.
69. Pisani RJ, Rosenow EC. Pulmonary oedema associated with tocolytic therapy. Ann Intern Med 1989;110:714–8.
70. Demakis JG, Rahimtoola SH. Peripartum cardiomyopathy. Circulation 1971;44: 964–8.
71. Elkayam U, Akhter MW, Singh HS, et al. Pregnancy-associated cardiomyopathy: clinical characteristics and a comparison between early and late presentation. Circulation 2005;111:2050–5.
72. Elkayam U, Akhter MW, Singh HS, et al. Peripartum cardiomyopathies: a review. Am J Obstet Gynecol 1984;148:805–18.
73. Brar SS, Khan SS, Sandhu GK, et al. Incidence, mortality, and racial differences in peripartum cardiomyopathy. Am J Cardiol 2007;100:302–4.
74. Hameed AB, Chan K, Ghamsary M, et al. Longitudinal changes in the B-type natriuretic peptide levels in normal pregnancy and post partum. Clin Cardiol 2009;32:E60–2.
75. Garrison E, Hibbard JU, Studee L, et al. Brain natriuretic peptide as a marker for heart disease in pregnancy. Am J Obstet Gynecol 2005;193:S83.
76. Troughton RW, Frampton CM, Yandle TG, et al. Treatment of heart failure guided by plasma aminoterminal brain natriuretic peptide (N-BNP) concentrations. Lancet 2000;355:1126–30.
77. Mueller C, Scholer A, Laule-Kilian K, et al. Use of B type natriuretic peptide in the evaluation and management of acute dyspnea. N Engl J Med 2004;350:647–54.
78. Hunt SA, Abraham WT, Chin MH, et al. 2009 Focused update incorporated into the ACC/AHA 2005 guidelines for the diagnosis and management of heart failure in adults: a report of the American College of Cardiology Foundation/ American Heart Association Task Force on Practice Guidelines. Circulation 2009;119:e391–479.
79. Di Bella G, de Gregorio C, Minutoli F, et al. Early diagnosis of focal myocarditis by cardiac magnetic resonance. Int J Cardiol 2007;117:280–1.
80. Mahrholdt H, Goedecke C, Wagner A, et al. Multimedia article. Cardiovascular magnetic resonance assessment of human myocarditis: a comparison to histology and molecular pathology. Circulation 2004;109:1250–8.
81. Cooper LT, Baughman KL, Feldman AM, et al. The role of endomyocardial biopsy in the management of cardiovascular disease: a scientific statement from the American Heart Association, the American College of Cardiology, and the European Society of Cardiology. Endorsed by the Heart Failure Society of America and the Heart Failure Association of the European Society of Cardiology. Eur Heart J 2007;28:3076–93.
82. Abboud J, Murad Y, Chen-Scarabelli C, et al. Peripartum cardiomyopathy: a comprehensive review [review]. Int J Cardiol 2007;118:295–303.
83. Chapa JB, Heiberger B, Weinert L, et al. Prognostic value of echocardiography in peripartum cardiomyopathy. Obstet Gynecol 2005;105:1303–8.
84. Hibbard J, Lindheimer M, Lang R. A modified definition for peripartum cardiomyopathy and prognosis based on echocardiography. Obstet Gynecol 1999; 94(2):311–6.

85. Taylor AL, Ziesche S, Yancy C, et al. Combination of isosorbide dinitrate and hydralazine in blacks with heart failure. N Engl J Med 2004;351:2049–57.

86. Ahmed A, Rich MW, Love TE, et al. Digoxin and reduction in mortality and hospitalization in heart failure: a comprehensive post hoc analysis of the DIG Trial. Eur Heart J 2006;27:178–86.

87. Rathore SS, Curtis JP, Wang Y, et al. Association of serum digoxin concentration and outcomes in patients with heart failure. JAMA 2003;289:871–8.

88. Dunkman WB, Johnson GR, Carson PE, et al. Incidence of thromboembolic events in congestive heart failure. Circulation 1993;87:VI94–101.

89. Dries DL, Rosenberg YD, Waclawiw MA, et al. Ejection fraction and risk of thromboembolic events in patients with systolic dysfunction and sinus rhythm. Evidence for gender differences in the studies of LV dysfunction trials. J Am Coll Cardiol 1997;29:1074–80.

90. Freudenberger RS, Hellcamp AS, Halperin JL. Risk of thromboembolism in heart failure: analysis of the sudden cardiac death in heart failure trial (SCD-HEFT). Circulation 2007;115:2637–41.

91. Goland S, Modi K, Bitar F, et al. Clinical profile and predictors of complications in peripartum cardiomyopathy. J Card Fail 2009;15:645–50.

92. Cibils LA, Pose SV, Zuspan FP. Effect of *l*-norepinephrine infusion on uterine contractility and cardiovascular system. Am J Obstet Gynecol 1962;84:307.

93. Habedank D, Kuhnle Y, Elgeti T, et al. Recovery from peripartum cardiomyopathy after treatment with bromocriptine. Eur J Heart Fail 2008;10:1149–51.

94. Hopp L, Weisse AB, Iffy L. Acute myocardial infarction in a healthy mother using bromocriptine for mild suppression. Can J Cardiol 1996;12:415–8.

95. Sliwa K, Skudicky D, Candy G, et al. The addition of pentoxyfylline to conventional therapy improves outcome in patients with peripartum cardiomyopathy. Eur J Heart Fail 2002;4:305–9.

96. Bozkurt B, Villaneuva FS, Holubkov R, et al. Intravenous immune globulin in the therapy of peripartum cardiomyopathy. J Am Coll Cardiol 1999;34:177–80.

97. McNamara DM, Holubkov R, Starling RC, et al. Controlled trial of intravenous immune globulin in recent-onset dilated cardiomyopathy. Circulation 2001;103:2254–9.

98. Zimmermann O, Kochs M, Zwaka TP, et al. Myocardial biopsy based classification and treatment in patients with dilated cardiomyopathy. Int J Cardiol 2005;104:92–100.

99. Fett JD. Monitoring subsequent pregnancy in recovered peripartum cardiomyopathy mothers. Criti Pathw Cardiol 2009;8:172–4.

100. Fleisher LA, Beckman JA, Brown KA, et al. ACC/AHA 2007 guidelines on perioperative cardiovascular evaluation and care for noncardiac surgery: a report of the American College of Cardiology/American Heart Association Task Force on Practice Guidelines (Writing Committee to Revise the 2002 Guidelines on Perioperative Cardiovascular Evaluation for Noncardiac Surgery). J Am Coll Cardiol 2007;50:e159–241.

101. Amos AM, Jaber WA, Russell SD. Improved outcomes in peripartum cardiomyopathy with contemporary. Am Heart J 2006;152:509–13.

102. Elkayam U, Tummala PP, Rao K, et al. Maternal and fetal outcomes of subsequent pregnancies in women with peripartum cardiomyopathy. N Engl J Med 2001;344:1567–71.

103. Fett JD, Fristoe KL, Welsh SN. Risk of heart failure relapse in subsequent pregnancy among peripartum cardiomyopathy mothers. Int J Gynaecol Obstet 2010;109(1):34–6.

of noradrenaline and serotonin). Of all these options, only bariatric surgery provides durable and significant reductions in body weight (>60% long-term excess weight loss), correction of comorbid conditions, and improved survival.[9–12] Indications for bariatric surgery include a trial of medical therapy for at least 6 months, and a BMI equal to or more than 40 kg/m^2 or 35 kg/m^2 with obesity-related comorbidities. The number of bariatric surgeries done in the United States has increased significantly (from 13,365 in 1996 to 72,177 in 2002), and women represent 84% of all patients undergoing this procedure.[13]

Types of Bariatric Surgery

There are several different types of bariatric surgery, including the Roux-en-Y gastric bypass (RYGBP), biliopancreatic diversion (BPD), BPD with duodenal switch (BPD-DS), laparoscopic adjustable gastric banding (LAGB), and vertical banded gastroplasty (VBG). The main difference in the types of surgery is whether weight loss occurs as a result of restriction, malabsorption, or a combination of both (**Table 1**). LAGB is a purely restrictive surgery whereby an inflatable band is placed below the gastroesophageal junction leaving a gastric pouch of 10 to 15 mL. These gastric dimensions can be adjusted by adding or removing fluid from the band through a subcutaneous port. The RYGBP creates a small gastric pouch ($\leq$30 mL), which is then connected to the Roux limb (a part of the jejunum where the food travels). The duodenum and proximal jejunum, which contain bile and pancreatic secretions, later join the Roux limb to form a common limb. The BPD and BPD-DS have greater malabsorption components compared with the RYGBP. The jejunoileal bypass (JIB), a procedure whereby the proximal jejunum is joined to the distal ileum, was the first type of malabsorptive bariatric surgery performed. Because of the severe long-term morbidities attributed to extreme malabsorption of all types of calories and vitamins, this procedure is no longer performed today. The type of procedure chosen for each patient depends on several criteria including their preoperative BMI and comorbidities, but also varies among institutions depending on available facilities and surgical expertise. The RYGBP and LAGB are the most common procedures performed in the United States.

OBESITY IN PREGNANCY

Amidst an epidemic of obesity in the United States, obesity among pregnant women has also risen dramatically. The prevalence of obesity among pregnant women ranges from 10% to 35%.[14–17] The combination of obesity and pregnancy creates additional risk factors for adverse perinatal outcomes (**Table 2**).[15–33] This increased perinatal morbidity associated with maternal obesity has caught the attention of obstetricians and gynecologists.[34] Long-term adverse outcomes of maternal obesity including

Table 1
Types of bariatric surgeries

Malabsorption	Restrictive	Combination
Jejunoileal bypass[a]	Laparoscopic adjustable banding	Roux-en-Y gastric bypass
	Vertical gastric banding	Biliopancreatic diversion
		Biliopancreatic diversion with duodenal switch

[a] No longer performed today.

85. Taylor AL, Ziesche S, Yancy C, et al. Combination of isosorbide dinitrate and hydralazine in blacks with heart failure. N Engl J Med 2004;351:2049–57.

86. Ahmed A, Rich MW, Love TE, et al. Digoxin and reduction in mortality and hospitalization in heart failure: a comprehensive post hoc analysis of the DIG Trial. Eur Heart J 2006;27:178–86.

87. Rathore SS, Curtis JP, Wang Y, et al. Association of serum digoxin concentration and outcomes in patients with heart failure. JAMA 2003;289:871–8.

88. Dunkman WB, Johnson GR, Carson PE, et al. Incidence of thromboembolic events in congestive heart failure. Circulation 1993;87:VI94–101.

89. Dries DL, Rosenberg YD, Waclawiw MA, et al. Ejection fraction and risk of thromboembolic events in patients with systolic dysfunction and sinus rhythm. Evidence for gender differences in the studies of LV dysfunction trials. J Am Coll Cardiol 1997;29:1074–80.

90. Freudenberger RS, Hellcamp AS, Halperin JL. Risk of thromboembolism in heart failure: analysis of the sudden cardiac death in heart failure trial (SCD-HEFT). Circulation 2007;115:2637–41.

91. Goland S, Modi K, Bitar F, et al. Clinical profile and predictors of complications in peripartum cardiomyopathy. J Card Fail 2009;15:645–50.

92. Cibils LA, Pose SV, Zuspan FP. Effect of *l*-norepinephrine infusion on uterine contractility and cardiovascular system. Am J Obstet Gynecol 1962;84:307.

93. Habedank D, Kuhnle Y, Elgeti T, et al. Recovery from peripartum cardiomyopathy after treatment with bromocriptine. Eur J Heart Fail 2008;10:1149–51.

94. Hopp L, Weisse AB, Iffy L. Acute myocardial infarction in a healthy mother using bromocriptine for mild suppression. Can J Cardiol 1996;12:415–8.

95. Sliwa K, Skudicky D, Candy G, et al. The addition of pentoxyfylline to conventional therapy improves outcome in patients with peripartum cardiomyopathy. Eur J Heart Fail 2002;4:305–9.

96. Bozkurt B, Villaneuva FS, Holubkov R, et al. Intravenous immune globulin in the therapy of peripartum cardiomyopathy. J Am Coll Cardiol 1999;34:177–80.

97. McNamara DM, Holubkov R, Starling RC, et al. Controlled trial of intravenous immune globulin in recent-onset dilated cardiomyopathy. Circulation 2001; 103:2254–9.

98. Zimmermann O, Kochs M, Zwaka TP, et al. Myocardial biopsy based classification and treatment in patients with dilated cardiomyopathy. Int J Cardiol 2005; 104:92–100.

99. Fett JD. Monitoring subsequent pregnancy in recovered peripartum cardiomyopathy mothers. Criti Pathw Cardiol 2009;8:172–4.

100. Fleisher LA, Beckman JA, Brown KA, et al. ACC/AHA 2007 guidelines on perioperative cardiovascular evaluation and care for noncardiac surgery: a report of the American College of Cardiology/American Heart Association Task Force on Practice Guidelines (Writing Committee to Revise the 2002 Guidelines on Perioperative Cardiovascular Evaluation for Noncardiac Surgery). J Am Coll Cardiol 2007;50:e159–241.

101. Amos AM, Jaber WA, Russell SD. Improved outcomes in peripartum cardiomyopathy with contemporary. Am Heart J 2006;152:509–13.

102. Elkayam U, Tummala PP, Rao K, et al. Maternal and fetal outcomes of subsequent pregnancies in women with peripartum cardiomyopathy. N Engl J Med 2001;344:1567–71.

103. Fett JD, Fristoe KL, Welsh SN. Risk of heart failure relapse in subsequent pregnancy among peripartum cardiomyopathy mothers. Int J Gynaecol Obstet 2010; 109(1):34–6.

Pregnancy After Bariatric Surgery

Michelle A. Kominiarek, MD

KEYWORDS

• Pregnancy • Obesity • Perinatal outcomes • Bariatric surgery

According to the World Health Organization (WHO) guidelines, normal weight is defined as a body mass index (BMI) of 18.5 to 24.9 kg/m^2, overweight as a BMI of 25 to 29.9 kg/m^2, and obesity as a BMI of 30 kg/m^2 or more.[1] Obesity then can be further categorized by BMI into class 1 (30–34.9 kg/m^2), class 2 (35–39.9 kg/m^2), and class 3 ($\geq$40 kg/m^2), also termed morbid obesity. In the United States, approximately 68% of adults were either overweight or obese in the period 2005 to 2006.[2] Obesity has become an epidemic in the United States. The Centers for Disease Control has been tracking this information for over 2 decades. In 2008, only one state (Colorado) had a prevalence of obesity less than 20% compared with 1990 when no state had a prevalence of more than 14%.[2] Taking a further look at the demographics of obesity, it affects a greater proportion of women than men, and African Americans have the highest prevalence of all races (35.7%).[3] Not only does obesity have a significant negative impact on health through increased rates of hypertension, diabetes, heart disease, cerebral vascular accidents, degenerative joint disease, and depression, it is also associated with increased mortality.[4,5] The economic impact of obesity on medical costs was estimated at $75 billion in 2003.[6] The United States is expected to spend $344 billion on health care costs attributed to obesity in 2018.[7,8] Behavioral and lifestyle factors likely account for the alarming increase in obesity rates over the past 20 years; however, environmental, social, economic, and genetic factors are also intertwined in its etiology.[5]

MANAGEMENT OF OBESITY

Of all diseases in medicine, obesity is likely one of the most difficult to treat and manage. Although obesity prevention should be the focus of clinical care, there are several treatment options for obesity including behavioral changes (diet, exercise), pharmacotherapy, and bariatric surgery. Unfortunately, conventional behavioral and dietary approaches are not successful primarily due to ineffectiveness and weight regain. Currently available drugs are orlistat (a lipase inhibitor that reduces the absorption of fat) and sibutramine (a centrally acting appetite suppressant that inhibits uptake

Department of Obstetrics and Gynecology, University of Illinois at Chicago, 840 South Wood Street, M/C 808, Chicago, IL 60612, USA
E-mail address: Mkomin1@uic.edu

Obstet Gynecol Clin N Am 37 (2010) 305–320
doi:10.1016/j.ogc.2010.02.010
0889-8545/10/$ – see front matter © 2010 Elsevier Inc. All rights reserved.

of noradrenaline and serotonin). Of all these options, only bariatric surgery provides durable and significant reductions in body weight (>60% long-term excess weight loss), correction of comorbid conditions, and improved survival.[9–12] Indications for bariatric surgery include a trial of medical therapy for at least 6 months, and a BMI equal to or more than 40 kg/m² or 35 kg/m² with obesity-related comorbidities. The number of bariatric surgeries done in the United States has increased significantly (from 13,365 in 1996 to 72,177 in 2002), and women represent 84% of all patients undergoing this procedure.[13]

Types of Bariatric Surgery

There are several different types of bariatric surgery, including the Roux-en-Y gastric bypass (RYGBP), biliopancreatic diversion (BPD), BPD with duodenal switch (BPD-DS), laparoscopic adjustable gastric banding (LAGB), and vertical banded gastroplasty (VBG). The main difference in the types of surgery is whether weight loss occurs as a result of restriction, malabsorption, or a combination of both (**Table 1**). LAGB is a purely restrictive surgery whereby an inflatable band is placed below the gastroesophageal junction leaving a gastric pouch of 10 to 15 mL. These gastric dimensions can be adjusted by adding or removing fluid from the band through a subcutaneous port. The RYGBP creates a small gastric pouch (≤30 mL), which is then connected to the Roux limb (a part of the jejunum where the food travels). The duodenum and proximal jejunum, which contain bile and pancreatic secretions, later join the Roux limb to form a common limb. The BPD and BPD-DS have greater malabsorption components compared with the RYGBP. The jejunoileal bypass (JIB), a procedure whereby the proximal jejunum is joined to the distal ileum, was the first type of malabsorptive bariatric surgery performed. Because of the severe long-term morbidities attributed to extreme malabsorption of all types of calories and vitamins, this procedure is no longer performed today. The type of procedure chosen for each patient depends on several criteria including their preoperative BMI and comorbidities, but also varies among institutions depending on available facilities and surgical expertise. The RYGBP and LAGB are the most common procedures performed in the United States.

OBESITY IN PREGNANCY

Amidst an epidemic of obesity in the United States, obesity among pregnant women has also risen dramatically. The prevalence of obesity among pregnant women ranges from 10% to 35%.[14–17] The combination of obesity and pregnancy creates additional risk factors for adverse perinatal outcomes (**Table 2**).[15–33] This increased perinatal morbidity associated with maternal obesity has caught the attention of obstetricians and gynecologists.[34] Long-term adverse outcomes of maternal obesity including

Table 1		
Types of bariatric surgeries		
Malabsorption	**Restrictive**	**Combination**
Jejunoileal bypass[a]	Laparoscopic adjustable banding	Roux-en-Y gastric bypass
	Vertical gastric banding	Biliopancreatic diversion
		Biliopancreatic diversion with duodenal switch

[a] No longer performed today.

Table 2 Risks of maternal obesity	
Maternal	**Fetal**
Miscarriage	Stillbirth
Hypertension (gestational and preeclampsia)	Birth defects (neural tube, cardiac, and omphalocele)
Gestational diabetes	Indicated premature birth
Labor induction	Macrosomia
Cesarean delivery	Birth trauma
Postpartum hemorrhage	Childhood obesity
Decreased vaginal birth after cesarean success	
Operative infectious morbidity	
Thromboembolic events	

Refs.[15–33]

childhood obesity are unfortunately becoming well known.[23,35] Although it seems plausible that perinatal outcomes would be improved in patients with an optimal pre-pregnancy BMI, whether weight loss prior to pregnancy improves future pregnancy outcomes has only been studied with respect to bariatric surgery interventions.

REPRODUCTIVE ISSUES AFTER BARIATRIC SURGERY

Approximately half of all bariatric procedures are performed in women of childbearing age. Consequently, pregnancies occurring after these procedures are not uncommon, and it is important to address the reproductive issues that arise. The relationship between obesity and infertility is well established and is likely attributed to changes in hormone secretion resulting in oligo-ovulation and anovulation.[36,37] Improved ovulatory function in women that have bariatric surgery also impacts their fertility.[38–40] As such, many unplanned pregnancies occur after bariatric surgery, and contraception coun-seling should be incorporated in the preoperative and postoperative care of these patients.

Obesity is also associated with increased miscarriage rates.[18] The interpretation of miscarriage rates after bariatric surgery is limited due to small numbers; however, the available studies have conflicting outcomes. Bilenka and colleagues[41] compared pregnancies before and after VBG. Of 18 pregnancies prior to the operation, 7 ended in miscarriage (33%), whereas only 1 of 14 (7%) pregnancies conceived after the oper-ation was lost. Similarly, in a survey of 195 patients, miscarriages were reported in 33% of patients before RYGBP surgery and in only 6% afterwards, $P<.001$.[40] In contrast, miscarriages increased from 22% to 26% after BPD procedures (as reported in a self-questionnaire despite significant weight loss) and from 25% to 40% after VBG.[42,43] These 2 studies did not provide statistical analysis.

For those who desire to become pregnant, most experts recommend waiting at least 18 to 24 months before future conception.[44] This delay may help avoid the exposure of a developing fetus to a rapid weight loss environment and help optimize the patient's weight loss. However, if pregnancy does occur before this time frame, studies have shown that risk may not necessarily be increased.[45–48] For example, Dao and colleagues[46] compared 21 pregnancies that occurred within 1 year of surgery to 13 that occurred after 1 year. The early groups gained less weight (1.8 kg vs 15.5 kg), but the remainder of the perinatal outcomes were similar. Of note, other investigators report that the more severe neonatal outcomes occurred at least 2 years after BPD procedures, suggesting that complications can occur regardless of the timing of the procedure.[49]

PREGNANCY AFTER BARIATRIC SURGERY
Side Effects and Complications of Bariatric Surgery and Their Effects on Pregnancy

Nutrition and anemia

Bariatric surgery patients require lifelong follow-up of hematological and iron parameters because iron deficiency and iron deficiency anemia can be long-term complications occurring in 6% to 50% of patients after RYGBP.[50–52] The reasons for this include decreased dietary intake due to intolerance to certain foods (based on self-reported decrease in red-meat consumption), decreased gastric acid secretion (attributed to fewer parietal cells), and duodenal exclusion (bypass of absorption site).[52–55] Folic acid deficiency can occur as a result of decreased gastric production of hydrochloric acid, which ordinarily allows for absorption of folic acid in the upper third of the intestine. Folic acid deficiency is reported in up to 38% of patients after RYGBP.[56] Low iron and folic acid in addition to deficiencies of fat-soluble vitamins and vitamin B_{12} are perhaps the most important factors to consider in a pregnancy. In pregnancy, a mild anemia is expected as a result of hemodilution, with the nadir hemoglobin approaching 10.5 g/dL at 28 to 34 weeks. In addition, iron and other nutrient requirements increase in pregnancy, so the risk for clinically important deficiencies increases in pregnant bariatric surgery patients. Risks of anemia in pregnancy may include preterm delivery and low infant birth weight.[57] The potential increased risk for birth defects is discussed in a subsequent section.

Surgical complications

Some of the known surgical complications of bariatric surgery include internal hernias (1%–5%),[58] adhesive bands, incarcerated hernias, and anastomotic leaks. After restrictive surgeries stomal obstructions, esophageal and gastric pouch dilation, and band slippage or migration can occur. One study reported that band migration was more common during pregnancy, 2.4% over the 40-week time span of pregnancy compared with 6% over 10 years in nonpregnant patients.[59] The presenting symptoms of these problems may include decreased appetite, nausea, vomiting, abdominal pain, heartburn, and changes in bowel habits, all of which can occur in an otherwise normal pregnancy.

Several adverse outcomes including intestinal obstructions and band erosions during a pregnancy have been described in case reports. In many of these reports, the initial laboratory tests (liver function tests, amylase, lipase, and electrolytes) were normal.[60–62] Two recent cases of maternal deaths have been reported, one at 25 weeks with a midgut volvulus leading to perforation and death by septic shock[63] and the other at 31 weeks with 61 cm of gangrenous small bowel herniating through a mesenteric defect.[60] These deaths were attributed to delayed recognition of surgical complications. Pregnant women may be at increased risk of bowel obstruction due to increased abdominal pressure associated with an enlarging gravid uterus; however, some of these complications have been described in the first trimester.[60]

Perinatal Outcomes

Maternal outcomes

Several studies have shown that bariatric surgery may be associated with decreased obesity-related or gestational-related pregnancy complications, including diabetes and hypertensive disorders.[64–68] In a systematic review of pregnancies following bariatric surgery, 3 matched cohort studies had lower adverse maternal outcomes in pregnancies after LAGB and RYGBP compared with obese controls. There is conflicting information regarding the occurrence of cesareans after bariatric surgery. In one study, cesareans were higher in the bariatric surgery group compared with the general population (25.2% vs 12.2%; odds ratio [OR] 2.4, $P<.001$) and the risk persisted even after controlling for prior cesarean delivery, labor induction, BMI, diabetes, and infant birth weight.[69] Several other investigators have reported this finding,[47,70] but cesareans were lower in 2 case-control studies[43,65] and similar in several other reports.[47,48,64,67,68,71]

Neonatal outcomes
Birth defects and perinatal mortality It is well known that adequate maternal folate intake can prevent fetal neural tube defects.[72] Neural tube defects and folic acid deficiency after bariatric surgery have been described in case reports.[70,73,74] However, a larger population based study reported similar occurrences of birth defects (unspecified types) in women with and without prior bariatric surgery (mixed types) (5.0% vs 4.0%, $P = .355$).[69] In a study comparing 301 deliveries before and 507 after bariatric surgery, Weintraub and colleagues[75] found an increase in birth defects (unspecified type) after surgery (3.3% vs 7.9%, OR 2.5 95% confidence interval [CI] 1.2–5.1), but after controlling for maternal age, diabetes, and birth weight, the effect was no longer significant (OR 1.9, 95% CI 0.88–4.12). Furthermore, none of the 77 infants born to mothers after intestinal (not gastric) bypass surgery in the Swedish Birth Registry had birth defects.[76] Nevertheless, many bariatric surgery patients are not compliant with daily multivitamin supplementation (up to 85%) and therefore may enter a pregnancy with a serious nutritional deficiency that could increase the risk for birth defects.[45,77]

Perinatal mortality also appears to be similar in bariatric patients, based on data from 2 Israeli studies: 0.3% (after bariatric surgery) versus 1.5% (general population), $P = .102$; and 2.3% (before bariatric surgery) versus 1.0% (after bariatric surgery), $P = .11$.[69,75] However, in a cohort of 239 pregnancies after BPD there were more perinatal deaths (n = 4) and congenital malformations (n = 3).[70]

Birth weight Infant weight is directly correlated to maternal BMI, and the risk for macrosomia increases in obese patients.[15,78–82] Studies that examine weight of infants born of mothers after bariatric surgery describe the following trends: a decrease in the mean birth weight, more appropriately grown neonates (AGA), more small for gestational age (SGA) neonates, fewer large for gestational age (LGA) neonates, and less macrosomia.[42,47,64–66,68] Although the occurrence of more SGA infants is concerning, the percentages of such birth weights were still within the normal birth weight distributions (ie, <10% were SGA). However, some studies have found no differences in birth weight.[43,67]

Other neonatal issues Even after delivery, issues related to nutrition continue to predominate in the care of both the mother and infant. Close monitoring of vitamin levels during this time comes from several case reports that describe vitamin B_{12} deficiency and failure to thrive in breastfed infants.[83–86] Another case report attributed a fetal cerebral hemorrhage to vitamin K deficiency in a mother who experienced complications from a gastric banding procedure and required parenteral feeding for several weeks before delivery.[87] In another case series, severe intracranial neonatal bleeding occurred in an additional 3 infants born to mothers after bariatric surgery (2 LAGB, 1 BPD).[88] Although not substantiated by laboratory testing, the presumed cause was maternal vitamin K deficiency. Usually pregnancies after LAGB are not associated with nutrient or vitamin deficiencies, but the investigators cautioned to screen for vitamin K deficiency in women with food intolerance and vomiting during pregnancy.

Long-Term Outcomes and the Offspring of Bariatric Surgery Patients

According to the Barker hypothesis, fetal nutrition begets adult diseases and the intra-uterine environment has a significant impact on susceptibility to obesity.[89–92] It is also known that parenteral obesity is a risk for childhood obesity, potentially as a result of an obesity-prone genotype.[93–95] One of the reasons to improve maternal morbidity related to obesity is the potentially positive effect on infant and childhood outcomes. A single center has published 3 studies on the long-term outcomes of infants born to mothers after bariatric surgery. The first investigation involved a questionnaire mailed to patients who had a BPD between 1984 and 1995. The range of the children's ages was 0.5 to 16 years at the time of the questionnaire. Of 88 children older than 4 years, all attended school at the appropriate level and there was a significant increase in weight categories from birth (6% macrosomia) to the time of the survey (23.8% >90th percentile for weight), $P<.01$.[42] More favorable results were later reported in a study that compared weight outcomes in 172 children born to obese mothers (mean BMI 31 $\pm$ 9 kg/m^2) after BPD or BPD-DS compared with 45 same-age siblings born before the surgery (mean maternal BMI 48 $\pm$ 8 kg/m^2). Comparing the offspring born before and after BPD, obesity and severe obesity (defined as a BMI >2 kg/m^2 above the cutoff point for obesity, equivalent to a BMI of 35 kg/m^2 in adults) decreased by 52% ($P = .005$) and 45% ($P = .04$), respectively. Furthermore, 16% of the children aged 6 to 18 years born after BPD were overweight,[71] which the investigators thought was comparable to the local population standards.

In a follow-up study of 111 children (54 before BPD and 57 after BPD) aged 2.5 to 26 years, cardiometabolic risk factors were assessed. In children born to women after BPD, there was greater insulin sensitivity (insulin resistance index [fasting glucose $\times$ fasting insulin/22.5] of 3.4 $\pm$ 0.3 vs 4.8 $\pm$ 0.5, $P = .02$), improved lipid profiles (total cholesterol/high-density lipoprotein cholesterol ratio 1.5 $\pm$ 0.05 vs 1.35 $\pm$ 0.05 mmol/L, $P = .04$), lower C-reactive protein levels (0.88 $\pm$ 0.17 vs 2.00 $\pm$ 0.34 μg/mL, $P = .004$), lower leptin levels (11.5 $\pm$ 1.5 vs 19.7 $\pm$ 2.5 ng/mL, $P = .005$) and increased ghrelin levels (a marker of satiety) (1.28 $\pm$ 0.06 vs 1.03 $\pm$ 0.06 ng/mL, $P = .005$) than in children born to women before BPD. The children born after BPD were also less likely to have severe obesity (11% vs 35%, $P = .004$).[96] The differences in body weight alone were insufficient to explain the differences in insulin resistance and dyslipidemia. These findings are promising in that offspring of mothers after bariatric surgery are less likely to be obese and may also have improvements in metabolic status.

Bariatric Surgery and Adolescents

The epidemic of obesity in the United States has also affected adolescents. For those aged 12 to 19 years, the prevalence of obesity has increased from 5.0% to 17.6% over the past 20 years.[97]

Obesity in the pregnant adolescent population carries similar perinatal risks, with increased rates of gestational diabetes, preeclampsia, induction, macrosomia, and cesarean deliveries.[98] Adolescents are also candidates for bariatric surgery if they have a BMI greater than 40 kg/m^2, comorbid conditions, and have failed nonoperative weight loss options. In addition, skeletal maturity ($\geq$13 years for girls and $\geq$15 years for boys) is also a prerequisite.[99] Adolescents also require a multidisciplinary team with additional expertise in pediatric or adolescent medicine. Given the increase in childhood obesity, it is expected that the number of adolescents having bariatric surgery will also continue to increase. The 282 procedures done in 2003 (an increase from 51 procedures in 1997) were performed on predominantly female patients (70%) with a mean age of 16 years.[100,101]

Although this is a unique population with concerns for both weight loss and perinatal outcomes, clinical management is linked due to the few studies on the topic.[102] Papadia and colleagues[103] reported on 52 girls and 16 boys who had a BPD at a mean age of 16.8 years and a follow-up of 2 to 23 years. Twenty percent required reoperations and 16% developed protein malnutrition. The mean percentage of excess weight loss at each patient's longest follow-up was 78%. Similar to adults, comorbidities such as hypertension (from 49% to 8.8%), lipid abnormalities (from 16% to 0%), and diabetes (from 2.9% to 0%) decreased. There were 18 females who delivered 28 healthy infants 4 to 23 years after BPD. However, 3 additional patients had severe complications after the pregnancy. One did not have nutrient supplements during pregnancy, and her infant was later diagnosed with mental retardation. The other 2 mothers died of protein malnutrition some time after the delivery.[102,103] Roehrig and colleagues[104] described 6 healthy term pregnancies in 47 adolescent female patients who had an RYGBP 10 to 22 months before conception.[105] Although there were no reported pregnancy complications, the investigators were impressed with their pregnancy rate (12.8%), which was significantly higher than the national pregnancy rates for adolescents. The reason for this is unclear, but it underscores the importance of contraceptive counseling before surgery, especially with adolescents. The recommendation to wait at least 1 year postoperatively before conception is also found in the adolescent bariatric surgery literature.[99]

Long-Term Maternal Outcomes Related to Bariatric Surgery

Many patients desire to become pregnant after having bariatric surgery. In a survey of women younger than 45 years given to patients less than 30 days before their bariatric surgery, 30% stated that a future pregnancy was important, and was more important to women having a LAGB than RYGPB (OR 1.75, 95% CI 1.03–2.98).[100,106] The best choice for a bariatric surgery procedure (ie, RYGBP vs LAGB vs BPD) for patients who desire future pregnancies is also not known. Although no study has prospectively evaluated this, the reversibility of the LAGB may make it a more appropriate approach for women considering future pregnancies. The higher occurrences of anemia after RYGBP, and malnutrition and other deficiencies after BPD are additional factors to take into consideration. Sheiner and colleagues[107] were the first to compare perinatal outcomes in purely restrictive surgeries (202 LAGB, 136 SRVG [silastic ring vertical gastroplasty], and 56 VBG) to RYGBP (n = 55). Pregnancies after LAGB had greater weight gains during the pregnancy (13.1 ± 9.6 kg) compared with the SRVG group (8.8 ± 7.4 kg), the VBG group (8.5 ± 8.0 kg), and the RYGBP group (11.6 ± 9.6 kg), P<.001. Although infant birth weight was higher in the RYGBP (3332.9 ± 475.5 g) compared with the restrictive group as a whole (3111.7 ± 533 g), there was no difference in low birth weight or macrosomia. All types of surgery had comparable outcomes with respect to gestational diabetes, hypertension, anemia, and perinatal mortality.[101,107]

The long-term effects of a pregnancy after bariatric surgery on maternal weight loss and comorbid conditions are unknown. However, one can look at the amount of weight gain during pregnancy as a potential marker. Patients gained less weight in a pregnancy after RYGBP (12.7 kg) compared with the pre-RYGBP group (20.4 kg), and most women lost all the weight gained during the pregnancy within 5 weeks postpartum.[64] Similar findings were also reported with respect to weight gain in pregnancies after LAGB[66,67] and BPD (6.6 ± 8.9 kg after BPD vs 13.4 ± 12.3 kg before BPD), $P<.0001$.[96] Weight gain appears to be diminished in pregnancies after bariatric surgery, but whether patients continue to lose or gain weight is not known.

RECOMMENDATIONS FOR CARE DURING PREGNANCY
Nutritional

In general, there are no evidence-based guidelines or consensus statements regarding nutritional management for a pregnancy after bariatric surgery, so recommendations for diagnosis and treatment are similar to the nonpregnant bariatric population. However, even in bariatric surgery literature, guidelines for specific vitamin doses have been poorly studied and are largely theoretical.[102] Furthermore, most of these recommendations come from RYGBP literature. Nutrient deficiencies are less common after purely restrictive procedures but can occur, especially in patients who have specific food intolerances or consume excess calories in a liquid form. Protein deficiencies are less common with the bariatric procedures performed today. Box 1 and Table 3 are the suggested approaches to the diagnosis and treatment of nutrient deficiencies after bariatric surgery with modifications for pregnant patients.[105] Many patients are not compliant with the daily multivitamin recommended by the bariatric surgery team and as such enter a pregnancy with nutrient deficiencies.[45,77]

These tests should be done at the initial prenatal visit, and if normal, repeated periodically (ie, once a trimester).

In pregnancy, iron deficiency can be diagnosed in the usual manner with a low hemoglobin, low mean corpuscular volume, and abnormal iron studies (low serum iron, high total iron-binding capacity, and a low serum ferritin). If iron deficiency anemia is diagnosed, then treatment and follow-up testing is recommended as in any other pregnant patient. Because they are more readily absorbed, only ferrous iron formulations should be prescribed (ie, ferrous sulfate 325 mg, ferrous fumarate 200 mg; both of which provide 65 mg of elemental iron per tablet). Once or twice daily dosing is sufficient to prevent iron deficiency, and 3 or 4 times daily dosing is recommended to restore iron. Iron should be taken on an empty stomach and not in close proximity

---

Box 1
Laboratory testing recommended for patients after RYGBP in pregnancy[a]

Complete blood count

Electrolytes

Glucose

Iron studies, ferritin

Vitamin B_{12}

25-Hydroxyvitamin D[a]

[a] Annual laboratory testing for nonpregnant patients also includes liver functions and lipid profile.

Data from Mechanick JI, Kushner RF, Sugerman HJ, et al. American Association of Clinical Endocrinologists, The Obesity Society, and American Society for Metabolic and Bariatric Surgery medical guidelines for clinical practice for the perioperative nutritional, metabolic, and nonsurgical support of the bariatric surgery patient. Perioperative bariatric guidelines. Obesity (Silver Spring) 2009;17:s1–70.

Table 3
Routine nutrient supplementation after bariatric surgery

Nonpregnant Population	During Pregnancy
Multivitamin 1–2 daily	One prenatal vitamin daily
Calcium citrate (1200–2000 mg/d) with vitamin D (400–800 U/d)	Calcium citrate (1200 mg/d) with vitamin D (400–800 U/d)
Folic acid 400 μg/d in multivitamin	Folic acid 400 μg/d in prenatal vitamin, replace with additional doses if deficiency confirmed
Elemental iron with vitamin C 40–65 mg/d	Elemental iron 40–65 mg/d plus prenatal vitamin, replace with additional doses if deficiency confirmed
Vitamin B_{12} ≥350 μg/d orally or 1000 μg/mo intramuscularly or 3000 μg every 6 mo intramuscularly or 500 μg every wk intranasally	Vitamin B_{12} ≥350 μg/d orally, replace with additional doses if deficiency confirmed

Data from Mechanick JI, Kushner RF, Sugerman HJ, et al. American Association of Clinical Endocrinologists, The Obesity Society, and American Society for Metabolic and Bariatric Surgery medical guidelines for clinical practice for the perioperative nutritional, metabolic, and nonsurgical support of the bariatric surgery patient. Perioperative bariatric guidelines. Obesity (Silver Spring) 2009;17:s1–70.

to teas and calcium. Concomitant vitamin C ingestion may help increase iron absorption and ultimately improve hematological parameters.[108] Although some studies recommend 2 multivitamins daily during pregnancy,[46,64] this should not be the case in pregnant patients because excess doses of vitamin A can be teratogenic. The usual calcium requirements for pregnancy are 1200 mg per day, and this dose is also appropriate for bariatric surgery patients. For protection against fetal neural tube defects and other congenital anomalies, 400 μg of folic acid daily is recommended. After LAGB, the pill size for any supplement or other oral medication should be less than 11 mm so that it can fit through the restricted area. The recommendation for protein intake is the same regardless of bariatric surgery status: 60 g daily. Patients with BPD or BPD-DS require closer monitoring for protein malnutrition. Finally, there is no consensus in the literature on total caloric intake during a pregnancy after bariatric surgery, but weight loss during pregnancy has never been recommended.

Role of the Bariatric Surgeon

If it has been more than a year since the patient has seen a member of the bariatric surgery team, then a consultation either with the surgeon and/or nutritionist is recommended during the pregnancy. Because the stoma size can be adjusted via a subcutaneous port to allow food to pass through more quickly or slowly, some unique issues arise in pregnancies after LAGB. In pregnancy, one recommendation is to remove all the fluid upon the diagnosis of pregnancy and then return fluid after 14 weeks depending on weight gain. Several investigators have described "active band management" whereby fluid from the gastric band is removed or lessened during a pregnancy so as to restore the normal gastric dimensions, allowing for greater caloric intake.[67,109–111] Removing fluid from the gastric band has also been done in 20% to 60% of patients to relieve nausea and vomiting during the first trimester.[65,109–111] In general, most pregnancies were well tolerated, but those who had all the fluid removed from the band had excessive weight gains. Some have recommended removing a minimal amount of fluid from the band if the patient is still obese at the time of conception so as to minimize weight gain, and adjusting the band volume for nonobese women with the aim of achieving a normal maternal weight gain.[67] However, there is no consensus on the management of an LAGB during pregnancy. Early consultation with a bariatric surgeon is recommended in these pregnancies.

When a pregnant patient with a history of bariatric surgery presents with nausea or vomiting or has an abnormal abdominal examination, one should be careful to include bariatric surgical complications in the differential diagnosis regardless of the timing or type of bariatric surgery. The evaluation may involve obtaining additional tests, imaging, and even consulting the bariatric surgery team. As described in aforementioned case reports, the symptoms and signs may not be diagnostic. In these cases, an exploratory laparotomy or diagnostic laparoscopy can provide a diagnosis and potentially improve perinatal outcomes. In summary, a high margin of suspicion and a low threshold for surgical exploration are recommended.

Other Considerations

Dumping syndrome can occur after the RYGBP procedure. During this process, foods high in simple sugars cause a sudden fluid shift into the gut in response to a high osmotic load directly in the small intestine. This fluid shift leads to symptoms including watery diarrhea, abdominal pain and cramping, and "hypotensive" symptoms such as nausea, light-headedness, tachycardia, diaphoresis, and syncope. The 50 g glucola commonly administered in the second trimester to screen for gestational diabetes can precipitate this syndrome. There are alternative ways to screen for diabetes. For example, the patient can check her fasting and 2-hour postprandial blood sugars

---

Box 2
Recommendations for care of the pregnant bariatric surgery patient

Provide contraception counseling

Nutritional monitoring and supplementation

  Identify and treat deficiencies in:

    Iron

    Folate

    Vitamin B_{12}

    Calcium

    Vitamin D

Screening for gestational diabetes

  Use alternative methods for patients with RYGBP

Concurrent obesity

  Counsel on risks of obesity in pregnancy

Multidisciplinary team

  Bariatric surgeons, nutritionists, other medical specialists

Surgical complications

  Have a high index of suspicion and low threshold to intervene

at home for 1 week during the 24- to 28-week period. A glycosylated hemoglobin level may also help direct prenatal care.

Even after having bariatric surgery, many patients (up to 80%)[48,109,111] still remain obese. As such, these pregnancies are at risk for complications (see **Table 2**), and patients should be counseled about this. Although several studies report increased cesareans after bariatric surgery,[47,69,70] cesareans should be done for the standard obstetric indications in patients with a pregnancy after bariatric surgery. Nonsteroidal anti-inflammatory drugs, which are commonly used in postpartum obstetric patients, should be avoided in bariatric surgery patients because they have been implicated in the development of anastomotic ulcerations.[104,105] **Box 2** summarizes these recommendations.

LIMITATIONS OF THE CURRENT LITERATURE

The literature on pregnancy after bariatric surgery is limited primarily by the small numbers reported in the retrospective studies (case-control and cohort) and case reports. The control groups are also heterogeneous in that some match to a pregnancy before surgery and others match to patients with a similar BMI or parity without surgery. There is also bias in the surveys conducted on patients whose pregnancies occurred several years prior. Moreover, many studies do not describe the type of surgery performed. More importantly, the studies are underpowered to detect significant differences in outcomes, especially birth defects and perinatal mortality. Long-term outcomes for both the mother and her offspring are still needed. When reading the literature on pregnancy after bariatric surgery, one should keep these issues in mind.

REFERENCES

1. World Health Organization Obesity: preventing and managing a global epidemic. Report of a WHO consultation. World Health Organ Tech Rep Ser 2000;894:1–253, i–xii.
2. National Center for Health Statistics. Prevalence of overweight, obesity and extreme obesity among adults: United States, trends 1976–80 through 2005–2006. Available at: http://www.cdc.gov/nchs/data/hestat/overweight/overweight_adult.pdf. Accessed December 20, 2009.
3. Pan L, Galuska DA, Sherry B. Differences in prevalence of obesity among black, white, and Hispanic adults—United States, 2006–2008. MMWR Morb Mortal Wkly Rep 2009;58:740–4. Available at: http://www.cdc.gov/mmwr/preview/mmwrhtml/mm5827a2.htm. Accessed December 20, 2009.
4. Allison DB, Fontaine KR, Manson JE, et al. Annual deaths attributable to obesity in the United States. JAMA 1999;282:1530–8.
5. National Heart, Lung, and Blood Institute. Clinical guideline on the identification, evaluation, and treatment of overweight and obesity in adults: the evidence report. Bethesda (MD): US Department of Health and Human Services, National Institutes of Health, National Heart, Lung, and Blood Institute; 1998. Available at: http://www.nhlbi.nih.gov/guidelines/obesity/ob_gdlns.htm. Accessed December 20, 2009.
6. Wald N, Sneddon J, Densem J, et al. Prevention of neural tube defects: Results of the medical research council vitamin study. Lanat 1991;338:131–7.
7. Finkelstein EA, Fiebelkorn IC, Wang G. State-level estimates of annual medical expenditures attributable to obesity. Obes Res 2004;12:18–24.
8. Thorpe KE. A collaborative report from United Health Foundation, the American Public Health Association and Partnership for prevention based on research by Kenneth E. Thorpe, Ph.D. of Emory University and Executive Director, Partnership

to Fight Chronic Disease. Updated November 2009. Available at: http://www.americashealthrankings/2009/spotlight.aspx. Accessed December 20, 2009.

9. Buchwald H, Avidor Y, Braunwald E, et al. Bariatric surgery: a systematic review and meta-analysis. JAMA 2004;292:1724–37.

10. Christou NV, Sampalis JS, Liberman M, et al. Surgery decreases long-term mortality, morbidity, and healthcare use in morbidly obese patients. Ann Surg 2004;240:416–23.

11. Adams TD, Gress RE, Smith SC, et al. Long term mortality after gastric bypass surgery. N Engl J Med 2007;357:753–61.

12. Sjostrom L, Narbro K, Sjostrom CD, et al. Swedish Obese Subjects Study. Effects of bariatric surgery on mortality in Swedish obese subjects. N Engl J Med 2007;357:741–52.

13. Santry HP, Gillen DL, Lauderdale DS. Trends in bariatric surgical procedures. JAMA 2005;294:1909–17.

14. Kim SY, Morrow B, Callaghan WM, et al. Trends in pre-pregnancy obesity in nine states, 1993–2003. Obesity (Silver Spring) 2007;15:986–93.

15. Baeten JM, Bukusi EA, Lambe M. Pregnancy complications and outcomes among overweight and obese nulliparous women. Am J Public Health 2001; 91:436–40.

16. Ogunyemi D, Hullett S, Leeper J, et al. Prepregnancy body mass index, weight gain during pregnancy, and perinatal outcome in a rural black population. J Matern Fetal Med 1999;7:190–3.

17. Young TK, Woodmansee B. Factors that are associated with cesarean delivery in a large private practice: the importance of prepregnancy body mass index and weight gain. Am J Obstet Gynecol 2002;187:312–20.

18. Lashen H, Fear K, Sturdee DW. Obesity is associated with increased risk of first trimester and recurrent miscarriage: matched case-control study. Hum Reprod 2004;19:1644–6.

19. Watkins ML, Rasmussen SA, Honein MA, et al. Maternal obesity and risk for birth defects. Pediatrics 2003;111:1152–8.

20. Anderson JL, Waller DK, Canfield MA, et al. Maternal obesity, gestational diabetes, and central nervous system birth defects. Epidemiology 2005;16: 87–92.

21. Cnattingus S, Bergstrom R, Lipworth L, et al. Prepregnancy weight and the risk of adverse pregnancy outcomes. N Engl J Med 1998;338:147–52.

22. Stephansson O, Dickman PW, Johansson A, et al. Maternal weight, pregnancy weight gain, and the risk of antepartum stillbirth. Am J Obstet Gynecol 2001; 184:463–9.

23. Whitaker RC. Predicting preschooler obesity at birth: the role of maternal obesity in early pregnancy. Pediatrics 2004;114:e29–36.

24. Bianco AT, Smilen SW, Davis Y, et al. Pregnancy outcome and weight gain recommendations for the morbidly obese women. Obstet Gynecol 1998;91: 97–102.

25. Chu SY, Callaghan WM, Kim SY, et al. Maternal obesity and risk of gestational diabetes mellitus. Diabetes Care 2007;30:2070–6.

26. Hibbard JU, Gilbert S, Landon MB, et al. Trial of labor or repeat cesarean delivery in women with morbid obesity and previous cesarean delivery. Obstet Gynecol 2006;108:125–33.

27. James AH, Jamison MG, Brancazio LR. Venous thromboembolism during pregnancy and the postpartum period: Incidence, risk factors, and mortality. Am J Obstet Gynecol 2006;194:1311–5.

28. Larsen CE, Serdula KM, Sullivan MK. Macrosomia: influence of maternal over-weight among a low-income population. Am J Obstet Gynecol 1990;162:490–4.

29. Myles TD, Gooch J, Santolaya J. Obesity as an independent risk factor for infectious morbidity in patients who undergo cesarean delivery. Obstet Gynecol 2002;100:959–64.

30. Naef RW, Chauhan SP, Chevalier SP, et al. Prediction of hemorrhage at cesarean delivery. Obstet Gynecol 1994;83:923.

31. O'Brien TE, Ray JG, Chan WS. Maternal body mass index and the risk of preeclampsia: a systematic overview. Epidemiology 2003;14:368–74.

32. Salsberry PJ. Taking the long view: the prenatal environment and early adolescent overweight. Res Nurs Health 2007;30:297–307.

33. Vermillion ST, Lamoutte C, Soper DE, et al. Wound infection after cesarean: effect of subcutaneous tissue thickness. Obstet Gynecol 2000;95:923–6.

34. Reece EA. Perspectives on obesity, pregnancy and birth outcomes in the United States: the scope of the problem. Am J Obstet Gynecol 2008;198:23–7.

35. Boney C, Vohr BR, Verma A, et al. Metabolic syndrome in childhood: association with birth weight, maternal obesity, and gestational diabetes mellitus. Pediatrics 2005;115:290–6.

36. Pathi A, Esen U, Hildreth A. A comparison of complications of pregnancy and delivery in morbidly obese and nonobese women. J Obstet Gynaecol 2006; 26:527–30.

37. Loret de Mola JR. Obesity and its relationship to infertility in men and women. Obstet Gynecol Clin North Am 2009;36:333–46.

38. Merhi ZO. Weight loss by bariatric surgery and subsequent fertility. Fertil Steril 2007;87:430–2.

39. Eid GM, Cottam DR, Velcu LM, et al. Effective treatment of polycystic ovarian syndrome with Roux-en-Y gastric bypass. Surg Obes Relat Dis 2005;1:77–80.

40. Teitelman M, Grotegut CA, Williams NN, et al. The impact of bariatric surgery on menstrual patterns. Obes Surg 2006;16:1457–63.

41. Bilenka B, Ben-Shlomo I, Cozacov C, et al. Fertility, miscarriage and pregnancy after vertical banded gastroplasty operation for morbid obesity. Acta Obstet Gynecol Scand 1995;74:42–4.

42. Marceau P, Kaufman D, Biron S, et al. Outcome of pregnancies after biliopancreatic diversion. Obes Surg 2004;14:318–24.

43. Deitel M, Stone E, Kassam HA, et al. Gynecologic-obstetric changes after loss of massive excess weight following bariatric surgery. J Am Coll Nutr 1988;7: 147–53.

44. American College of Obstetricians and Gynecologists. Practice Bulletin #105. Bariatric surgery and pregnancy 2009.

45. Rand CS, Macgregor AM. Adolescents having obesity surgery: a 6-year follow-up. South Med J 1994;87:1208–13.

46. Dao T, Kuhn J, Ehmer D, et al. Pregnancy outcomes after gastric-bypass surgery. Am J Surg 2006;192:762–6.

47. Patel JA, Patel NA, Thomas RL, et al. Pregnancy outcomes after laparoscopic Roux-en-Y gastric bypass. Surg Obes Relat Dis 2008;4:39–45.

48. Wax JR, Cartin A, Wolff R, et al. Pregnancy following gastric bypass surgery for morbid obesity: maternal and neonatal outcomes. Obes Surg 2008;18: 540–4.

49. Cools M, Duval EL, Jespers A. Adverse neonatal outcome after maternal biliopancreatic diversion operation: report of nine cases. Eur J Pediatr 2006;165: 199–202.

50. Simon SR, Zemel R, Betancourt S, et al. Hematologic complications of gastric bypass for morbid obesity. South Med J 1989;82:1108–10.
51. Alvarez-Cordero R, Aragon-Viruette E. Post-operative complications in a series of gastric bypass patients. Obes Surg 1992;2:87–9.
52. Halverson JD. Micronutrient deficiencies after gastric bypass for morbid obesity. Am Surg 1986;52:594–8.
53. Halverson JD, Zuckerman GR, Koehler RE, et al. Gastric bypass for morbid obesity. A medical-surgical assessment. Ann Surg 1981;194:152–60.
54. Crowley LV, Seay J, Mullin G. Late effects of gastric bypass for obesity. Am J Gastroenterol 1984;79:850–60.
55. Avinoah E, Ovate A, Charuzi I. Nutritional status seven years after Roux-en-Y gastric bypass surgery. Surgery 1992;111:137–42.
56. Brolin RE, Gorman JH, Gorman RC, et al. Are vitamin B12 and folate deficiency clinically important after roux-en-Y gastric bypass? J Gastrointest Surg 1998;2:436–42.
57. Ramussen K. Is there a causal relationship between iron deficiency or iron deficiency anemia and weight at birth, length of gestation and prenatal mortality? J Nutr 2001;131:590s–601s.
58. Paroz A, Calmes JM, Giusti V, et al. Internal hernia after laparoscopic Roux-en-Y gastric bypass for morbid obesity: a continuous challenge in bariatric surgery. Obes Surg 2006;16:1482–7.
59. Bar-Zohar D, Azem F, Klausner J, et al. Pregnancy after laparoscopic adjustable gastric banding: perinatal outcome is favorable also for women with relatively high gestational weight gain. Surg Endosc 2006;20:1580–3.
60. Moore KA, Ouyang DW, Whang EE. Maternal and fetal deaths after gastric bypass surgery for morbid obesity. N Engl J Med 2004;351:721–2.
61. Kakarla N, Dailey C, Marino T, et al. Pregnancy after gastric bypass surgery and internal hernia formation. Obstet Gynecol 2005;105:1195–8.
62. Charles A, Domingo S, Goldfadden A, et al. Small bowel ischemia after Roux-en-Y gastric bypass complicated by pregnancy: a case report. Am Surg 2005;71:231–4.
63. Loar PV 3rd, Sanchez-Ramos L, Kaunitz AM, et al. Maternal death caused by midgut volvulus after bariatric surgery. Am J Obstet Gynecol 2005;193:1748–9.
64. Wittgrove AC, Jester L, Wittgrove P, et al. Pregnancy following gastric bypass for morbid obesity. Obes Surg 1998;8:461–4 [discussion: 465–6].
65. Ducarme G, Revaux A, Rodrigues A, et al. Obstetric outcome following laparoscopic adjustable gastric banding. Int J Gynaecol Obstet 2007;98:244–7.
66. Dixon JB, Dixon ME, O'Brien PE. Birth outcomes in obese women after laparoscopic adjustable gastric banding. Obstet Gynecol 2005;106:965–72.
67. Skull AJ, Slater GH, Duncombe JE, et al. Laparoscopic adjustable banding in pregnancy: safety, patient tolerance and effect on obesity-related pregnancy outcomes. Obes Surg 2004;14:230–5.
68. Richards DS, Miller DK, Goodman GN. Pregnancy after gastric bypass for morbid obesity. J Reprod Med 1987;32:172–6.
69. Sheiner E, Levy A, Silverberg D, et al. Pregnancy after bariatric surgery is not associated with adverse perinatal outcome. Am J Obstet Gynecol 2004;190:1335–40.
70. Friedman D, Cuneo S, Valenzano M, et al. Pregnancies in an 18-year follow-up after biliopancreatic diversion. Obes Surg 1995;5:308–13.
71. Kral JG, Biron S, Simard S, et al. Large maternal weight loss from obesity surgery prevents transmission of obesity to children who were followed from 2 to 18 years. Pediatrics 2006;118:1644–9.

72. Anonymous. Prevention of neural tube defects: results of the medical research council vitamin study. MRC Vitamin Study Research Group. Lancet 1991;338: 131–7.
73. Moliterno JA, Diluna ML, Sood SA, et al. Gastric bypass: a risk factor for neural tube defects? J Neurosurg Pediatr 2008;1:406–9.
74. Haddow JE, Hill LE, Kloza EM, et al. Neural tube defects after gastric bypass. Lancet 1986;1:1330.
75. Weintraub AY, Levy A, Levi I, et al. Effect of bariatric surgery on pregnancy outcome. Int J Gynaecol Obstet 2008;103:246–51.
76. Knudsen LB, Källén B. Gastric bypass, pregnancy, and neural tube defects. Lancet 1986;2:227.
77. Dixon JB, Dixon ME, O'Brien PE. Elevated homocysteine levels with weight loss after lap-band surgery: higher folate and vitamin B12 levels required to maintain homocysteine level. Int J Obes 2001;25:219–27.
78. Perlow JH, Morgan MA. Massive maternal obesity and perioperative cesarean morbidity. Am J Obstet Gynecol 1994;170:560–5.
79. Sebire NJ, Jolly M, Harris JP, et al. Maternal obesity and pregnancy outcome: a study of 287,213 pregnancies in London. Int J Obes Relat Metab Disord 2001;25:1175–82.
80. Kumari AS. Pregnancy outcome in women with morbid obesity. Int J Gynaecol Obstet 2001;73:101–7.
81. Lu GC, Rouse DJ, DuBard M, et al. The effect of the increasing prevalence of maternal obesity on perinatal morbidity. Obstet Gynecol 2001;185:845–9.
82. Ehrenberg HM, Mercer BM, Catalano PM. The influence of obesity and diabetes on the prevalence of macrosomia. Am J Obstet Gynecol 2004;191:964–8.
83. Grange DK, Finlay JL. Nutritional vitamin B_{12} deficiency in a breastfed infant following maternal gastric bypass. Pediatr Hematol Oncol 1994;11: 311–8.
84. Campbell CD, Ganesh J, Ficicioglu C. Two newborns with nutritional vitamin B12 deficiency: challenges in newborn screening for vitamin B12 deficiency. Haematologica 2005;90:ECR45.
85. Wardinsky TD, Montes RG, Friederich RL, et al. Vitamin B_{12} deficiency associated with low breast-milk vitamin B_{12} concentration in an infant following maternal gastric bypass surgery. Arch Pediatr Adolesc Med 1995;149: 1281–4.
86. Martens WS, Martin LF, Berlin CM. Failure of a nursing infant to thrive after the mother's gastric bypass for morbid obesity. Pediatrics 1990;86:777–8.
87. VanMieghem T, VanSchoubroeck D, Depiere M, et al. Fetal cerebral hemorrhage caused by vitamin K deficiency after complicated bariatric surgery. Obstet Gynecol 2008;112:434–6.
88. Eerdekens A, Debeer A, Van Hoey G, et al. Maternal bariatric surgery: adverse outcomes in neonates. Eur J Pediatr 2010;169:191–6.
89. Catalano PM. Obesity and pregnancy—the propagation of a viscous cycle? J Clin Endocrinol Metab 2003;88:3505–6.
90. Barker DJ, Osmond C, Golding J, et al. Growth in utero, blood pressure in childhood and adult life, and mortality from cardiovascular disease. BMJ 1989;298:564.
91. Barker DJ. In utero programming of cardiovascular disease. Theriogenology 2000;53:555.
92. Oken E, Gillman MW. Fetal origins of obesity. Obes Res 2003;11:496–506.

93. Lee JH, Reed DR, Price RA. Familial risk ratios for extreme obesity: implications for mapping human obesity genes. Int J Obes 1997;21:935–40.
94. Silventoinen K, Kapria J, Lahelma E, et al. Assortative mating by body height and BMI: Finnish twins and their spouses. Am J Hum Biol 2003;15:620–7.
95. Herman KM, Craig CL, Gauvin L, et al. Tracking of obesity and physical activity from childhood to adulthood: the physical activity longitudinal study. Int J Pediatr Obes 2009;4:281–8.
96. Smith J, Cianflone K, Biron S, et al. Effects of maternal surgical weight loss in mothers on intergenerational transmission of obesity. J Clin Endocrinol Metab 2009;94:4275–83.
97. NHANES data on the prevalence of overweight among children and adolescents: United States, 2003–2006. CDC National Center for Health Statistics, Health E-Stat.
98. Sukalich S, Mingione MJ, Glantz JC. Obstetric outcomes in overweight and obese adolescents. Am J Obstet Gynecol 2006;195:851–5.
99. Inge TH, Krebs NF, Garcia VF, et al. Bariatric surgery for overweight adolescents: concerns and recommendations. Pediatrics 2004;114:217–23.
100. Schilling PL, Davis MM, Albanese CT, et al. National trends in adolescent bariatric surgical procedures and implications for surgical centers of excellence. J Am Coll Surg 2008;206:1–12.
101. Tsai WS, Inge TH, Burd RS. Bariatric surgery in adolescents: recent national trends in use and in-hospital outcome. Arch Pediatr Adolesc Med 2007;161: 217–21.
102. Beard JH, Bell RL, Duffy AJ. Reproductive considerations and pregnancy after bariatric surgery: current evidence and recommendations. Obes Surg 2008;18: 1023–7.
103. Papadia FS, Adami GF, Marinari GM, et al. Bariatric surgery in adolescents: a long-term follow-up study. Surg Obes Relat Dis 2007;3:465–8.
104. Roehrig HR, Xanthakos SA, Sweeney J, et al. Pregnancy after gastric bypass surgery in adolescents. Obes Surg 2007;17:873–7.
105. Mechanick JI, Kushner RF, Sugerman HJ, et al. American Association of Clinical Endocrinologists, the Obesity Society, and American Society for Metabolic and Bariatric Surgery medical guidelines for clinical practice for the perioperative nutritional, metabolic, and nonsurgical support of the bariatric surgery patient. Perioperative bariatric guidelines. Obesity (Silver Spring) 2009;17:s1–70.
106. Gosman GG, King WC, Schrope B, et al. Reproductive health of women electing bariatric surgery. Fertil Steril 2009. [Epub ahead of print].
107. Sheiner E, Balaban E, Dreiher J, et al. Pregnancy outcome in patients following different types of bariatric surgeries. Obes Surg 2009;19:1286–92.
108. Rhode BM, Shustik C, Christou NV, et al. Iron absorption and therapy after gastric bypass. Obes Surg 1999;9:17–21.
109. Dixon JB, Dixon ME, O'Brien PE. Pregnancy after Lap-Band surgery: management of the band to achieve healthy weight outcomes. Obes Surg 2001;11: 59–65.
110. Martin L, Chavez GF, Adams MJ, et al. Gastric bypass surgery as maternal risk factor for neural tube defects. Lancet 1988;1:640–1.
111. Weiss HG, Nehoda H, Lubeck B, et al. Pregnancies after adjustable gastric banding. Obes Surg 2001;11:303–6.

Selected Viral Infections in Pregnancy

Britta Panda, MD[a], Alexander Panda, MD, MPH[b,c],
Laura E. Riley, MD[d],*

KEYWORDS

- Influenza • Hepatitis A • Hepatitis B • Hepatitis C

Epidemics of influenza typically occur from October to April and have been respon-sible for an average of 36,000 deaths per year in the United States. Influenza viruses cause disease among all age groups; however, rates of serious illness and death are highest among persons older than 65 years, children younger than 2 years, pregnant women, and persons of any age who have medical conditions that place them at increased risk for complications from influenza.[1] Influenza A is a single-stranded nega-tive sense RNA virus that encodes 8 major genes, including 2 major surface antigens: hemagglutinin (HA) (16 subtypes) and neuraminidase (NA) (9 subtypes). Seasonal influ-enza poses a major global health burden annually that is magnified when potential strains create pandemics through point mutations in genes encoding HA and NA (anti-genic drift) or viral genomic reassortment of subtypes (especially during interspecies transmission), often resulting in the introduction of novel influenza strains into the human population (antigenic shift).[2,3]

A novel H1N1 Type A influenza virus is responsible for the current pandemic.[4] This novel virus was initially termed "swine flu" because many of its genes appeared very similar to those in viruses that infect North American pigs; however, further studies reveal that this new virus is in fact more complex. The novel H1N1 influenza virus represents quadruple reassortment of 1 human, 1 avian, and 2 swine strains (North American and Eurasian) of influenza virus.[4]

[a] Division of Maternal Fetal Medicine, Massachusetts General Hospital, 55 Fruit Street, Founders 450, Boston, MA 02210, USA
[b] Division of Pulmonary and Critical Care Medicine, Yale University, 333 Cedar Street, TAC–441 South, PO Box 208057, New Haven, CT 06512, USA
[c] Division of Infectious Diseases, Yale University, 333 Cedar Street, TAC–441 South, PO Box 208057, New Haven, CT 06512, USA
[d] Division of Maternal Fetal Medicine, Founders 4-414, Massachusetts General Hospital, Boston, MA 02114, USA
* Corresponding author.
E-mail address: lriley@partners.org

Obstet Gynecol Clin N Am 37 (2010) 321–331
doi:10.1016/j.ogc.2010.02.009
0889-8545/10/$ – see front matter © 2010 Elsevier Inc. All rights reserved.

CLINICAL PRESENTATION/MATERNAL-FETAL TRANSMISSION

The 2009 pandemic declared in July 2009 by the World Health Organization (WHO) with the H1N1 virus often presents with similar symptoms to seasonal influenza with body aches, fatigue, chills, rhinorrhea, conjunctivitis, shortness of breath, headache, and gastrointestinal symptoms. Unlike with seasonal influenza, the gastrointestinal symptoms such as diarrhea and vomiting appear more frequently in patients with H1N1 infection.[4]

The severity of this influenza strain is particularly high in pregnant women. Pregnant women with the 2009 H1N1 virus were 4 times more likely to be hospitalized than the general public when infected with this strain.[5] Of 45 deaths reported early in the pandemic, 6 patients were pregnant. All developed viral pneumonia and acute respiratory distress syndrome requiring mechanical ventilation. None had evidence of secondary bacterial infection or hemorrhage.[5] In a large series of pregnant and postpartum patients who were hospitalized with or died from 2009 H1N1 influenza, 95% of the pregnant patients were infected in the second or third trimester, and almost one-fifth required intensive care. One-third of these patients had preexisting medical conditions that were recognized risk factors for complications from influenza. Eight patients who were hospitalized had onset of symptoms within 2 weeks postpartum; half of those required intensive care and 2 died, highlighting the continued high-risk period immediately after delivery. In this surveillance study, pregnant women were less likely to have underlying medical conditions than nonpregnant women hospitalized with 2009 H1N1 virus. Although these pregnant women frequently presented with mild or moderate symptoms, many had a rapid clinical progression and deterioration.[6]

Little is known regarding the direct effects of the influenza virus on the fetus. Viremia is believed to occur infrequently[7] and thus vertical transmission appears to be rare.[8] Highly pathogenic strains of influenza virus, such as avian influenza A (H5N1), are more likely to be transmitted across the placenta.[9] During previous pandemics, infected pregnant women, particularly those with pneumonia, had remarkably high rates of spontaneous abortion and preterm birth.[10] It is hypothesized that maternal hyperthermia may account for these adverse outcomes.[11,12] There is no evidence that influenza viruses are teratogenic.

Diagnosis

A number of effective laboratory tests exist: direct antigen detection tests, virus isolation in cell culture, and detection of influenza-specific RNA by real-time reverse transcriptase–polymerase chain reaction (rRT-PCR). Culture has limited clinical application because of its long turnaround time. The sensitivity of the direct antigen test for detecting this novel virus compared with RT-PCR ranges from 10% to 70%.[13] The Centers for Disease Control and Prevention (CDC) recommends rRT-PCR swine flu panel assay to be performed to confirm the diagnosis.[4] Although rapid influenza tests are widely available and can be completed within 15 minutes, reliance on rapid test results might have contributed to treatment delays. In the surveillance study of pregnant and postpartum patients who were hospitalized with or died from 2009 H1N1 influenza, 38% of patients who underwent testing had false negative results; less than 30% of the pregnant women with false negative results received antiviral treatment within 48 hours after symptom onset, and 5 of the patients who died had false negative results.[6] Therefore, during this pandemic the CDC issued a health advisory alerting clinicians to the poor sensitivity of these rapid test results and recommending that clinical decisions about the treatment of influenza should not be guided or delayed by negative results on rapid testing.[14]

Treatment

Women with suspected or confirmed influenza who are pregnant or who have delivered within the previous 2 weeks should receive aggressive antiviral treatment and undergo close monitoring regardless of the results of rapid antigen tests. Because pregnant women and their fetuses may require specialized care and monitoring, early consideration should be given to the transfer of critically ill pregnant and postpartum women to tertiary care facilities that can provide specialized services such as neonatal intensive care or extracorporeal membrane oxygenation.

The benefit of treatment with antiviral medications outweighs its theoretical risk because pregnant women are at increased risk for severe complications from the H1N1 virus infection.[15] Early treatment with antiviral medication is recommended for pregnant women with suspected novel H1N1 infection regardless of the gestational age. Clinicians should not wait for test results, as these medications are most effective when started within the first 48 hours of the onset of symptoms.[16] Nonetheless, data from seasonal influenza studies indicate benefit for hospitalized patients even if treatment is initiated more than 48 hours after the onset of symptoms. Therefore, antiviral medications are recommended for high-risk patients (patients with chronic metabolic diseases [including diabetes mellitus], renal dysfunction, hemoglobinopathies, or immunosuppression [including immunosuppression caused by medications or by HIV]; adults and children who have any condition [eg, cognitive dysfunction, spinal cord injuries, seizure disorders, or other neuromuscular disorders] that can compromise respiratory function or the handling of respiratory secretions or that can increase the risk for aspiration), particularly pregnant women requiring hospitalization, even if presenting more than 48 hours after onset of symptoms.[1,17]

The 2009 novel influenza H1N1 is sensitive to neuraminidase inhibitors zanamivir (Relenza) and oseltamivir (Tamiflu), but resistant to adamantanes.[13] Oseltamivir (75 mg orally) and zanamivir (10 mg intranasal) are administered twice a day for 5 days.[18] Because of its systemic activity, the drug of choice for treatment of pregnant women is oseltamivir. For seasonal flu or influenza B, adamantanes are most effective.[1]

Prevention

The CDC recommends that all pregnant women receive seasonal influenza vaccination. Inactivated influenza A or B strains may be incorporated into the vaccine. Multidose vials generally contain trace thimerisol, which has not been linked to neonatal adverse outcomes. There have been at least 11 cohort studies of seasonal influenza vaccination in pregnancy with no evidence of excess adverse maternal or fetal outcomes.

Maternal vaccination also provides a benefit to the newborn infant, with a decreased risk of respiratory infections related to influenza in both the mother and infant during the first 6 months after delivery.[19]

Pregnant and postpartum women should be counseled about the importance of vaccination.[19–21] Pregnant women were a top-priority group for immunization against 2009 H1N1 influenza. Because the 2009 H1N1 monovalent vaccine is manufactured according to the same processes that are used for the seasonal influenza vaccine, its safety profile among pregnant women is expected to be similar to that of the seasonal influenza vaccine.[22] Preliminary results from a trial of 2009 H1N1 nonadjuvanted vaccine showed a robust immune response in pregnant women, similar to the response in nonpregnant adults, and no safety concerns were identified.[23]

Prophylaxis after exposure to a person with confirmed, probable, or suspected H1N1 infection is indicated for patients at high risk of complications from influenza (eg, pregnancy) and for health care workers who were not using appropriate personal protective equipment. Either oseltamivir (75 mg orally) or zanamivir (10 mg intranasal) may be used once daily for 10 days from the time of last exposure.[20,24]

The risk of transmission of H1N1 through breast milk is unknown.[25,26] The probability that H1N1 will cross into breast milk is low because H1N1 viremia is low. Therefore, infected mothers may breastfeed.[25,26] The decision to separate infected mothers from their newborns is individualized. If feasible, infected women should express their breast milk for bottle feeding by a healthy family member. Alternatively, women should wear a face mask while breastfeeding and providing care to their babies to minimize exposure. In the midst of a pandemic, there may be additional benefit from the immune protection provided by breastfeeding.[25,26]

In summary, influenza viruses appear to pose particular risks to pregnant women in the second and third trimesters of pregnancy. The virulence of the 2009 H1N1 pandemic has mirrored the seriousness of influenza in pregnancy seen in the pandemics of 1918 and 1957, both of which reported excess death and morbidity for pregnancy.[13] Given the severity of illness for pregnant women and neonates, further use of the best prevention strategy to date, vaccination for pregnant women, is paramount.[1]

HEPATITIS A VIRUS
Background

Every year, approximately 10 million people worldwide are infected with the hepatitis A virus (HAV).[27] HAV is a picornavirus and contains a single-stranded RNA. It is most commonly transmitted by the fecal-oral route via contaminated food or drinking water. The distribution of HAV is global; however, in developing countries, and in regions with poor hygiene standards, the incidence of infection with HAV is high and the illness is usually contracted in early childhood. In industrialized countries on the other hand, the infection is contracted primarily by adults traveling to countries with a high incidence of the disease.[27]

Clinical Presentation/Maternal-Fetal Transmission

The symptoms of hepatitis A infection include fatigue, malaise, fever, nausea, and anorexia, but some infected persons, particularly children, exhibit no symptoms at all. Pregnant women who are infected experience similar symptoms, whereas others may present with significant weight loss.[28] The classic picture of icterus and hepatosplenomegaly becomes apparent within 10 days of systemic symptoms. Liver function abnormalities, typically characterized by elevations in alanine aminotransferase (ALT) and aspartate aminotransferase (AST), peak before the appearance of jaundice. ALT and AST may remain elevated for more than a month. A chronic carrier state for HAV does not exist.[28,29] The course of hepatitis A infection is unaffected by pregnancy and pregnant women infected with HAV should be reassured that no adverse fetal outcome has been linked to viral hepatitis.[30] If a neonate is born within 2 weeks of acute maternal illness with HAV, immunoglobulin is recommended for the newborn. If the exposure is more than 2 weeks before birth, the immunoglobulin does not appear to be effective.[31]

Diagnosis

The diagnosis is made by the detection of HAV-specific immunoglobulin M (IgM) antibodies in the blood by enzyme-linked immunosorbent assay (ELISA). IgM antibody is present in the blood only following an acute hepatitis A infection. It is detectable from 1 to 2 weeks after the initial infection and persists for up to 14 weeks. The presence of

IgG antibody in the blood means that the acute stage of the illness is past and the person is immune to future infection.[31]

Treatment

There is no specific treatment for hepatitis A infection. Other than supportive care, patients should be advised to rest, eat a well-balanced diet, and stay hydrated. Approximately 6% to 10% of people diagnosed with hepatitis A may experience one or more symptomatic relapse(s) for up to 40 weeks after contracting the disease.[29]

Prevention

Hepatitis A infection can be prevented by vaccination, and good hygiene and sanitation. The recombinant vaccine contains inactivated hepatitis A virus providing active immunity against a future infection and is recommended for all people traveling to endemic areas, including pregnant women. The vaccine is given in 2 doses—the first dose provides protection 2 to 4 weeks after initial vaccination; the second booster dose, given 6 to 12 months later, provides protection for up to 20 years in approximately 90% of vaccinated persons.[31] Twinrix, a combined hepatitis A and B vaccine is also available. The seroconversion after 3 doses is nearly 100%.[31]

HEPATITIS B VIRUS
Background

In 2005, approximately 51,000 people became infected with hepatitis B in the United States and about 1.25 million people in the United States have chronic hepatitis B virus (HBV) infection. Each year about 3000 to 5000 people die from cirrhosis or liver cancer caused by HBV.[31] HBV is a double-stranded DNA virus in the Hepadnaviridae family.[32] HBV is found in highest concentrations in the blood, and lower concentrations in semen and vaginal secretions. Sexual transmission accounts for most adult HBV infections in the United States. Approximately 25% of the regular sexual contacts of infected individuals will themselves become seropositive.[32]

Clinical Presentation/Maternal-Fetal Transmission

Patients with an acute infection are either asymptomatic or present with loss of appetite, nausea, vomiting, fever, abdominal pain, and jaundice. Most patients with chronic hepatitis B are asymptomatic, but some have nonspecific symptoms such as fatigue.[32]

Hepatitis B infection during pregnancy does not increase maternal mortality or morbidity. There is also no association between maternal HBV infection and adverse fetal outcome in an otherwise healthy mother. Chronic HBV infection is usually mild in pregnant women, but may flare shortly after delivery.[33] Approximately 10% to 20% of women who are seropositive for hepatitis B surface antigen (HBsAg) transmit the virus to their neonates only in the absence of immunoprophylaxis.[34] Of mothers who are positive for HBsAg and hepatitis B e antigen (HBeAg), approximately 90% of infants will become infected if no immunoprophylaxis is given.[34] Transmission rates with primary infection are much higher in the third trimester (80%–90%) compared with the first trimester (10%).[34] In the event of preterm premature rupture of membranes, the decision to continue with conservative management versus immediate delivery should be individualized based on gestational age. Theoretically, the risk of transmission is higher with prolonged rupture of membranes; however, in some cases the morbidity associated with prematurity may be greater. There is no evidence that the small dose of steroids given for fetal lung maturity will have a negative impact on the course of the infection.

After an acute infection, 2% to 6% of adults are not able to eliminate the virus and develop chronic hepatitis. On the other hand, 90% of neonates who become infected develop a chronic infection and approximately 60% of infected children younger than 5 develop a chronic infection.[35]

Diagnosis

The diagnosis of acute hepatitis B is based on the detection of HBsAg and IgM anti-hepatitis B core (HBc). The diagnosis of chronic HBV infection is based on the persistence of HBsAg for more than 6 months.[32] HBeAg is a viral protein that is found in the blood only in the setting of active infection and is used as a marker for infectivity. The core antigen is found on virus particles but disappears early in the course of infection. The HBc antibody is produced during and after an acute HBV infection and is usually found in chronic HBV carriers as well as those who have cleared the virus, and it usually persists for life. Anti-HBs indicates previous exposure to HBV, but the virus is no longer present and the person is no longer infectious. This antibody also protects the body from future HBV infection. In addition to exposure to HBV, the anti-HBs can also be acquired from successful vaccination.[36]

Treatment

The treatment for acute HBV infection in pregnant and nonpregnant individuals is supportive care. The immune system controls the infection and eliminates the virus within about 6 months in most healthy adults.[36,37] In recent years, more treatment options for chronic hepatitis B infection or severe acute hepatitis B infections have become available. Pregnant women have been treated with lamivudine during acute, fulminant infections with HBV with improved maternal and fetal outcomes.[38,39] In addition, pregnant women with high viral loads (>10^9 copies/mL in serum) may be given lamivudine to reduce perinatal transmission.[38,39]

Newborns born to HBsAg-positive mothers should receive hepatitis B immunoglobulin within 12 hours after birth concurrently with the first pediatric dose of the vaccine. Vaccination series should be completed at 1 and 6 months.[36,37]

Prevention

Hepatitis B vaccination is the most effective measure to prevent HBV infection and its consequences. HBsAg is the recombinant antigen used for hepatitis B vaccination; therefore, it can be given safely in all trimesters of pregnancy and during breastfeeding.[32,33] Neonatal HBV infection can be prevented by vaccinating pregnant patients at risk for HBV infection, safe-sex practices of the mother, antenatal screening of all patients for HBV, treatment and prophylaxis of the newborn after delivery if indicated, and vaccination of all newborns. Thus, it is imperative to vaccinate pregnant women who have multiple sex partners, intravenous (IV) drug users, household contacts of people infected with HBV, health care workers, and women with chronic kidney and liver disease, and complete the series for those who have initiated the series before pregnancy.[31]

HEPATITIS C VIRUS
Background

An estimated 270 to 300 million people are infected with the hepatitis C virus (HCV) worldwide. It is the most common chronic blood-borne infection in the United States.[40] Hepatitis C is a single-stranded RNA virus related to the family Flaviridae that is characterized by striking genetic heterogeneity, including 6 major genotypes and numerous subtypes.[41] This heterogeneity and the rapid mutation rate of HCV present multiple challenges in the development of a vaccine against HCV infections.[41] HCV is transmitted through exposure to infected blood, sexual contact, or mother-to-infant (vertical) transmission.[42] It is estimated that 60% to 80% of IV drug users are infected with HCV.[40] Among HIV-infected nonpregnant women the prevalence is as high as 17% to 54%.[40] After implementing routine screening of all blood products for HCV in 1992, the CDC reports that the risk of HCV infection from a unit of transfused blood in the United States is less than 1 per 100,000 transfused units. Sexual transmission appears to be relatively low, on the order of 0% to 4%.[43] Among the pregnant population, it is estimated that approximately 1% is HCV positive, which corresponds to approximately 40,000 births to HCV-infected mothers annually.[44]

Clinical Presentation/Maternal-Fetal Transmission

Of patients with acute HCV infection, 65% to 75% are asymptomatic, 25% are icteric, and 10% show symptoms of acute illness with fatigue, nausea, vomiting, and abdominal pain. Symptoms usually develop 4 to 12 weeks after infection. After an acute infection, only 15% to 25% of persons clear the infection, whereas 75% to 85% develop chronic hepatitis C. Most patients with chronic hepatitis C are asymptomatic or have mild fatigue and are identified incidentally in the course of evaluation for unexplained elevated ALT and AST or after blood donation.[42,43] Of patients with chronic HCV infection, 20% to 30% will develop liver cirrhosis and/or liver cancer in their lifetimes.[43]

Pregnancy does not affect the course of acute or chronic hepatitis C infection, although several studies have shown temporary improvement of biochemical markers of liver damage in HCV-positive women during pregnancy.[45,46] Conversely, chronic hepatitis does not appear to have an adverse effect on the pregnancy. The rate of spontaneous miscarriage, growth restriction, preterm delivery, and obstetric complications, such as gestational diabetes or hypertension, were similar in patients with HCV infection and healthy controls.[47]

There are several factors that influence mother-to-infant transmission of HCV. Vertical transmission is greater with a higher maternal viral load of HCV. If the mother is anti-HCV positive but HCV RNA negative, the risk for transmission to the baby is approximately 1% to 3%. If the mother is HCV RNA positive, the risk for transmission is approximately 4% to 6%.[44,48] The highest reported transmission rates occur in infants born to mothers who are HCV positive and HIV positive, with rates as high as 36%.[49,50] The mode of delivery does not seem to influence transmission rates; however, invasive procedures, such as fetal scalp blood sampling or internal electronic fetal heart rate monitoring via scalp electrode should be avoided.[51] Some observations suggest that prolonged rupture of fetal membranes increases the risk for vertical transmission; therefore, early artificial rupture of membranes should be avoided if possible.[51] In the event of preterm premature rupture of membranes in patients infected with HCV, the decision to continue with conservative management versus immediate delivery should be individualized based on gestational age. The risk of transmission seems to be higher with prolonged rupture of membranes; however, in some cases the morbidity associated with prematurity may be greater. There is no association between gestational age at delivery and the risk of vertical transmission.[52] There is no evidence that the small dose of steroids given for fetal lung maturity will have a negative impact on the course of the infection.

Amniocentesis in women infected with hepatitis C does not appear to significantly increase the risk of vertical transmission, but women should be counseled that very few studies have properly addressed this possibility.[53] No cases of HCV transmission through breastfeeding are known; therefore, hepatitis C infection is not a contraindication to breastfeeding.[54]

Diagnosis

The diagnosis of HCV infection can be made by detecting either anti-HCV by enzyme immunoassay (EIA) or HCV RNA using the reverse-transcriptase polymerase chain reaction (RT-PCR). If the HCV RNA result is negative in a woman with anti-HCV antibody, supplemental testing should be performed. The CDC recommends confirmation of a positive EIA with supplemental recombinant immunoblot assay (RIBA) or RT-PCR for HCV RNA.[40]

Treatment

At present, no HCV vaccine is available. Treatment for chronic HCV infection includes alpha interferon alone or in combination with the oral agent ribavirin. Interferon does not appear to have an adverse affect on the fetus; however, the data are limited, and the potential benefits of interferon use during pregnancy should clearly outweigh potential hazards. Because there are no large studies of ribavirin use during human pregnancy, and ribavirin is teratogenic in multiple animal species, the use of ribavirin during pregnancy is contraindicated.[55]

Prevention

There is currently no available therapy to prevent vertical transmission of HCV. Routine screening of all mothers is unwarranted. Current screening guidance suggests checking hepatitis C antibodies only in pregnant women with a current or past history of IV drug use; women who received clotting factor concentrates produced before 1987, or a blood transfusion or an organ transplant before 1992; women who were ever on chronic hemodialysis; women with persistently abnormal liver function tests; or health care workers after needle sticks or mucosal exposures to HCV-positive blood. Infants of infected mothers should be tested for anti-HCV at 1 year and followed for the development of hepatitis.[43]

REFERENCES

1. Fiore AE, Shay DK, Broder K, et al. Prevention and control of seasonal influenza with vaccines: recommendations of the Advisory Committee on Immunization Practices (ACIP), 2009. MMWR Recomm Rep 2009;58:1.
2. Khiabanian H, Trifonov V, Rabadan R. Reassortment patterns in Swine influenza viruses. PLoS One 2009;4(10):e7366.
3. Neumann G, Noda T, Kawaoka Y. Emergence and pandemic potential of swine-origin H1N1 influenza virus. Nature 2009;459(7249):931–9.
4. Novel Swine-Origin Influenza A (H1N1) Virus Investigation Team. Emergence of a novel swine-origin influenza A (H1N1) virus in humans. N Engl J Med 2009; 361:1.
5. Jamieson DJ, Honein MA, Rasmussen SA, et al. Novel Influenza A (H1N1) Pregnancy Working Group. H1N1 2009 influenza virus infection during pregnancy in the USA. Lancet 2009;374(9688):451–8.
6. Louie J, Acosta M, Jamieson D, et al. Severe 2009 H1N1 influenza in pregnant and postpartum women in California. N Engl J Med 2010;362(1):27–35.
7. Zou S. Potential impact of pandemic influenza on blood safety and availability. Transfus Med Rev 2006;20(3):181–9.

8. Irving WL, James DK, Stephenson T, et al. Influenza virus infection in the second and third trimesters of pregnancy: a clinical and seroepide-miological study. BJOG 2000;107(10):1282–9.

9. Shu Y, Yu H, Li D. Lethal avian influenza A (H5N1) infection in a pregnant woman in Anhui Province, China. N Engl J Med 2006;354(913):1421–2.

10. Nuzum JW, Pilot I, Stangl FH, et al. 1918 pandemic influenza and pneumonia in a large civil hospital. IMJ Ill Med J 1976;150(6):612–6.

11. Moretti ME, Bar-Oz B, Fried S, et al. Maternal hyperthermia and the risk for neural tube defects in offspring: systematic review and meta-analysis. Epidemiology 2005;16(2):216–9.

12. Coffey VP, Jessop WJ. Maternal influenza and congenital deformities. A follow-up study. Lancet 1963;1(7284):748–51.

13. Fiore AE, Shay DK, Broder K, et al. Prevention and control of influenza: recommendations of the Advisory Committee on Immunization Practices (ACIP), 2008. MMWR Recomm Rep 2008;57(RR–7):1–60.

14. Idem. CDC Health Alert Network (HAN) info service message: recommendations for early empiric antiviral treatment in persons with suspected influenza who are at increased risk of developing severe disease. Available at: http://www.cdc.gov/H1N1flu/HAN/101909.htm. Accessed January 8, 2010.

15. Ellis JS, Zambon MC. Molecular diagnosis of influenza. Rev Med Virol 2002;12: 375.

16. Rasmussen SA, Jamieson DJ, Macfarlane K, et al. Pandemic influenza and pregnant women: summary of a meeting of experts. Am J Public Health 2009; 99(Suppl 2):S248–54.

17. Allen UD, Aoki FY, Silver HG. The use of antiviral drugs for influenza: recommended guidelines for practitioners. Can J Infect Dis Med Microbiol 2006;17(5): 273–84.

18. Centers for Disease Control and Prevention (CDC). Interim guidance of antiviral recommendations for patients with novel influenza A (H1N1) virus infection and their close contacts. Available at: http://www.cdc.gov/h1n1flu/recommendations. htm. Accessed January 8, 2010.

19. World Health Organization. Experts advise WHO on pandemic vaccine policies and strategies. Pandemic (H1N1) 2009 briefing note 14. Available at: http://www.who.int/csr/disease/swineflu/notes/briefing_20091030/en/index.html. Accessed January 8, 2010.

20. Centers for Disease Control and Prevention (CDC). Novel influenza A (H1N1) virus infections in three pregnant women—United States, April–May 2009. [published erratum appears in MMWR Morb Mortal Wkly Rep 2009;58:541]. MMWR Morb Mortal Wkly Rep 2009;58(18):497–500.

21. Centers for Disease Control and Prevention. 2009 H1N1 influenza vaccine and pregnant women: information for healthcare providers. Available at: http://www.cdc.gov/h1n1flu/vaccination/providers_qa.htm. Accessed January 8, 2010.

22. Zaman K, Roy E, Arifeen SE, et al. Effectiveness of maternal influenza immunization in mothers and infants. N Engl J Med 2008;359:1555–64.

23. Tamma PD, Ault KA, Del Rio C, et al. Safety of influenza vaccination during pregnancy. Am J Obstet Gynecol 2009;201(6):547–52.

24. National Institute of Allergy and Infectious Diseases. H1N1 vaccine clinical studies in pregnant women. Available at: http://www3.niaid.nih.gov/topics/Flu/H1N1/ClinicalStudies/PregnantWomen.htm. Accessed January 8, 2010.

25. Centers for Disease Control and Prevention (CDC). Interim pre-pandemic planning guidance: community strategy for pandemic influenza mitigating in the United

States—early, targeted, layered use of nonpharmaceutical interventions. Available at: http://www.pandemicflu.gov/plan/community/community_mitigation.pdf. Accessed January 8, 2010.

26. Centers for Disease Control and Prevention. Pregnant women and novel influenza A (H1N1): considerations for clinicians. Available at: http://www.cdc.gov/h1n1flu/clinician_pregnant.htm. Accessed January 8, 2010.

27. Hepatitis A: fact sheet. Center for Disease Control. Available at: http://www.cdc.gov/hepatitis/hav/havfaq.htm. Accessed September 8, 2009.

28. Routenberg JA, Dienstag JL, Harrison WO, et al. A food-borne outbreak of hepatitis A: clinical and laboratory features of acute and protracted illness. Am J Med Sci 1979;278:123–37.

29. Inman RD, Hodge M, Johnston MEA, et al. Arthritis, vasculitis and cryoglobulinemia associated with relapsing hepatitis A virus infection. Ann Intern Med 1986; 105:700–3.

30. Tong MJ, Thursby M, Rakela J, et al. Studies on the maternal-infant transmission of the viruses which cause acute hepatitis. Gastroenterology 1981;80: 999–1004.

31. CDC. Protection against viral hepatitis. Recommendations of the Immunization Practices Advisory Committee (ACIP) MMWR Recomm Rep 2008;39(RR–2):1–26

32. Dienstag JL. Hepatitis B virus infection. N Engl J Med 2008;359:1486–500.

33. Hieber JP, Dalton D, Shorey J, et al. Hepatitis and pregnancy. J Pediatr 1977;91: 545.

34. Shapiro CN. Epidemiology of hepatitis B. Pediatr Infect Dis J 1993;12:433–7.

35. Lok A, Mcmahon B. Chronic hepatitis B. Hepatology 2007;45:507–39.

36. NIH Consensus Development Conference 2008. Management of hepatitis B. Available at: http://consensus.nih.gov/2008/2008HepatitisBCDC120main.htm. Accessed January 15, 2010.

37. Fiore S, Savasi V. Treatment of viral hepatitis in pregnancy. Expert Opin Pharmacother 2009;10:2801–9.

38. Potthoff A, Rifai K, Wedemeyer H, et al. Successful treatment of fulminant hepatitis B during pregnancy. Z Gastroenterol 2009;47(7):667–70.

39. Xu WM, Cui YT, Wang L, et al. Lamivudine in late pregnancy to prevent perinatal transmission of hepatitis B virus infection: a multicentre, randomized, double-blind, placebo-controlled study. J Viral Hepat 2009;16(2):94–103.

40. National Institute of Health (NIH). Management of hepatitis C [review]. NIH Consens State Sci Statements 2002;19(3):1–46.

41. Zein NN, Persing DH. Hepatitis C genotypes: current trends and future implications. Mayo Clin Proc 1996;71:458–62.

42. Dienstag JL. Non-A, non-B hepatitis I. Recognition, epidemiology, and clinical features. Gastroenterology 1983;85:439–62.

43. Recommendations for prevention and control of hepatitis C virus (HCV) and HCV-related chronic disease Centers for Disease Control and Prevention. MMWR Morb Mortal Wkly Rep 1998;47:1–39.

44. Wejstal R, Widell A, Mansson AS, et al. Mother to infant transmission of hepatitis C virus. Ann Intern Med 1992;117:887–90.

45. Conte D, Fraquelli M, Prati D, et al. Prevalence and clinical course of chronic hepatitis C virus (HCV) infection and the rate of vertical transmission in a cohort of 15,250 women. Hepatology 2000;31:751–5.

46. Gervais A, Bacq Y, Bernaunau J, et al. Decrease in serum ALT and increase in serum HCV RNA during pregnancy in women with chronic hepatitis C. J Hepatol 2000;32:293–9.

47. Simms J, Duff P. Viral hepatitis in pregnancy. Semin Perinatol 1993;17:384–93.
48. Zanetti AR, Tanzi E, Newell ML. Mother-to-infant transmission of hepatitis C virus. J Hepatol 1999;3(Suppl 1):S96–100.
49. Thomas DL, Villano SA, Riester KA, et al. Perinatal transmission of hepatitis C virus from human immunodeficiency virus type 1-infected mothers. J Infect Dis 1998;177:480–8.
50. Tovo PA, Palomba E, Ferraris G. Increased risk of maternal–infant hepatitis C virus transmission for women coinfected with HIV type 1. Clin Infect Dis 1997;25: 1121–4.
51. European Paediatric Hepatitis C Virus Network. Effects of mode of delivery and infant feeding on the risk of mother-to-child transmission of hepatitis C virus. BJOG 2001;108:371–7.
52. Eriksen NL. Perinatal consequences of hepatitis C. Clin Obstet Gynecol 1999;42: 121–33.
53. Minola E, Maccabruni A, Pacati I, et al. Amniocentesis as a possible risk factor for mother-to-infant transmission of HCV. Hepatology 2001;33:1341–2.
54. Polywka S, Schroter M, Feucht HH, et al. Low risk of vertical transmission of hepatitis C virus by breast milk. Clin Infect Dis 1999;29:1327–9.
55. Pelham J, Berghella V. Alpha interferon use in pregnancy. Obstet Gynecol 2004; 103:77S.

Thromboprophylaxis in Pregnancy: Who and How?

Sarah M. Davis, MD, D. Ware Branch, MD*

KEYWORDS

- Pregnancy • Thrombophilia • Screening • Prophylaxis

Venous thrombosis and embolism (VTE) is one of the most common, serious complications associated with pregnancy, and now ranks as a leading cause of maternal morbidity and mortality in developed countries.[1] Information regarding the association of VTE with acquired and heritable thrombophilias has greatly expanded in the last 20 years, adding a new layer of complexity to decisions about thromboprophylaxis. The objective of this review is to detail which patients are at clinically important increased risk for VTE, are candidates for thrombophilia screening, and warrant thromboprophylaxis. Suggested management schemes for use in specific patient subgroups are also provided.

EPIDEMIOLOGY

Pregnancy and the postpartum period carry an increased risk of VTE, with an incidence between 0.61 and 1.72 per 1000 deliveries.[2,3] Compared with nonpregnant women, pregnant and postpartum women are approximately 4 to 5 times more likely to develop VTE.[4] Roughly equal proportions of clinically apparent, pregnancy-related venous thromboembolic events are diagnosed in the antepartum and postpartum periods.[3] The risk of antepartum VTE was highest in the third trimester in one study.[5] In contrast, others found an increased risk in early pregnancy.[6,7] Overall, in these studies the risk of antepartum VTEs were evenly distributed throughout each trimester.[6,7]

In general, deep venous thrombosis (DVT) is more commonly diagnosed than pulmonary embolism (PE) in pregnancy. When DVT presents during pregnancy, it is more likely to be in the left lower extremity.[2,8] Predominance of left lower extremity clot formation may be due to compression of the left common iliac vein by the enlarging gravid uterus.[9] Pelvic venous thrombosis is a rare manifestation of deep venous thrombosis in nonpregnant individuals, and has been cited in a large prospective registry of DVT in the United States as accounting for less than 1% of DVTs.[10] Obstetricians should be

Department of Obstetrics and Gynecology, University of Utah Health Sciences Center, 30 North 1900 East, Salt Lake City, UT 84132, USA
* Corresponding author.
E-mail address: wareb@aol.com

Obstet Gynecol Clin N Am 37 (2010) 333–343
doi:10.1016/j.ogc.2010.02.004
0889-8545/10/$ – see front matter © 2010 Elsevier Inc. All rights reserved.

aware that pelvic venous thrombosis is more common in pregnancy, occurring in approximately 11% to 13% of venous thrombotic cases.[7,11]

Of importance is that PE is more likely to be diagnosed in the postpartum period.[2–4] This, coupled with the relatively higher incidence of VTE in the postpartum period, is cause for appropriate deliberation regarding postpartum thromboprophylaxis in at-risk patients.

PATHOPHYSIOLOGY AND RISK FACTORS

Virchow's triad describes 3 elements that contribute to the development of thrombosis: (1) stasis, (2) vascular trauma, and (3) hypercoagulability. These elements are all present during pregnancy and the postpartum period. Lower extremity venous stasis has been demonstrated during pregnancy.[12] Venous flow velocity decreases with advancing gestation, and is lower in the left compared with the right lower extremity. In addition, venous distention has been demonstrated, which may result in endothelial damage and prothrombotic changes in the endothelium.[13] Macklon and Greer[14] found that lower extremity venous flow velocity increased and vessel diameter decreased between 4 and 42 days postpartum. Venous flow velocity and diameter returned to levels observed in early pregnancy at the 42-day measurement.[13,14] In addition to mechanical compression of pelvic veins, increased circulating levels of estrogen and local production of prostacyclin and nitric oxide increase deep venous capacitance during pregnancy.[15]

Vascular trauma in the form of endothelial damage may occur due to venous distention during pregnancy,[13] or may occur during conditions such as preeclampsia where vascular endothelial activation is present.[16] During normal delivery, venous compression may occur. Operative and assisted deliveries are thought to contribute to vascular trauma, also possibly contributing to the risk of thrombosis in the postpartum period; this is especially true for cesarean delivery.

Normal pregnancy is accompanied by changes in the hemostatic system that would seem to result in a hypercoagulable state for the prevention of hemorrhage at the time of delivery. Overall, most clotting factors increase, some anticoagulants decrease, and fibrinolytic activity decreases. Regarding specific factors, factors II, VII, VIII, IX, XII, and von Willebrand factor increase throughout pregnancy.[17] Fibrinogen levels increase to levels that are almost twice that of the nonpregnant state.[17,18] Anticoagulant changes include decreased free and total protein S antigen levels, as well as decreased activity, occurring very early in pregnancy. Although protein C levels remain unchanged,[17,19] an overall increase in activated protein C resistance is present, with the degree of resistance dependent on several modifiers, including the presence of the Factor V Leiden mutation (FVLM), thrombin generation, and the presence of antiphospholipid antibodies.[20] Fibrinolysis is decreased, predominantly due to diminished tissue plasminogen activator activity. Increases have been noted in plasminogen activator inhibitor-1 and -2, and thrombin activatable fibrinolysis inhibitor. Other markers of a hypercoagulable state include increased thrombin-antithrombin complexes, prothrombin fragments 1 and 2, peak thrombin generation, and increased D-dimer levels.[17–19]

CLINICAL RISK FACTORS

Specific clinical risk factors have been identified that impact the likelihood of VTE. Not surprisingly, these are typically related to the elements of Virchow's triad and include such factors as bed rest (ie, stasis), operative delivery (ie, vascular trauma), and heritable thrombophilias (ie, hypercoagulability). Maternal age 35 years or older and cesarean delivery confer significant risk. Complications of pregnancy and delivery that increase the odds of VTE include critical illness, transfusion, and postpartum infection.[3] **Table 1**, modified from the work of James and colleagues,[3] shows the odds ratios associated with pertinent risk factors regarding risk of VTE.

Also shown in **Table 1** are the odds ratios associated with several common antenatal and postnatal risk factors both alone and in combination; these are modified from the work of Jacobsen and colleagues.[21] For example, the risk of VTE is substantially increased with the combination of antepartum bed rest and an increased body mass index (weight in kilograms divided by height in meters squared), or with postpartum infection following cesarean delivery.[21]

ACQUIRED AND HERITABLE THROMBOPHILIAS

The overall VTE risk associated with specific thrombophilias is well described in a systematic literature review by Robertson and colleagues in 2005.[22] Odds ratios were increased to varying degrees for FVLM (homozygous and heterozygous),

Table 1	
Clinical risk factors for venous thrombosis or embolism	
Condition	**Odds Ratio (95% Confidence Interval)**
Medical Complications	
Hypertension	1.8 (1.4–2.3)
Heart disease	7.1 (6.2–8.3)
Thrombophilia	51.8 (38.7–69.2)
History of thrombosis	24.8 (17.1–36.0)
Antiphospholipid syndrome	15.8 (10.9–22.8)
Sickle cell disease	6.7 (4.4–10.1)
Lupus	8.7 (5.8–13.0)
Diabetes	2.0 (1.4–2.1)
Obesity	4.4 (3.4–5.7)
Antepartum risk	
Body mass index (BMI) >25	1.8 (1.3–2.4)
Antepartum immobilization	7.7 (3.2–19.0)
BMI >25 and antepartum immobilization	62.3 (11.5–337.6)
Smoking (10–30 cigarettes/d)	2.1 (1.3–3.4)
Spontaneous twin gestation	2.6 (1.1–6.2)
ART twin gestation	6.6 (2.1–21.0)
Postpartum risk	
Smoking (10–30 cigarettes/d)	3.4 (2.0–5.5)
Hemorrhage (without surgery)	4.1 (2.3–7.3)
Hemorrhage (with surgery)	12.0 (3.9–36.9)
Infection (vaginal delivery)	20.2 (6.4–63.5)
Infection (cesarean delivery)	6.2 (2.4–16.2)
Planned cesarean	1.3 (0.7–2.2)
Acute cesarean	2.7 (1.8–4.1)

Data from James AH, Jamison MG, Brancazio LR, et al. Venous thromboembolism during pregnancy and the postpartum period: incidence, risk factors, and mortality. Am J Obstet Gynecol 2006;194:1311–5; and Jacobsen AF, Skjeldestad FE, Sandset PM. Ante- and postnatal risk factors of venous thrombosis: a hospital-based case-control study. J Thromb Haemost 2008;6:905–12.

prothrombin gene mutation (PGM) (homozygous and heterozygous), antithrombin deficiency, protein C and protein S deficiency, and antiphospholipid antibodies (**Table 2**). Of note, the C677T methylene tetrahydrofolate reductase mutation was not significantly associated with VTE.

The 2 most common heritable thrombophilias, heterozygosity for FVLM and PGM, have been examined in prospective observational studies and have not been found to pose a clinically important risk of VTE in otherwise healthy pregnant women with no history of thrombosis.[23–25] Deficiency of antithrombin, protein C, or protein S and antiphospholipid antibodies have not been studied in the same way, largely due to their infrequency.

THE ROLE OF THROMBOPHILIA TESTING

While the association between thrombophilias and VTE is apparent, the utility and cost-effectiveness of screening pregnant women for these disorders is not. Most experts agree that universal screening of asymptomatic women is not cost effective.[26–28] Obstetricians are left with the question of who should be screened. When considering thrombophilia screening, it may be helpful to think of candidate patients as falling into 1 of 4 categories: (1) those with acute VTE, (2) those with recurrent VTE (2 or more events), (3) those with a personal history of a single, prior VTE, or (4) those with a family history of VTE but without a personal history of VTE.

Acute VTE is not the subject of this review, but clinicians should recognize that testing for heritable thrombophilias in the setting of a first episode of VTE is controversial,[29] largely because the findings are not likely to change management and certainly will not alter the usual acute management with heparin and transition to warfarin (in nonpregnant patients). In addition, the heritable thrombophilias most commonly found, heterozygosity for FVLM or PGM, are not indications for long-term anticoagulation. Testing for antiphospholipid syndrome (via lupus anticoagulant, anticardiolipin, and anti–β_2-glycoprotein I) is common practice in a first-episode VTE because patients with antiphospholipid syndrome should be considered for long-term anticoagulation.[30]

Most women with *recurrent VTE* will have been screened for thrombophilias, and hence will not require consideration of screening. Regardless, the risk in women with recurrent VTE is generally sufficient to warrant long-term anticoagulation. Such

Table 2 Thrombophilia risk factors for venous thrombosis or embolism	
Thrombophilia[22]	**Odds Ratio (95% Confidence Interval)**
Factor V Leiden homozygous	34.40 (9.86–120.05)
Factor V Leiden heterozygous	8.32 (5.44–12.70)
Prothrombin G20210A homozygous	26.36 (1.24–559.29)
Prothrombin G20210A heterozygous	6.80 (2.46–18.77)
Antithrombin deficiency	4.69 (1.30–16.96)
Protein C deficiency	4.76 (2.15–10.57)
Protein S deficiency	3.19 (1.48–6.88)

Data from Robertson L, Wu O, Langhorne P, et al. Thrombophilia in pregnancy: a systematic review. Br J Haematol 2005;132:171–96.

patients are typically candidates for full anticoagulation, rather than thromboprophylaxis, during pregnancy.

Many women with a *personal history of a single, prior VTE and who are not on long-term anticoagulants* will have been tested for heritable and acquired thrombophilias by physicians other than their obstetricians. When considering pregnancy, those women with a single prior VTE episode previously tested for and known to be positive for a thrombophilia should be managed according to guidelines outlined later in this discussion. However, for many clinicians it is the patients who have *not* been previously tested for thrombophilias that are most confusing, especially because the current American College of Obstetrician and Gynecologists (ACOG) practice guidelines suggest that these women should be "offered testing, especially if such testing would affect management."[26]

One way in which thrombophilia testing might alter pregnancy management is in determining which women with a single, prior VTE can be managed without antepartum thromboprophylaxis. In the only credible study of its type, Brill-Edwards and colleagues[31] followed 125 women with a single prior VTE without using heparin thromboprophylaxis during the pregnancy. (Readers should take careful note that all subjects were treated with postpartum anticoagulation for 6 weeks.) All subjects were tested for FVLM, PGM, protein C deficiency and protein S deficiency, antithrombin deficiency, and antiphospholipid antibodies. Some subjects were tested for protein S deficiency during pregnancy, and a free protein S level of less than 24% was considered to indicate protein S deficiency. Overall, 2.5% of the subjects had an antepartum thrombosis. However, none of 44 women who (1) tested negative for thrombophilias and (2) had their prior thrombosis in association with a temporary risk factor, including pregnancy or oral contraceptives, had a recurrent VTE during the antepartum period.[31] Although not all experts agree, these results can be interpreted to allow selected women to avoid antepartum thromboprophylaxis. However, it must be kept in mind that the number of women in this subgroup was too small to conclude that there is no risk of VTE in these women.

In this light, and though the evidence is by no means robust, a reasonable approach to the woman with a single prior VTE episode who has not been tested for thrombophilias and is considering pregnancy or is in early pregnancy is as follows:

- Rule out antiphospholipid syndrome, as this diagnosis would alter pregnancy care as well as be an indication for heparin use.
- In the infrequent circumstance of a family history of antithrombin deficiency, test for antithrombin deficiency, as this diagnosis would be an indication for anticoagulation during pregnancy.
- As a general rule, there is no need for heritable thrombophilia testing in a woman whose single prior VTE was truly idiopathic in nature, that is, not associated with a temporary risk factor (including pregnancy or oral contraceptives), because current evidence suggests the patient should be treated with thromboprophylaxis regardless of the results of heritable thrombophilia testing.
- If after counseling regarding the risks of VTE in pregnancy, the patient with a single prior VTE episode associated with a transient risk factor and who is not on long-term anticoagulants would like to avoid using heparin during pregnancy (antepartum thromboprophylaxis), it is reasonable to do so if she is negative for FVL, PGM, protein C and protein S deficiency (<24% free protein S), antithrombin deficiency, and antiphospholipid antibodies.[31] However, if the patient views antepartum heparin use in her best interest, thrombophilia testing is unnecessary.

The fourth category of patients, those with a *family history of VTE but without a personal history of VTE*, is particularly difficult. The ACOG admits this when they state "it is controversial whether to test women who do not have a history of thrombosis but have a family history of thrombosis."[26] Patients with a first-degree relative with antithrombin deficiency should certainly be tested for the same. It would also seem reasonable to test women with a first-degree relative with homozygosity for FVLM or PGM or compound heterozygosity for FVLM and PGM for these mutations.

If thrombophilia screening is deemed necessary, the authors suggest testing for the thrombophilias shown in **Box 1**. The preferred method for testing for each is also shown. Deciding whether to modify the list of tests ordered should be based on the clinical scenario of each patient and the potential impact on thromboprophylaxis treatment. It is also important that normal physiologic changes in the hemostatic system during pregnancy can alter results for protein C and S testing. Physicians should be aware that testing for antithrombin, and proteins C and S might have falsely low results in the setting of anticoagulant therapy or significant clotting.[26]

THROMBOPROPHYLAXIS

Heparin is the anticoagulant drug of choice during pregnancy. Heparin does not cross the placenta and is widely considered safe for the embryo-fetus. Of the 2 clinically available forms, the low molecular weight heparin (LMWH) preparations offer some advantages over unfractionated heparin (UFH). Both UFH and LMWH act primarily by binding to antithrombin to catalyze the molecule binding to and altering the activity of serine protease procoagulants. UFH enhances the activity of antithrombin for Factor Xa and thrombin, whereas the predominant effect of LMWH is via antithrombin-mediated anti-Factor Xa activity.

UFH has complex pharmacokinetics that ultimately leads to a somewhat unpredictable anticoagulant response. Also, the bioavailability of the UFH after subcutaneous (SC) injection is reduced compared with intravenous infusion. LMWH, in contrast, is less likely to bind nonspecifically to various circulating protein or cell surfaces and so has improved pharmacokinetics and bioavailability when given SC. In addition, LMWH is less likely than UFH to cause heparin-induced thrombocytopenia (HIT) and osteoporosis, though the latter is very infrequent in women treated during pregnancy.[9,15] For the most part, the longer half-life of LMWH is seen as an advantage because it allows once- or twice-daily dosing regimens to be used.

Box 1
Thrombophilia testing

Lupus anticoagulant and anticardiolipin antibodies (personal history of VTE only)

Factor V Leiden mutation

Prothrombin G20210A mutation

Antithrombin activity levels

Protein C activity levels

Protein S activity levels

Most experts prefer postpartum thromboprophylaxis be accomplished with warfarin, though LMWH is also considered acceptable. Like the heparin compounds, warfarin is regarded as safe for breastfeeding.

The most highly regarded guidelines for pregnancy thromboprophylaxis are those of the American College of Chest Physicians (eighth edition),[32] and the recommendations provided herein are in agreement with these except where specifically noted. The guidelines specifically define UFH, LMWH, and warfarin regimens, as detailed in **Table 3**.

General Categories of At-risk Patients

In an effort to provide a simple and clinically acceptable approach for the obstetrician, the authors suggest that women being considered for thromboprophylaxis be categorized into different clinical scenarios as follows:

- Acute VTE within several months of conception or during pregnancy
- Recurrent VTE (2 or more prior VTEs)
- Single, prior VTE episode and not on long-term anticoagulants
  Without transient risk factor
  With transient risk factor
- Antiphospholipid syndrome without prior VTE (diagnosed because of obstetric event(s)
- High-risk thrombophilia
- Low-risk thrombophilia without prior VTE.

Table 3
Thromboprophylaxis regimens

Unfractionated heparin (UFH)	
Prophylactic UFH	UFH 5000 units SC every 12 h
Intermediate-dose UFH	UFH SC every 12 h, adjust dose to target an anti-Xa level of 0.1–0.3 U/mL
Adjusted-dose UFH	UFH SC every 12 h, adjust dose to target a mid-interval activated partial thromboplastin time (aPTT) into the therapeutic range
Low molecular weight heparin (LMWH)[a]	
Prophylactic LMWH	Enoxaparin 40 mg SC every 24 h, dose may be modified pending body weight per standard recommendations
Intermediate-dose LMWH	Enoxaparin 40 mg SC every 12 h
Adjusted-dose LMWH	Enoxaparin 1 mg/kg SC every 12 h, weight-adjusted, full treatment dose per standard recommendations
Postpartum anticoagulation	
Warfarin	Goal INR of 2.0–3.0 for 4–6 wk, overlap UFH or LMWH until INR is ≥2.0
Prophylactic LMWH[a]	Enoxaparin 40 mg SC every 24 h for 4–6 wk

Abbreviations: INR, international normalized ratio; SC, subcutaneously.
[a] Enoxaparin used as an example; may use other formulations of LMWH.
Data from Bates SM, Greer IA, Pabinger I, et al. Venous thromboembolism, thrombophilia, antithrombotic therapy, and pregnancy: American College of Chest Physicians Evidence-Based Clinical Practice Guidelines (8th edition). Chest 2008;133:844–66.

Acute VTE within several months of conception or during pregnancy
Such patients should be fully anticoagulated with an adjusted-dose UFH or LMWH regimen (see **Table 3**) for at least 6 months from the initial presentation with VTE. Women who are on warfarin should discontinue the warfarin before 6 weeks of gestation. Some clinicians favor discontinuing the warfarin when the patient initiates attempting to conceive, replacing it with UFH or LMWH.

If the patient reaches 6 months of anticoagulation during the pregnancy, consideration of reducing the degree of anticoagulation (eg, to prophylactic UFH or LMWH) is reasonable, especially in preparation for epidural anesthesia. Following delivery, the UFH or LMWH should be restarted and bridged to warfarin.

Recurrent VTE (2 or more prior VTEs)
Such patients should be fully anticoagulated during pregnancy using an adjusted-dose regimen (see **Table 3**). Following delivery, the UFH or LMWH should be restarted and bridged to warfarin.

Single, prior VTE episode and not on long-term anticoagulants
Patients whose single, prior VTE occurred without provocation should receive either prophylactic or intermediate-dose UFH or LMWH during pregnancy (see **Table 3**). Patients whose single, prior VTE was associated with a transient risk factor and who do not have a thrombophilia are candidates to avoid treatment during pregnancy, but must be cautioned regarding the signs and symptoms of VTE and what measures to take to decrease risk. In addition, the physician must take the entire clinical picture, for example, obesity or bed rest, into account. Patients with a single, prior VTE should be given postpartum thromboprophylaxis.

Antiphospholipid syndrome without prior VTE
Women without prior VTE and diagnosed with antiphospholipid syndrome because of pregnancy morbidity should receive either prophylactic or intermediate-dose UFH or LMWH during pregnancy. In the setting of definite antiphospholipid syndrome, the authors and others have suggested prophylactic UFH be 7500 to 10,000 units SC every 12 hours and LMWH to be given in an every 12-hour regimen.[33] Following delivery, postpartum thromboprophylaxis with warfarin or LMWH is indicated.

High-risk thrombophilia
Though uncommon, antithrombin deficiency, homozygosity for FVLM or PGM, heterozygosity for FVLM and PGM, and persistent positive antiphospholipid antibodies are considered by most experts as being at high risk for thrombosis during pregnancy even if the patient has not previously had a VTE. The American College of Chest Physicians guidelines recommends more aggressive management than with other thrombophilias and careful clinical surveillance for VTE. Prophylactic-dose UFH or LMWH may be employed during pregnancy with pharmacologic postpartum thromboprophylaxis. The authors are skeptical regarding the efficacy of prophylactic-dose UFH or LMWH in women with antithrombin deficiency, and favor either intermediate-dose or adjusted-dose UFH or LMWH (with anti-Factor Xa levels monitored). Some women with antithrombin deficiency may need antithrombin concentrate during the pregnancy or peripartum period.[34]

Low-risk thrombophilia without prior VTE
Women without a prior VTE who have heterozygosity for FVLM or PGM, protein C deficiency, or protein S deficiency can be managed without antepartum thromboprophylaxis if an individualized risk assessment proves acceptable. The role of postpartum thromboprophylaxis also will have to be individualized. Regarding the ACOG, specific

treatment recommendations are not made for the asymptomatic patients with low-risk thrombophilia.[26]

Cesarean delivery

Cesarean delivery has been cited as a risk for VTE.[3,21] Recommendations for thromboprophylaxis are made by Bates and colleagues[32] for women following cesarean section. It is suggested that those with one additional risk factor (such as those in **Table 1**) in addition to pregnancy and cesarean delivery receive thromboprophylaxis with prophylactic LMWH or UFH, or by mechanical prophylaxis with lower extremity compression devices while hospitalized. For those with multiple risk factors, both pharmacologic and mechanical prophylaxis should be employed for the same duration of time. Patients with persistent risk factors for VTE following cesarean delivery should have pharmacologic prophylaxis extended for 4 to 6 weeks following delivery. The authors agree with these recommendations.

Peripartum Heparin Management

Heparin management during the peripartum period is important to understand, as the risk of hemorrhage is compounded by anticoagulation. Low- to moderate-risk patients on LMWH can be transitioned to UFH at 36 to 37 weeks' gestation in an effort to improve the likelihood of epidural anesthesia if preterm labor occurs. Patients should be advised that if they suspect spontaneous labor, heparin should be discontinued. For induction or scheduled cesarean, adjusted-dose heparin and intermediate-dose LMWH should be discontinued 24 hours before the scheduled admission. Prophylactic heparin should be discontinued at least 12 hours prior. For high-risk patients, for example, those with a recent VTE, reasonable options include reducing the heparin dose to 5000 units SC twice a day or using a judiciously applied continuous infusion of heparin during labor, with discontinuation when delivery is estimated to be 1 to 2 hours away.

In most cases, heparin should be restarted 6 to 8 hours following delivery or cesarean section. Regarding high-risk patients, continuous infusion should be restarted after delivery when the risk of bleeding has decreased (usually 2 to 4 hours after delivery).

The American Society of Regional Anesthesia (ASRA) has made recommendations regarding anticoagulation and regional anesthesia. Regional anesthesia is contraindicated in patients less than 24 hours from their last dose of twice-daily LMWH. For prophylactic LMWH, regional anesthesia can be placed 10 to 12 hours' duration from the last dose of LMWH heparin. The neuraxial catheter should be removed 2 hours before the first LMWH dose. Intravenous heparin can be initiated 1 hour following neuraxial anesthesia, with catheter removal 2 to 4 hours after the last heparin dose. SC heparin dosed twice daily with a total dose less than 10,000 units of UFH per day is not a contraindication to neuraxial anesthesia. However, neuraxial anesthesia at doses greater than 10,000 units of UFH or dosing at a frequency greater than twice-daily dosing has not been established to be safe.[35]

SUMMARY

It is evident that obstetricians and gynecologists have the capacity to be uniquely instrumental in the prevention of VTE in the obstetric patient. Attaining the ability to identify patients at risk for VTE, determine who is a candidate for thrombophilia screening, and who may warrant thromboprophylaxis is important to this end. In addition, it is valuable to understand various thromboprophylaxis regimens and peripartum anticoagulant management, as detailed in this review.

REFERENCES

1. Chang J, Elam-Evans LD, Berg CJ, et al. Pregnancy-related mortality surveillance—United States, 1991–1999. In: Surveillance summaries. MMWR Surveill Summ 2003;52(No. SS-2):1–8.
2. Gherman RB, Goodwin TM, Leung B, et al. Incidence, clinical characteristics, and timing of objectively diagnosed venous thromboembolism during pregnancy. Obstet Gynecol 1999;94:730–4.
3. James AH, Jamison MG, Brancazio LR, et al. Venous thromboembolism during pregnancy and the postpartum period: incidence, risk factors, and mortality. Am J Obstet Gynecol 2006;194:1311–5.
4. Heit JA, Kobbervig CE, James AH, et al. Trends in the incidence of venous thromboembolism during pregnancy or postpartum: a 30-year population-based study. Ann Intern Med 2005;143:697–706.
5. Pomp ER, Lenselink AM, Rosendaal FR, et al. Pregnancy, the postpartum period and prothrombotic defects: risk of venous thrombosis in the MEGA study. J Thromb Haemost 2008;6:632–7.
6. Ginsberg JS, Brill-Edwards P, Burrows RF, et al. Venous thrombosis during pregnancy: leg and trimester of presentation. Thromb Haemost 1992;67:519–20.
7. James AJ, Tapson VF, Goldhaber SZ. Thrombosis during pregnancy and the postpartum period. Am J Obstet Gynecol 2005;193:216–9.
8. Ray JG, Chan WS. Deep vein thrombosis during pregnancy and the puerperium: a meta-analysis of the period of risk and the leg of presentation. Obstet Gynecol Surv 1999;54:256–71.
9. Bourjeily G, Paidas M, Khalil H, et al. Pulmonary embolism in pregnancy. Lancet 2009 Nov 3. DOI:10.1016/S0140-6736(09)60996-X.
10. Goldhaber SZ, Tapson VF. A prospective registry of 5,451 patients with ultrasound-confirmed deep vein thrombosis. Am J Cardiol 2004;93:259–62.
11. James KV, Lohr JM, Deshmukh RM, et al. Venous thrombotic complications of pregnancy. Cardiovasc Surg 1996;4(6):777–82.
12. Rabhi Y, Charras-Arthapignet C, Gris J, et al. Lower limb vein enlargement and spontaneous blood flow echogenicity are normal sonographic findings during pregnancy. J Clin Ultrasound 2000;28:407–13.
13. Macklon NS, Greer IA, Bowman AW. An ultrasound study of gestational and postural changes in the deep venous system of the leg in pregnancy. Br J Obstet Gynaecol 1997;104:191–7.
14. Macklon NS, Greer IA. The deep venous system in the puerperium: an ultrasound study. Br J Obstet Gynaecol 1997;104:198–200.
15. Pettker CM, Lockwood CJ. Thromboembolic disorders. In: Gabbe SG, Niebyl JR, Simpson JL, editors. Obstetrics: normal and problem pregnancies. 5th edition. Philadelphia: Churchill Livingstone; 2007. p. 1064–76.
16. Rousseau A, Favier R, Van Dreden P. Elevated circulating soluble thrombomodulin activity, tissue factor activity and circulating procoagulant phospholipids: new and useful markers for pre-eclampsia? Eur J Obstet Gynecol Reprod Biol 2009; 146(1):46–9.
17. Franchini M. Haemostasis and pregnancy. Thromb Haemost 2006;95:401–13.
18. Kjellberg U, Anderson NE, Rosen S, et al. APC resistance and other haemostatic variables during pregnancy and puerperium. Thromb Haemost 1999;81:527–31.
19. Rosenkranz A, Hiden M, Leschnik B, et al. Calibrated automated thrombin generation in normal uncomplicated pregnancy. Thromb Haemost 2008;99:331–7.

20. Clark P, Walker I. The phenomenon known as acquired activated protein C resistance. Br J Haematol 2001;114:767–73.
21. Jacobsen AF, Skjeldestad FE, Sandset PM. Ante- and postnatal risk factors of venous thrombosis: a hospital-based case-control study. J Thromb Haemost 2008;6:905–12.
22. Robertson L, Wu O, Langhorne P, et al. Thrombophilia in pregnancy: a systematic review. Br J Haematol 2005;132:171–96.
23. Dizon-Townson D, Miller C, Sibai B, et al. The relationship of the factor V Leiden mutation and pregnancy outcomes for mother and fetus. Obstet Gynecol 2005; 106:517–24.
24. Said JM, Higgins JR, Moses EK, et al. Inherited thrombophilia polymorphisms and pregnancy outcomes in nulliparous women. Obstet Gynecol 2010;115: 5–13.
25. Silver RM, Zhao Y, Spong CY, et al. Prothrombin gene G20210A mutation and obstetric complications. Obstet Gynecol 2010;115:14–20.
26. The American College of Obstetricians and Gynecologists (ACOG). Thromboembolism in pregnancy. Practice Bulletin 19. Washington, DC: ACOG; 2000.
27. Lussana F, Dentali F, Abbate R, et al. Screening for thrombophilia and antithrombotic prophylaxis in pregnancy: Guidelines of the Italian Society for Haemostasis and Thrombosis (SISET). Thromb Res 2009;124:e19–25.
28. Royal College of Obstetricians and Gynaecologists (RCOG). Reducing the risk of thrombosis and embolism during pregnancy and the puerperium. Green-top Guideline No. 37. London: RCOG; 2009.
29. Bates SM, Ginsberg JS. Clinical practice. Treatment of deep-vein thrombosis. N Engl J Med 2004;351(3):268–77.
30. Dalen JE. Should patients with venous thromboembolism be screened for thrombophilia? Am J Med 2008;121(6):458–63.
31. Brill-Edwards P, Ginsberg JS, Gent M, et al. Safety of withholding heparin in pregnant women with a history of venous thromboembolism. N Engl J Med 2000;343: 1439–44.
32. Bates SM, Greer IA, Pabinger I, et al. Venous thromboembolism, thrombophilia, antithrombotic therapy, and pregnancy: American College of Chest Physicians evidence-based clinical practice guidelines (8th edition). Chest 2008;133: 844–66.
33. Branch DW, Khamashta MA. Antiphospholipid syndrome: obstetric diagnosis, management, and controversies. Obstet Gynecol 2003;101(6):1333–44.
34. Rodgers GM. Role of antithrombin concentrate in treatment of hereditary antithrombin deficiency. An update. Thromb Haemost 2009;101(5):806–12.
35. Horlocker TT, Wedel DJ, Rowlingson JC, et al. Regional anesthesia in the patient receiving antithrombotic or thrombolytic therapy. American Society of Regional Anesthesia and Pain Medicine Evidence-Based Guidelines (Third edition). Reg Anesth Pain Med 2010;35:64–101.

Ethical Issues
in Obstetrics

Laura M. DiGiovanni, MD[a,b,c,d],*

KEYWORDS

- Medical ethics • Ethics in obstetrics • Maternal-fetal conflict
- Obstetrics • Preeclampsia • Patient autonomy
- Informed consent • Surrogate decision making

Sound ethical reasoning and moral judgment are essential to the work of a physician. Obstetricians make ethically complex decisions on a daily basis. Clinical medical ethics is a discipline that provides a structured approach for identifying, analyzing, and resolving ethical issues in clinical medicine. Obstetricians must become comfortable addressing the ethical issues involved in clinical obstetrics and therefore must have an understanding of the key elements of clinical medical ethics. Balancing the principles of medical ethics can guide clinicians toward solutions to ethical dilemmas encountered in the care of pregnant women. In situations that seem to pit the interests of pregnant women against the interests of their fetuses, clinicians must be prepared to identify the key issues and relevant ethical aspects in cases encountered to find a solution in the mother-fetus dyad. This article is not intended to turn the reader into an expert on medical ethics. The purpose of this article is to review the ethical foundations of clinical practice, recognize the ethical issues obstetricians face every day in caring for patients, and facilitate decision making. This article discusses the relevant ethical principles, identifies unique features of obstetric ethics, examines ethical principles as they apply to the mother and fetus, and thereby, provides a conceptual framework for considering ethical issues and facilitating decision making in clinical obstetrics.

ETHICAL DIMENSIONS UNIQUE TO OBSTETRICS AND PERINATAL MEDICINE

Obstetrical ethics can be considered a branch of medical ethics pertaining to the particular aspects and unique ethical issues specific to obstetrics. The obstetrician

The author has nothing to disclose.
[a] The Fetal Center, University of Chicago, 5841 South Maryland Avenue, MC 2050, Chicago, IL 60637, USA
[b] The MacLean Center of Clinical Medical Ethics, University of Chicago, 5841 South Maryland Avenue, MC 2050, Chicago, IL 60637, USA
[c] Ultrasound Division, Department of Obstetrics and Gynecology, University of Chicago, 5841 South Maryland Avenue, MC 2050, Chicago, IL 60637, USA
[d] Division of Maternal-Fetal Medicine Department of Obstetrics and Gynecology, University of Chicago, 5841 South Maryland Avenue, MC 2050, Chicago, IL 60637, USA
* Division of Maternal-Fetal Medicine Department of Obstetrics and Gynecology, University of Chicago, 5841 South Maryland Avenue, MC 2050, Chicago, IL 60637.
E-mail address: ldigiovanni@uchicago.edu

Obstet Gynecol Clin N Am 37 (2010) 345–357
doi:10.1016/j.ogc.2010.02.005
0889-8545/10/$ – see front matter © 2010 Elsevier Inc. All rights reserved.

obgyn.theclinics.com

has two interwoven patients whose interests at times may be at odds. There is the uniqueness of pregnant patients and the essential tie between pregnant women and the developing fetuses. There is the vulnerability of patients undergoing various diagnostic, therapeutic, and surgical procedures. They are often under regional or general anesthesia during delivery or surgery, and this aspect of trust in their physician is one of the cornerstones of the doctor-patient relationship in obstetrics. The obstetrician, as in other surgical fields, must be able to develop patient trust rapidly over a short time, often meeting patients only once they are pregnant and without a preexisting or long-standing doctor-patient relationship.

Most ethical issues in obstetrics, emergent and non-emergent, revolve around the maternal-fetal relationship. With information and support, most pregnant women strive to improve their chance of having a healthy baby. There are situations where the interests of the mother do not correspond with fetal interests; therefore, the concept of the maternal-fetal conflict may arise.[1] At the center of the maternal-fetal conflict is the concept of the fetus as a patient and a pregnant woman's autonomy. The 'maternal-fetal conflict' is often not a conflict between the mother and her fetus, but rather a conflict between the woman's autonomy and the physician's judgment of what is best for her fetus. The term maternal-fetal conflict implies divergent rather than shared interest of the pregnant woman and her fetus. In the vast majority of cases, the interests of the pregnant woman and fetus actually converge. Obstetrics, maternal-fetal medicine, and neonatology are rapidly evolving with new technologic advances and innovations, with patients often wanting 'everything done'. With these new advances in treatment, new and unique aspects of obstetric ethics have evolved.

Although obstetricians deal with ethical issues on a daily basis, ethics education in obstetric training is currently inadequate. Professionalism is one of the core competencies as defined by the Accreditation Council for Graduate Medical Education that all residents must demonstrate. Ethics is at the center of professionalism and therefore ethics education is central to the competency. A recent study on ethics education by Grossman and Angelos revealed that over the last 35 years, published articles on ethics education in residency training in obstetrics and gynecology lagged significantly behind internal medicine, pediatrics, family medicine, general surgery, and psychiatry. Obstetrics and gynecology had less than eight such articles. The only field with a lower number of articles on ethics education than obstetrics and gynecology was radiology.[2] The principle goal of teaching clinical ethics is to improve the quality of patient care in both the process and medical outcome. There are two main reasons for teaching medical ethics. First, it provides students with essential and practical knowledge on issues that frequently arise in patient care and are necessary for appropriate medical decision making. These key issues include respect for autonomy; informed consent; truthful communication; end-of-life issues; and particular to obstetrics, beginning-of-life issues. Second, the key principles of medical ethics are essential aspects of the doctor-patient relationship that continue to be centrally important to medicine, delivering health care and improving cost effectiveness and quality of care (Mark Siegler, MD personal communication, Jan 2010). It is time to recognize the importance of ethics in obstetrics and gynecology and to take time to teach it.

ETHICAL FRAMEWORK: THE FOUR BASIC PRINCIPLES

There are four basic principles regarded as the cornerstones of medical ethics to guide medical decision making: beneficence, nonmaleficence, respect for autonomy, and justice.[3] Beneficence requires acting for the benefit of others and obligates the physician to seek the greater balance of clinical good over harm for each patient.

Nonmaleficence is the duty to first do no harm, *primum non nocere*. The principle of justice concerns the fair distribution of health resources and the decision of who gets what treatment (fairness and equality). Respect for autonomy is central to clinical medicine. Autonomy is the "right to choose and follow one's own plan of life and action." It is the "personal rule of the self that is free both from controlling interferences from others and from limitations that prevent meaningful choice, such as inadequate understanding."[4] Respect for autonomy requires the physician to respect the patient's values and beliefs and the patient's decisions made in the informed consent process. Therefore, essential to patient autonomy is the process of informed consent.

Informed consent is the "willing acceptance of a medical intervention by a patient who has decisional capacity (the ability to make decisions) after disclosure by the physician of the nature of the intervention with its risks and benefits, as well as the alternatives with their risks and benefits"[5] It is a *process* of communication and negotiation between patient and physician that helps patients make a decision that is right for them. It is *not* signing a consent form; the signing of a consent form merely *documents* the informed consent process. A consent form may be legally necessary but it is not ethically or legally sufficient unless the informed consent process has occurred. Informed consent is a cornerstone of the ethical practice of medicine. It is integral to the principle of respect for autonomy. It requires communication and time, and patients should be given the full range of options.

There are three important elements of informed consent: (1) disclosure, which is communication that requires risk and benefit disclosure to satisfy what a reasonable person in the patient's situation would want to know; (2) comprehension; and (3) free consent, which involves freedom of choice to voluntarily consent or decide not to consent.[6] At the heart of medical ethics is the dynamic process of communication between doctor and patient. Communication should be truthful and based on facts. How much do patients really want to know? Should a physician tell the patient how poor the prognosis is and does telling eliminate hope? Should they be given detailed information and statistics if the numbers are bleak? Patients want necessary medical information and honest assessments of what to expect with clear acknowledgment of uncertainties. Recent studies demonstrate the limitations of obstetric estimation of neonatal outcome in extremely premature neonates.[7,8] Predicting outcomes, survival, and morbidity are often uncertain, such as in cases of medical complications of pregnancy, extreme prematurity, certain fetal anomalies, preterm premature rupture of membranes, intrauterine growth restriction (IUGR), and intrauterine infection. Honesty is more important than protecting hope and not dwelling on negativity. Sir William Osler described clinical medicine as "a science of uncertainty and an art of probability."[6] The practice of medicine is not an exact science and part of the disclosure is to be honest about medical uncertainty. Medical knowledge has limitations and medical judgment is fallible. Truthful and open communication requires acknowledging uncertainty when it exists. It is the duty of the physician to teach the patient about her condition, including treatment risks, benefits and alternatives, the range of possible outcomes, including the possibility of undesired outcomes, and answer questions to ensure patients understand their medical condition and all the options. Only then can the patient make a meaningful decision to give her informed consent or decide not to consent. It is important to the communication process to keep it dynamic, revisit decisions, and allow for reconsideration, on the part of both patients and obstetricians.

According to Beauchamp and Childress, none of the four principles should be hierarchically ordered above the others.[3] These four ethical principles are *prima facie*, binding, but not absolute or exceptionless.[9] The resolution of an ethical issue should be attained by balancing principles through compromise and negotiation. Balancing these principles provides a useful framework for understanding and resolving conflicts.

Reality mandates a practical paradigm for ethics case analysis to identify what is at issue and the best course of action. The commonly used method is the application and balancing of the ethical principles described earlier. Another method is the "4 boxes" approach developed by Jonsen, Siegler, and Winslade as a structured approach to ethics case analysis to work through difficult cases.[6,10] Ethical dilemmas are framed as a case workup that takes into account four topics that are intrinsic to every clinical encounter: medical indications, patient preferences, quality of life, and contextual features. Using this approach, clinicians are able to identify the relevant issues and the best course of action. However, the "4 boxes" framework fails to take account of the uniqueness of pregnant patients, which would require subdividing two boxes (medical indications and quality of life) to consider fetal and maternal interests. For more on this method, the reader should refer to *Clinical Ethics*.[6,10]

In treating actual patients and applying the principles elaborated by Beauchamp and Childress, Mahowald has proposed the following maxims or prioritizing guidelines on how to apply the principles in specific ethical conflicts[11]:

1. The interests of the patient count most (interests = autonomy + beneficence + nonmaleficence).
2. Respect for patient autonomy trumps beneficence and nonmaleficence.
3. The interests of others may outweigh respect for patient autonomy.
4. If harms and benefits are proportionate, nonmaleficence outweighs beneficence.

Maxim 3 refers to cases where the interests of the family or physicians may be more compelling. For example, if a patient requests treatment that is not medically indicated, the physician is not obligated to provide it. Maxim 4 takes into account that exceptions should consider benefits lost through the avoidance of harm. For example, whether an obstetrician should perform a cesarean section for the benefit of the fetus depends not only on the expected benefit to the fetus but also on the amount of risk the surgery involves for the pregnant woman.

THE CONCEPT OF THE FETUS AS A PATIENT

The concept of the fetus as a patient is an essential concept in perinatal medicine. Developments in fetal diagnosis and management to optimize fetal outcomes are now widely accepted and have promoted this concept. Chervenak and McCullough emphasize the two principles of beneficence and respect for autonomy as essential for understanding the ethical concept of the fetus as a patient.[12–14] According to Chervenak and McCullough, the fetus is a patient "when it is presented to the physician and there exist medical interventions, whether diagnostic or therapeutic, that are reliably expected to result in a greater balance of clinical good over harm for the fetus and the child it is expected to become."[15] The previable fetus is not a patient independent of the pregnant woman's autonomy. It is only a patient as a function of the pregnant woman's autonomy. The pregnant woman is free to withhold, confer, or withdraw the patient status from her previable fetus according to her values and beliefs. In contrast, a viable fetus is a patient independent of the pregnant woman's autonomy to confer this status. For the purpose of this discussion, viability occurs at approximately 23 weeks gestation and applies to the ability of the fetus to live *ex utero*, with technologic support if needed, and subsequently become a child.[14,15] Although the fetus can be a patient, the term 'fetal rights' has no meaning and no application in obstetrical ethics.[12]

The principle of beneficence obligates the obstetrician to protect and promote the pregnant woman's health-related interests. The principle of respect for autonomy obligates the physician to respect the woman's right to choose what happens to her. The woman's autonomous decisions are based on her own set of values and preferences. The fetus, however, "does not possess its own values and beliefs or a perspective on its interests; therefore, there is no autonomy-based obligation to the fetus."[12] There is, however, a beneficence-based obligation to the fetus. Chervenak and McCullough have identified principle-based obligations to the pregnant woman and the fetus. The physician has maternal autonomy-based and maternal beneficence-based obligations as well as fetal beneficence-based obligations. The pregnant woman's autonomy has priority. The physician is equally obligated to promote the medical interests of the mother and fetus; however, if the medical interest of the woman and fetus are at odds (eg, severe preeclampsia at a gestational age of periviable or extreme prematurity) treatment of the one most at risk should be given priority.[16] However, if maternal autonomy (part of her interests) is at odds with fetal interests, then her interests, which include her autonomy, still trump fetal interests even if the fetus is at increased risk. The most common ethical issues that arise in managing the medical complications of pregnancy require the physician to navigate these principles and obligations. The clinical consequences of the concept of the fetus as a patient are that the obstetrician must balance the autonomy-based and beneficence-based obligations to the pregnant woman with the beneficence-based obligations to the fetus.

MATERNAL DECISION MAKING AND THE MATERNAL FETAL CONFLICT
Shared Decision Making

In the past four decades medical ethics and decision making has undergone a rapid metamorphosis from beneficence-focused decision making to autonomy-focused decision making. Historically, medical decision making was based on paternalism, in which the physician determined what was in the patient's best interest. This shift from physician paternalism to a paradigm of shared decision making evolved over the last four decades, and medical decisions are now based on patient autonomy, and respect for the patient's wishes even when they conflict with doctor's recommendations. The information, alternatives, and options are presented to the patient and the patient makes the ultimate decision.

The current model of shared decision making assumes a physician and patient work together as partners and have the same goals. This concept of a partnership is central to the doctor-patient relationship and is an accurate description of the vast majority of doctor-patient encounters. Potential barriers to successful shared decision making include failure to communicate, fear or pain, lack of trust, lack of shared goals, and decisional incapacity. Shared decision making is the ideal. It is a collaboration and negotiation in which physicians share medical knowledge and opinions and patients share goals, values, and preferences. The patient is the ultimate decision maker, with doctor serving as critical interpreter of information and reliable guide toward reasonable decisions. It is an exchange with the patient making the final decision.

Pregnant patients are very capable of making complex medical decisions when provided relevant medical information and guidance by physicians. With biomedical and technological advances and their application in perinatal medicine, there are new and expanding ethical challenges for obstetricians and patients. The first-trimester risk assessment currently offered to all pregnant women has demonstrated that pregnant women are capable of making complex and sophisticated decisions about risk-assessment information and subsequent decisions about invasive testing and diagnosis.[17] Pregnant women, given information and an appropriate informed consent process, would be expected to make similarly complex and sophisticated decisions about assessment of the fetus and other complex decisions during pregnancy.[18]

The Maternal-Fetal Conflict

Case one: A 39-year-old G1P0 at 30 weeks gestation with chronic hypertension, diabetes, end stage renal disease, and completely intact decisional capacity, is likely to die within 2 weeks from renal failure. She refuses life-saving dialysis or delivery at this time for what she repeatedly states are personal reasons. The patient has a blood pressure of 162/94, ultrasound estimated fetal weight less than fifth percentile, and an amniotic fluid index of 4.2 cm with elevated umbilical artery Doppler values.

This is a case of treatment refusal of potentially life-sustaining treatment, for the mother and fetus, in a patient with decisional capacity. This case raises ethical concerns for respect for autonomy, informed consent, communication, the maternal-fetal conflict, and the physician's obligations to the mother and the fetus. At issue is the maternal-fetal conflict that arises when a pregnant woman rejects medical advice or interventions necessary to avert fetal complications or death to herself or her fetus. That is, the conflict is between the physician's recommendation and the pregnant woman's autonomous decision to reject it. Does a clinician's obligation of beneficence to the pregnant woman and her fetus outweigh the obligation to respect patient autonomy? Following the ethical principle of respect for autonomy, the pregnant patient's decisions should be respected as long as she has decisional capacity to make informed medical decisions. The principles direct us to respect autonomy, but in this case it is difficult to do because her decision seems unfounded and harmful to herself and her fetus when there is good potential for survival for both. Also at issue in this case is beneficence and nonmaleficence. When it is treatable and the harm of not treating is great, the medical team feels uncomfortable. Is it ethical to examine her reasons for refusing even though she says they are personal? Yes, patient autonomy and informed consent are integral to patient choice. Therefore, it is essential to inquire about the reasons for her decision and ensure that her condition and range of options have been clearly explained, and that she comprehends these options and the risks and consequences to herself and her fetus. This inquiry is all part of respect for autonomy, the informed consent process, and shared decision making. In the context of this case, maternal autonomy trumps her medical interests and those of the fetus, despite how uncomfortable this makes the medical team.

Legal cases and decisions have revolved around refusal of treatment and the maternal-fetal conflict. In 1994, Mrs. Doe and her husband had religious objections to delivery by cesarean section that her doctors thought medically indicated because of IUGR and placental insufficiency. She was at 37-weeks gestation and clearly had decisional capacity. Doctors at St. Joseph Hospital in Chicago petitioned the Illinois courts to take wardship of the fetus to allow cesarean section. The appellate courts denied the petition, and the Illinois State Supreme Court denied review. She transferred to another hospital where the doctors agreed to respect this patient's decision regarding mode of delivery. Her pregnancy continued and 2 weeks later she had a vaginal delivery of a healthy baby boy. The 1994 court ruling in this case rejected court-ordered interventions in pregnancy stating that "The woman's decision, not the fetus's interest is the only dispositive factor. A woman's right to refuse invasive medical treatment, derived from her rights to privacy, bodily integrity and religious liberty is not diminished during pregnancy.... The potential impact upon the fetus is not legally relevant."[19] In this case and others, the courts now uphold maternal autonomy in the maternal-fetal conflict. The American College of Obstetrics and

Gynecology (ACOG) strongly opposes any coercive or legal approaches to the pregnant woman.[20]

When a pregnant woman's health condition is deemed hazardous to the fetus, or when the fetal condition requires some type of medical intervention, a 'maternal-fetal conflict' may arise. This conflict is usually between the pregnant woman's autonomous decisions, as determine by her, and the best interests of the fetus, as determined by her physician. The state of pregnancy does not deprive a woman of her right to decide what should happen to her body. Based on legal cases and precedent, the law recognizes the rights of all adults, pregnant or not, to informed consent and bodily integrity, regardless of the impact of the person's decision on others.[20,21] She has the right to refuse any lifestyle modification or medical intervention for the sake of the fetus. On the other hand, she also has a duty to promote the fetus' best interests. That is, mother and physician have principle-based obligations to the pregnant patient and fetus. One must consider the best interests of the pregnant woman, which are both maternal autonomy-based obligations and maternal beneficence-based obligations of the physician. At the same time, one must consider the best interests of the fetus, which are fetal beneficence-based obligations of the pregnant woman and the fetal beneficence-based obligations of the physician.[16] These types of maternal-fetal conflicts hinge on the pregnant woman's autonomy, the physician's autonomy, the physician's duty of beneficence to the pregnant woman and her fetus, as well as the pregnant woman's duty of beneficence to her fetus. For the pregnant woman, her duty of beneficence to the fetus may override her right to autonomy; however, the resolution of this conflict must be her choice. In the maternal-fetal conflict, the pregnant woman's autonomy takes center stage. In the context of Case one, if decisional capacity is present, ethics demands respecting maternal autonomy and choices, even 'bad' choices. A pregnant woman's autonomy and informed refusal should be respected.

SURROGATE DECISION MAKING

Case two: AB, a 28-year-old G2P1 at 20-weeks gestation with no prenatal care was brought into the emergency department (ED) by her boyfriend after "saying strange things and walking funny" for several days. The patient was confused and disoriented to person, place, and time, confabulated when questions were posed to her and exhibited new onset neurologic findings on physical examination. This patient's history was significant for several prior visits to multiple emergency departments for nausea and vomiting during which she reported a 30-pound weight loss since being pregnant, had a normal mental status before this admission, and a history of hyperemesis in her prior pregnancy that resolved by 12 weeks. A diagnostic workup revealed findings consistent with Wernicke's encephalopathy secondary to hyperemesis gravidarum, and that the patient did not have decisional capacity. The patient did not regain decisional capacity after inpatient treatment and the pregnancy continued. Who should make the medical decisions on this patient's behalf because she now clearly lacks decisional capacity?

Case three: HN is a 30-year-old G2P1 at 25-weeks gestation in previously good health with an uncomplicated pregnancy who was admitted from the ED because of worsening shortness of breath, cough, fever, and malaise. A chest radiograph revealed bilateral nodular infiltrates. Within 24 hours of admission she developed pneumonia and subsequent respiratory failure and acute respiratory distress syndrome requiring mechanical ventilation. Over the next several days, laboratory tests confirmed H1N1 influenza, her respiratory status worsened, and the family and boyfriend were informed of her rapidly worsening condition, possible maternal and fetal outcomes including death, and the urgent medical decisions that needed to be made for her and her fetus, including possible delivery.

These are two cases that illustrate the need for surrogate decision making on behalf of a pregnant patient. These cases raise issues of decisional capacity, surrogate decision making, autonomy, beneficence of mother and fetus, and beginning and end-of-life issues. Who should now make the medical decisions on this patient's behalf? When a patient is mentally incapacitated and lacks decisional capacity, medical decisions must be made by a surrogate decision maker, an authorized person acting on the patient's behalf.[6] Decisional capacity is the ability to comprehend the nature and consequences of a medical decision and to reach and communicate an informed decision. A surrogate decision maker is an adult individual who has decisional capacity, is available, and is willing to make medical decisions on behalf of a patient who lacks decisional capacity.[22]

In case two and three, the two most pressing relevant issues are who should now make the medical decisions on the patient's behalf and on what information should they base those decisions. Traditionally, family members have been considered the natural surrogates. In recent years, many states have enacted legislative statutes that give specific authority to family members and rank them in priority. The durable power of attorney for health care statutes provides for a designated surrogate decision maker, and this person would supersede any other party, including immediate family members. The usual order of priority for determining who is appointed the surrogate would be

1. Patient's legally appointed guardian or durable power of attorney for health care designated surrogate, if there is one
2. Patient's spouse
3. Any adult (18 years of age or older) son or daughter of the patient
4. Either parent of the patient
5. Adult brother or sister of the patient
6. Any adult grandchild of the patient
7. An adult close friend of the patient.

This priority list differs in various states and in some states this order is codified.[22] The surrogate decision makers, as identified by the attending physician, are then authorized to make medical decisions for patients who lack decisional capacity, including decisions regarding whether to forgo life-sustaining treatment on behalf of patients without court involvement. In the case of the partner of the pregnant woman as a surrogate, it would depend on whether he is the spouse or boyfriend. If he is not the pregnant woman's spouse, that would put him in the close-friend category.

Surrogate decision making on behalf of a pregnant patient is difficult and should strive to reach a decision that the patient would make if she had decisional capacity. The decisions of surrogates should be guided by the standards. First, when the patient's preferences are known, surrogates should use knowledge of the patient's preferences to make medical decisions on the patient's behalf. Second, when the patient's preferences are not known, the surrogate's judgment must promote the best interests of the patient.[6] When a surrogate relies on the patient's known preferences, it is called a "substituted judgment" standard. This substituted judgment standard is used when the patient previously expressed their preferences explicitly, either in writing or verbally, or where the surrogate can reasonably infer the patient's preferences based on past statements or actions. The goal is for the surrogate decision maker to use knowledge of these preferences in making medical decisions for patients. Courts typically apply this substituted judgment standard in cases where the patients' preferences are known. When the patient has not specifically stated what she would want in the situation, the surrogate should use knowledge of the patient's values and beliefs to make decisions for them. The goal of surrogate decision making is to reach a decision that the patient would reach. When asking the surrogate what he or she wants done, the question is not "what would you want?", but rather "what would the patient want?" Obviously this situation becomes even more complex in the surrogate decision making on behalf of pregnant patients with the additional considerations for the interests of the fetus.

In life-threatening obstetric emergencies, patients are often unable to give informed consent or express their preferences because they are in shock, hemodynamically unstable, or unconscious. In these life-threatening emergency situations, no surrogate may be immediately available and the physician may presume that the patients would give consent if they were able to do so, because they would prefer life over death. This is called "implied consent," which is really the physician presuming consent.[6] The physician should presume consent when emergency action is necessary to preserve the patient's life. Beneficence is the ethical principle justifying emergency treatment of incapacitated patients.

RETHINKING ETHICAL CONSIDERATIONS IN SCREENING AND PREDICTION OF PREECLAMPSIA

Preeclampsia (PE), a hypertensive complication in pregnancy with multisystem involvement, affects 3% to 5% of pregnant women and is associated with serious morbidity and mortality for mother and fetus. It is both a leading cause of maternal mortality, with more than 60,000 maternal deaths per year worldwide, and of premature birth.[23] As of early 2010, the only effective treatment is delivery of the placenta. The pathogenesis of preeclampsia has been mysterious and elusive, though this past decade has witnessed significant advances in our understanding of the pathophysiology of preeclampsia.[24–27] As discussed elsewhere in this issue, Karumanchi and colleagues[24] have demonstrated that two antiangiogenic factors, soluble fms-like tyrosine kinase 1 and soluble endoglin, are overproduced by the placenta in women who develop preeclampsia.[25] These proteins enter the maternal circulation, correlate with severity of disease, and appear responsible for several preeclampsia phenotypes.[24,26,27] More importantly, their levels in the maternal circulation rise weeks to months before overt symptoms and disease, and thus they have become the object of study as biomarkers that screen for or predict preeclampsia.[24,28]

Would it be beneficial to the mother and fetus to predict preeclampsia? Some investigators propose that reliable prediction of preeclampsia would allow closer prenatal monitoring, including referral to high-risk clinics; more aggressive intervention, such as restricting activity; and perhaps initiation of antihypertensive therapy and steroids to enhance fetal lung maturity when decisions of delivery to end the pregnancy are being considered.[29] Reliable prediction would also permit preventive and treatment regimens that are currently unavailable. Although there is no definitive treatment of preeclampsia, exciting possibilities are under investigation. A reliable biomarker to predict preeclampsia would certainly be of merit in exploring the value of new therapeutic approaches and their use when and if developed. Although some reports are exciting and promising, no single screening test has yet proven accurate enough to meet the requirements of acceptable positive and negative likelihood ratios that would permit their use in clinical practice. Focus is therefore currently on combining tests for better prediction.[29,30]

Because there is no known treatment for preeclampsia other than delivery of the placenta, the prediction of preeclampsia using angiogenic factors raises new ethical issues. To screen for a disease, the disease should have (1) an understood etiology, (2) early detection and treatment should lead to improvement of the condition, (3) early detection should not create undue anxiety, and (4) screening method should be acceptable to patients. A screening test should have use for all pregnant women; be rapid; noninvasive; inexpensive; easy to perform early in gestation; and have high sensitivity and high positive and low negative likelihood ratios, respectively, to reduce anxiety and prevent unnecessary interventions. In a recent study of first trimester screening of PE, Poon and colleagues[30] evaluated 7797 women with singleton pregnancies during weeks 11 to 13, 157 developed preeclampsia, 34 before 34-weeks gestation. Screening by history alone would identify only 30% of cases destined to develop early PE. A multiple marker algorithm test was used to predict patients that developed early PE with resultant sensitivity of the prediction for early PE of 94.1% and specificity of 94.3%. The likelihood ratio for a positive test was 16.5 and for a negative test was 0.06, easily fulfilling the criteria of the World Health Organization for a clinical prediction test. These are remarkably good results. However, prospective observational studies are required to assess the effectiveness of early prediction and perform cost-benefit analyses. Also, the mortality and morbidity of PE is far greater in developing nations where these tests are not readily available and the costs appear prohibitive.

A screening test for the first trimester prediction of early preeclampsia raises several ethical issues. Although it may now be possible to identify women at risk for early disease, since there is currently no definitive prevention or treatment of PE, how does early detection improve outcomes or minimize maternal and fetal complications of early PE?

Case four: EH, a 38-year-old G2P0100 currently at 9-weeks gestation and with a history of severe preeclampsia with HELLP in her previous pregnancy necessitating delivery at 26 weeks, then suffered a cerebrovascular accident, was intubated in the medical intensive care unit for 4 days and her infant expired from complications of extreme prematurity. She now requests first-trimester prediction tests for preeclampsia stating that although she very much desires a child, she does not want to continue this pregnancy if she is going to have early PE again along with all its complications.

If first trimester screening for PE becomes available in the United States, would it be useful to offer it to all pregnant patients, only to patients with a history of early or severe PE, or not offer it all because currently PE has no prevention or treatment? Case four illustrates, that although the intended purpose of first-trimester screening for PE is to determine a population to be referred for high-risk care and improve pregnancy outcomes, some women might use it in decisions to terminate the pregnancy, creating additional ethical dilemmas. Should she be offered first-trimester screening because of her history of early PE? The real dilemma in this case is that women with histories defining high risk are not in need of a screening test as they would be referred automatically by history. However, because history alone is not that reliable, it would seem that universal screening may be useful. Other ethical issues raised include patient autonomy, informed consent, disclosure, and innovation. It is also misleading to suggest that a new screening test for the prediction of PE is an improvement when there is no evidence that it improves outcomes. If it were available, the obstetrician should inform her that this is a new and innovative technology with no current evidence to show the use of the test results in better care and outcomes than current management. There are many ethical considerations in this new forefront of developing a predictive test for PE.

There is a general assumption that knowledge is good. With regards to a screening test for preeclampsia, it would also be difficult for the obstetrician to counsel patients for a condition that cannot be prevented. If the screening test could predict the likelihood that the patient will get the disease, what would the patient and obstetrician do with that information? One must evaluate why knowing is valuable when assessing the ethical considerations and implications of acquiring knowledge about a disease in pregnancy from a screening test.

MEDICAL FUTILITY

Futility often comes up in the management of medical complications of pregnancy for mother and fetus, especially surrounding interventions for the fetus, extreme prematurity, fetal anomalies, and neonatal treatment. Patients often request physicians to "do everything" for the baby regardless of risks for themselves or the ability to achieve the desired goal. Futility is included briefly here to warn against the use of the term. The meaning of this term and its use in clinical medicine has been ambiguous and hotly debated. Medical futility has been the topic of many articles in the literature and debate continues. It is a moving target that is subjective, not objective. And although much of the literature is on futility in end-of-life decision making, obstetricians deal with beginning-of-life ethical decision making with inherent uniqueness and uncertainties. Lantos and colleagues,[31] elegantly described the complexities of the illusion of futility and the obligations of physicians not to declare a situation futile and abandon one's patient. Helft and colleagues,[32] eloquently discuss the rise and fall of the futility movement and warn against using futility to swing the pendulum of decision making power back toward physicians. "Everything done" is often a misleading request or offer. When patients request "do everything" they usually mean do everything that is medically indicated. Physicians should discuss the patient's status and explore their goals and then the interventions that are medically indicated. The ACOG has cautioned against defining medical interventions as futile.[33] Invoking the term futility breaks down communication and patient care and should be avoided. Better to describe a treatment as medically or surgically inappropriate or not beneficial in meeting the desired goals. When there is a futility conflict regarding treatment options, the values of the patient and family and the default position of maintaining life ordinarily take priority. Doctors recognize situations in which interventions will not achieve the desired goal, and this should initiate the difficult task of discussing goals and realistic expectations with patients and explaining why it is believed further treatment will not attain the desired result. There is growing consensus that the use of the term medical futility may itself be futile.[34]

SUMMARY

Balancing ethical principles in clinical practice is often challenging. Obstetrics is further confounded by the integrally intertwined maternal-fetal dyad, making it an especially complex discipline. This article presents an overview of the salient ethical principles relevant to issues encountered in obstetrics that can help clinicians simultaneously consider the interests of the pregnant patient and her fetus. Decisions in obstetrics should be guided by balancing the principles of beneficence, nonmaleficence, and respect for autonomy, which are the cornerstones of medical ethics, along with concepts presented here, including informed consent, truth telling, shared decision making, the maternal-fetal conflict, surrogate decision making, and the fetus as a patient. These guidelines provide an ethical framework for identifying, analyzing, and resolving the complex ethical situations that arise in day-to-day clinical practice and promotes sound ethical judgment and medical decision making. The obstetrician who is familiar with the concepts of medical ethics will be able to apply these concepts, principles, and case precedents to ethical dilemmas in a structured approach to identify what is at issue and decide the best course of action to resolve real-life cases.

ACKNOWLEDGMENTS

The author gratefully acknowledges Marshall Lindheimer MD, Mary Mahowald PhD, and Peter Angelos MD, for their editorial assistance in this manuscript and their inspiration.

REFERENCES

1. van Bogaert LJ, Dhai A. Ethical challenges of treating the critically ill pregnant patient. Best Pract Res Clin Obstet Gynaecol 2008;22(5):983–96.
2. Grossman E, Posner M, Angelos P. Ethics education in surgical residency: past, present, and future. Surgery 2010;147:114–9.
3. Beauchamp TL, Childress JF. Principles of biomedical ethics. 6th edition. Oxford: Oxford University Press; 2009.
4. ACOG Committee Opinion, Number 390. Ethical decision making in obstetrics and gynecology, December 2007.
5. Siegler M, Collins ME, Cronin DC. Special challenges to the informed consent doctrine in the United States. J Clin Ethics 2004;15(1):38–47.
6. Jonsen AR, Siegler M, Winslade WJ. Clinical ethics: a practical approach to ethical decision in clinical medicine. 6th edition. New York: McGraw-Hill Medical Publishing; 2006.
7. Skupski DW, McCullough LB, Levene M, et al. Improving obstetric estimation of outcomes of extremely premature neonates: an evolving challenge. J Perinat Med 2010;38:19–22.
8. Meadow W, Frain L, Reen Y, et al. Serial assessment of mortality in the neonatal intensive care unit by algorithm and intuition: certainly, uncertainty, and informed consent. Pediatrics 2002;109:878–86.
9. Childress JF. The normative principles of medical ethics. In: Veatch RM, editor. Medical ethics. 2nd edition. Boston: Jones and Barlett Publishers; 1997. p. 29–46.
10. Sokol DK. The "four quadrant" approach to clinical case analysis; an application and review. J Med Ethics 2008;34:513–6.
11. Mahowald MB. Bioethics and women across the life span. New York: Oxford University Press; 2006.
12. Chervenak FA, McCullough LB. The fetus as a patient: an essential concept for the ethics of perinatal medicine. Am J Perinatol 2003;20(8):399–404.
13. McCullough LB, Chervenak FA. Ethics in obstetrics and gynecology. New Work: Oxford University press; 1994.
14. Chervenak FA, McCullough LB, Levene M. An ethically justified, clinically comprehensive approach to peri-viability: gynaecological, obstetric, perinatal and neonatal dimensions. J Obstet Gynaecol 2007;27(1):3–7.
15. Chervenak FA, McCullough LB. Ethical dimensions on non-aggressive fetal management. Semin Fetal Neonatal Med 2008;13:316–9.
16. Adams S, Mahowald M, Gallagher J. Refusal of treatment during pregnancy. Clin Perinatol 2003;30:127.

17. McCullough LB, Nicolaides KH, Chervenak FA, et al. Evidence-based obstetric ethics and informed decision-making by pregnant women about invasive diagnosis after first-trimester assessment of risk for trisomy 21. Am J Obstet Gynecol 2005;193(2):322–6.

18. Papp Z. Ethical challenges of genomics for perinatal medicine: the Budapest Declaration. Am J Obstet Gynecol 2009;201:336.

19. In re Baby Boy Doe vs. Mother Doe, 632 NE2d 326 (Ill App 1 Dist 1994).

20. ACOG Committee Opinion, Maternal decision making, ethics and the law. Number 321, November 2005.

21. Annas GJ. Foreclosing the use of force: A.C. reversed. Hastings Cent Rep 1990; 20(4):27–9.

22. Health Care Surrogate Act including amendments effective January 1998. Available at: http://gac.state.il.us/hcsa.html#3. Accessed May 6, 2010.

23. World Health Organization. World health report: make every mother and child count. Geneva (Switzerland): World health Org; 2005.

24. Wang A, Rana S, Karumanchi SA. Preeclampsia: the role of angiogenic factors in its pathogenesis. Physiology (Bethesda) 2009;147–58.

25. Levine RJ, Maynard SE, Qian C, et al. Circulating angiogenic factors and the risk of preeclampsia. N Engl J Med 2004;350:672–83.

26. Levine RJ, Lam C, Qian C, et al. Soluble endoglin and other circulating antiangiogenic factors in preeclampsia. N Engl J Med 2006;355:992–1005.

27. Park CW, Park JS, Shim SS, et al. An elevated maternal plasma, but not amniotic fluid soluble fms-like tyrosine kinase-1 (sFlt1) at the time of mid-trimester genetic amniocentesis is a risk factor for preeclampsia. Am J Obstet Gynecol 2005;193: 984–9.

28. Conde-Agudelo A, Romero R, Lindheimer MD. Test to predict preeclampsia. In: Lindheimer MD, Roberts JM, Cunningham FG, editors. Chesley's hypertensive disorders in pregnancy. 3rd edition. San Diego: Elsevier; 2009. p. 189–212.

29. Levine RJ, Lindheimer MD. First-trimester prediction of early preeclampsia: a possibility at last! Hypertension 2009;53:747–8.

30. Poon L, Kametas NA, Maiz N, et al. First trimester prediction of hypertensive disorders in pregnancy. Hypertension 2009;53:812–8.

31. Lantos JD, Singer PA, Walker RM, et al. The illusion of futility in clinical practice. Am J Med 1989;87:81–4.

32. Helft PR, Siegler M, Lantos J. The rise and fall of the futility movement. N Engl J Med 2000;343:293–6.

33. ACOG Committee Opinion. Medical futility. Number 362, March 2007.

34. Grossman E, Angelos P. Futility: what Cool Hand Luke can teach the surgical community. World J Surg 2009;33:1338–40.

Index

Note: Page numbers of article titles are in **boldface** type.

Obstet Gynecol Clin N Am 37 (2010) 359–368
doi:10.1016/S0889-8545(10)00054-9
0889-8545/10/$ – see front matter © 2010 Elsevier Inc. All rights reserved.

obgyn.theclinics.com

Moving?

Make sure your subscription moves with you!

To notify us of your new address, find your **Clinics Account Number** (located on your mailing label above your name), and contact customer service at:

Email: journalscustomerservice-usa@elsevier.com

800-654-2452 (subscribers in the U.S. & Canada)
314-447-8871 (subscribers outside of the U.S. & Canada)

Fax number: 314-447-8029

Elsevier Health Sciences Division
Subscription Customer Service
3251 Riverport Lane
Maryland Heights, MO 63043

*To ensure uninterrupted delivery of your subscription,
please notify us at least 4 weeks in advance of move.

Printed and bound by CPI Group (UK) Ltd, Croydon, CR0 4YY

03/10/2024

01040441-0006